DEBATING
HEALTH CARE
ETHICS

DEBATING HEALTH CARE ETHICS

Canadian Contexts

Second Edition

Patrick Findler, Doran Smolkin, and Warren Bourgeois

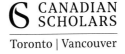

CANADIAN SCHOLARS

Toronto | Vancouver

Debating Health Care Ethics: Canadian Contexts, Second Edition
Patrick Findler, Doran Smolkin, and Warren Bourgeois

First published in 2019 by
Canadian Scholars, an imprint of CSP Books Inc.
425 Adelaide Street West, Suite 200
Toronto, Ontario
M5V 3C1

www.canadianscholars.ca

Library and Archives Canada Cataloguing in Publication

Title: Debating health care ethics : Canadian contexts / Patrick Findler, Doran Smolkin, and Warren Bourgeois.
Names: Smolkin, Doran, 1963- author. | Findler, Patrick, 1962- author. | Bourgeois, Warren, 1947- author.
Description: Second edition. | Revision of: Smolkin, Doran, 1963-. Debating health care ethics. | Includes bibliographical references and index.
Identifiers: Canadiana (print) 20190083794 | Canadiana (ebook) 20190083832 | ISBN 9781773381060 (softcover) | ISBN 9781773381077 (PDF) | ISBN 9781773381084 (EPUB)
Subjects: LCSH: Medical ethics—Canada—Textbooks. | LCGFT: Textbooks.
Classification: LCC R724 .S575 2019 | DDC 174.20971—dc23

Text design by Elisabeth Springate
Typesetting by Brad Horning
Cover design by Rafael Chimicatti
Cover image by pogonici, Shutterstock.com

Printed and bound in Ontario, Canada

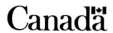

For my wife, Cara, and our children, Cashel and Reese,
who continue to amaze and inspire.
—*Patrick Findler*

I dedicate this work to my parents, Debby and Barry Smolkin,
to my wife, Julie Smolkin, and to my children, Elie Smolkin,
Kaytlin Carlson, Andrew Carlson, and Mischa Smolkin.
—*Doran Smolkin*

I dedicate this work to my wife, a compassionate and wise physician,
whose unflagging efforts on behalf of patients here and in Africa are an inspiration,
to my late mother for her constant faith in me, and to my sons
who keep me focused on making this world a better place.
—*Warren Bourgeois*

CONTENTS

About the Authors   *xiv*
Preface   *xv*

CHAPTER 1 ARGUMENTS AND METHODOLOGY   1

INTRODUCTION   1

ARGUMENTS   1
  What Is an Argument?   1
  Evaluating Arguments   3

PHILOSOPHICAL METHODOLOGY: COUNTEREXAMPLES AND THOUGHT
  EXPERIMENTS   9

COMMON FALLACIES   11
  Circularity (a.k.a. Begging the Question)   11
  False Dilemma   13
  Equivocation   13
  Appeal to Emotion   13
  Straw Man   14
  Ad Hominem   14

CONCLUSION   15

REVIEW QUESTIONS   15

NOTES   16

CHAPTER 2 PHILOSOPHICAL ETHICS: AN INTRODUCTION   17

INTRODUCTION   17

THREE TYPES OF ETHICAL INQUIRY   18

SKEPTICAL CONCERNS: ETHICAL RELATIVISM   21

NORMATIVE ETHICAL THEORY   24

CLASSICAL ACT UTILITARIANISM   24
  Objections to Utilitarianism   27
  Utilitarian Responses   30

RULE UTILITARIANISM   32

NON-CONSEQUENTIALISM AND DEONTOLOGY   34

KANT'S ETHICS   34
  The Idea of Moral Worth   34

The Categorical Imperative   35
The Universal Law Formulation of the Categorical Imperative   36
The Humanity Version of the Categorical Imperative   38
Objections to the Universal Law and Humanity Tests   40

PLURALISTIC DEONTOLOGY   43
Difficulties with Ross's Theory   45

SOCIAL CONTRACT THEORY   46

HOBBES'S SOCIAL CONTRACT THEORY   47
Objections to Hobbes's Social Contract Theory   48

RAWLS'S SOCIAL CONTRACT THEORY: JUSTICE AS FAIRNESS   49
Difficulties with Rawls's Social Contract Theory   51

ARISTOTLE'S VIRTUE THEORY   54
Objections to Virtue Theory   55

FEMINIST ETHICS   57

THE ETHICS OF CARE   58
Difficulties with the Ethics of Care   60
Status-Oriented Feminist Approaches   61

CONCLUSION   63

REVIEW QUESTIONS   63

NOTES   64

CHAPTER 3   OUR PHILOSOPHICAL APPROACHES   70

INTRODUCTION   70

DORAN'S PLURALISTIC APPROACH TO ETHICS   70
Leading Ethical Theories and Their Problems   71
Moral Pluralism   73

PATRICK'S VIRTUE-BASED APPROACH TO ETHICS   75
Metaethics   76
Normative Ethics   78
Some Objections and Responses   79

WARREN'S APPROACH TO ETHICS: PRACTICAL SOCIAL CONTRACT THEORY   82
The Main Contractarian Ideas for Warren's Purposes   82
The Committee Metaphor   84
The Video Game Metaphor   86
Warren's Use of Social Contract Theory   86
Cultural Relativism   87
Ethics Regarding Non-Humans   87
Social Contract Theory beyond Ethics   89

Warning   89

CONCLUSION   90

REVIEW QUESTIONS   90

NOTES   90

CHAPTER 4   AUTONOMY AND THE RIGHT TO REFUSE TREATMENT   92

INTRODUCTION   92

DRAMA   93

DEBATE   100
   Identifying Relevant Facts   100

MORAL ISSUES RAISED BY THE CASE   102
   Stating Our Positions   102

AN ARGUMENT FOR THE RIGHT TO IGNORE EXPERTS   104
   Clarifying Premise (3)   105
   Assuming Mr. Edwards Was Competent, Did His Health Care Team Err in Releasing Him from the Hospital When They Did?   108

OBJECTIONS TO PREMISE (5)   111
   Was Mr. Edwards Competent?   111
   The Gangrenous Foot Example   113
   Incompetence to Refuse Medical Care: Skepticism without Reason   114
   Competence and Psychiatric Evaluation   116
   Did Mr. Edwards Give a Valid Refusal?   120

OBJECTIONS TO PREMISE (7)   124
   Virtue May Overpower the Right to Refuse   124
   Doubt Justifies Delay   126

SUMMARY   129

REVIEW QUESTIONS   130

NOTES   131

CHAPTER 5   EUTHANASIA   132

INTRODUCTION   132

CASE DESCRIPTION   133
   Case Description: Tim Regan's Voluntary Active Euthanasia   133
   What Is Euthanasia?   134
   Different Kinds of Euthanasia   137

DECIDING WHICH ISSUES TO DEBATE   141

THE MORALITY OF VOLUNTARY ACTIVE EUTHANASIA   141

The Autonomy and Best Interest Argument for Voluntary Active Euthanasia   142

The Revised Autonomy and Best Interest Argument   144

The Sanctity of Life Objection to the Morality of Voluntary Active Euthanasia   145

Suicide and Hare's Lorry Driver—More Counterexamples to the Sanctity of Life
Principle   148

An Argument That the Moral Reasons against Killing Do Not Apply to Voluntary Active
Euthanasia   150

An Argument That Euthanasia Is Wrong Because It Destroys What Belongs
to God   150

A Counterexample to the Revised Autonomy and Best Interest Argument   152

THE MORALITY OF NON-VOLUNTARY ACTIVE EUTHANASIA   152

The Best Interest Argument for Non-Voluntary Active Euthanasia   153

Philippa Foot's Objection to Non-Voluntary Active Euthanasia   156

The Never-Best-Interest Objection to Non-Voluntary Active Euthanasia   157

SUMMARY   158

REVIEW QUESTIONS   159

NOTES   160

CHAPTER 6   ABORTION   161

INTRODUCTION   161

DRAMA   163

DEBATE   165

Clarifying the Case and Identifying Relevant Facts   165

MORAL ISSUES RAISED BY THE CASE   167

Stating Our Positions   168

LEADING ARGUMENTS AGAINST THE MORALITY OF ABORTION   169

Noonan's Argument   169

Marquis's Argument for the Wrongfulness of Abortion   173

The Argument That This Abortion Discriminates against the Disabled   177

Patrick's Virtue-Based Argument for Why Abortion Would Be Permissible in
This Case   180

The Right to Life Weighed against Marissa and Don's Virtues   181

DORAN'S ARGUMENT THAT MARISSA AND DON'S DECISION TO ABORT WAS MORALLY
PERMISSIBLE   185

The Rationality Criterion for a Right to Life   185

The Life Criterion   186

The Sentience Criterion   187

The Addition of Rationality to Sentience   188

Objections to Doran's Sentience-Based Criterion of a Right to Life   190

SUMMARY   196

REVIEW QUESTIONS   197

NOTES   197

CHAPTER 7   C-SECTION BY CHOICE   199

INTRODUCTION   199

DRAMA   200

DEBATE   205
    Clarifying the Case and Identifying Relevant Facts   205

MORAL ISSUES RAISED BY THE CASE   210
    Stating Our Positions   210

DORAN'S ARGUMENT FOR WHY WENDY'S DECISION IS MORALLY PERMISSIBLE   212

DO POTENTIAL HARMS MAKE WENDY'S AUTONOMOUS CHOICE WRONG?   214
    Harms to the Baby   215
    Harms to the Mother   222
    Harms to Others besides the Baby and the Mother   224

SUMMARY   227

REVIEW QUESTIONS   228

NOTES   228

CHAPTER 8   TWO-TIER HEALTH CARE   232

INTRODUCTION   232

DRAMA   234

DEBATE   236
    Clarifying the Case and Identifying Relevant Facts   236

MORAL ISSUES RAISED BY THE CASE   240
    Stating Our Positions   241

A LIBERTARIAN ARGUMENT   242
    The Wilt Chamberlain Example   244
    Is Redistributive Taxation Inherently Unjust?   245
    The Complicity Objection to the Second Premise   250
    The Compassion Objection to the Second Premise   251

AN EGALITARIAN ARGUMENT   253
    The Self-Respect Argument   255

TWO-TIER ARGUMENTS   257
    Is Two-Tier MRI Permissible If It Does Not Harm the Public Health Care
        System?   257

Is Two-Tier MRI Permissible If It Benefits the Public Health Care System?   258
Warren's Social Contract View on When Two-Tier MRI Is Justified   259
Patrick's Virtue-Based View on When Two-Tier MRI Is Justified   260

COMMENTS ON CANADA'S CURRENT PUBLIC HEALTH CARE SYSTEM   264

FROM THE POLITICAL TO THE INDIVIDUAL   264

CLOSING ARGUMENTS   266

SUMMARY   268

REVIEW QUESTIONS   269

NOTES   270

CHAPTER 9   MICROALLOCATION OF SCARCE RESOURCES   271

INTRODUCTION   271

DRAMA   272

DEBATE   276
Clarifying the Case and Identifying Relevant Facts   276

MORAL ISSUES RAISED BY THE CASE   277
Stating Our Positions   278

MICROALLOCATION RULES: CLINICAL CONSIDERATIONS   279
Warren's Argument for Fair Microallocation Rules: Worst First, First Come, and
    Hopeless Second   279
Doran's Objection to the Sympathy Metarule   282
Patrick's Objection to the Sympathy Metarule   286
Objection to the Sufficiency of Hopeless Second   287
Minimize YPLL (Minimize Years of Potential Life Lost)   288
Substantial Benefit   289
Fair Turn   290

MICROALLOCATION RULES: NON-CLINICAL CONSIDERATIONS   293
Moral Responsibility   293
Innocents First   294
Third-Party Interests   296
Public Interest   297
Medical Interests   298

COLLECTING OUR THOUGHTS   300

SUMMARY   301

REVIEW QUESTIONS   302

NOTES   303

CHAPTER 10 ALTERNATIVE MEDICATIONS AND PROFESSIONAL
RELATIONSHIPS   304

INTRODUCTION   304

DRAMA   306

DEBATE   310
Clarifying the Case and Identifying Relevant Facts   310

MORAL ISSUES RAISED BY THE CASE   313
Stating Our Positions   314

THE BEST INTEREST PRINCIPLE   314
Patrick's Frog Toxin Counterexample to the Best Interest Principle   317

THE AMPLE DISCRETION PRINCIPLE   318
Doran's Indeterminacy Objection to Warren's Principle   319

THE AMPLE DISCRETION PRINCIPLE REVISED: VALID CONSENT OF COMPETENT PATIENTS
ONLY   321
Ample Discretion, Patient Competence, and Valid Consent   322
Ample Discretion and Patient Autonomy   324

THE AMPLE DISCRETION PRINCIPLE REVISED (AGAIN): HARM AVOIDANCE   326

AGAINST THE REVISED AMPLE DISCRETION PRINCIPLE: THE DIVISION OF LABOUR
OBJECTION   329
The Psychic Surgery Counterexample   331
More Counterexamples to the Ample Discretion Principle: Prayer and Other
Unconventional Treatments   333

FINAL THOUGHTS   334

SUMMARY   336

REVIEW QUESTIONS   337

NOTES   337

Glossary   *339*
Index   *359*

ABOUT THE AUTHORS

Patrick Findler, PhD, received his PhD, with a specialization in ethics, from the University of California, Davis, in 2001. He has taught at UC Davis, Simon Fraser University, the University of British Columbia, and Capilano University. Patrick joined the Philosophy Department at Kwantlen Polytechnic University in 2002. His teaching and research interests are in ethics, metaphysics, and the philosophy of sport. His most recent publication addresses the question of whether kids should play football (or other similarly risky sports). Current projects include a paper on mountaineering ethics and the duty to rescue. Patrick is a co-founder and co-organizer of the PHILOsurfer Convergence, an annual conference for philosophy professors who share a passion for surfing.

Doran Smolkin, PhD, earned his BA at the University of British Columbia, and his MA and PhD at the University of Illinois at Chicago. Doran was an assistant professor at Kansas State University from 1992 to 1996. Since 1996, he has been a member of the Philosophy Department at Kwantlen Polytechnic University. Doran also teaches regularly in the Philosophy Department at the University of British Columbia. Doran enjoys working with students and he has received several awards in recognition of teaching excellence. His research interests are in moral and political philosophy, with article publications on whether speciesism is a prejudice, what makes a life fortunate or unfortunate, the nature of trust, the nature of our obligations to future generations, and the ethical obligations of physicians to treat patients with HIV.

Warren Bourgeois, PhD, received his BA at the University of Toronto and his PhD at the University of California, Irvine. He has taught at the University of Salzburg, Austria; the University of California, San Diego; and the University of British Columbia, and is now emeritus at Kwantlen Polytechnic University. He helped develop policies on academic freedom and research ethics. He chaired the Research Ethics Board through its challenging first five years of development. Among his published writings is the book *Persons: What Philosophers Say about You*, released in its second edition by Wilfrid Laurier University Press in 2003. From 1978 to 2018, he was a director of the BC Civil Liberties Association. He has helped to found and has served on two hospital ethics committees. In his most recent publication, he applied the theory he presents in this book to questions of environmental sustainability.

PREFACE

Debating Health Care Ethics: Canadian Contexts addresses both traditional and cutting-edge topics in health care ethics, with a special emphasis on issues of particular concern to Canadians. Many textbooks display the results of debates in ethics. This textbook shows *how* the debates are done.

Debating Health Care Ethics: Canadian Contexts provides the tools to examine issues critically and debate topics intelligently. This text provides students with background information about philosophical methods and ethical theories, and then shows how to defend these positions using these theories and methods.

Dramatized case studies on issues followed by a three-way debate by the textbook authors form the major thrust of this book. Positions emerge, are defended, and sometimes are revised or rejected in response to objections. Rather than confronting students with only the complex outcome of long discussion and thought, the text demonstrates *how* philosophical ethics is done.

Students need the tools to examine critically and to debate intelligently various topics in health care ethics. The textbook's structure reflects that goal, beginning with a chapter on **philosophical arguments and methods.** This first chapter serves as a brief introduction for students new to philosophy or as a refresher for more seasoned students.

The second chapter provides a very readable, yet in-depth introduction to the strengths and weaknesses of major **normative ethical theories.** Understanding the theories can be challenging, so the text attempts to make this material accessible. At the same time, the book does not gloss over the fact that every ethical theory is the object of serious debate: the authors present some of the most difficult objections confronting each ethical theory and suggest ways in which defenders of these theories may respond to these criticisms. In sum, the introduction to normative ethical theory aims to be clear and informative, and to give a sense of where the strengths and weaknesses of each theory are thought to lie, while avoiding the appearance that ethics is just a game of setting up views and knocking them down.

The third chapter briefly explains the particular ethical positions (**philosophical approaches**) of the three debaters—the authors of this text. In this chapter, the authors present and defend their own particular brand of three of the ethical theories discussed in chapter 2: deontological pluralism, contractarianism, and virtue ethics. After reading this chapter, students will understand how each of the text authors will approach various ethical issues throughout the rest of the book.

After laying the foundation for argumentation and theory, chapters 4 through 10 examine important ethical issues in health care. Each of these chapters begins with a brief drama or case study that introduces a particular set of moral problems. These dramas or cases will engage readers while bringing certain ethical issues in health care to light. In the debates following the dramas or cases, a philosophical discussion takes place: facts are clarified, questions for debate are identified, and arguments are advanced and critically examined.

The debate format has the advantage of demonstrating to students how philosophy is done. Students see a wide array of ethical theories applied to specific questions; they see arguments from a variety of perspectives carefully developed, criticized, and reformulated; they see how consensus can sometimes be reached; and they see how thoughtful disagreement can remain.

In addition to chapters on philosophical methods, normative ethical theory, and the authors' favoured philosophical approaches, the following ethical issues are examined in this text.

Autonomy and the Right to Refuse Treatment: A drama concerning an elderly patient who insists on being discharged from the hospital even though he is at high risk of choking leads to a philosophical discussion of the concepts of competence, autonomy, and valid consent.

Euthanasia: A straightforward description of a case of medical assistance in dying (MAID) reported on CBC motivates this debate on the moral permissibility of voluntary and non-voluntary active euthanasia.

Abortion: A couple, Don and Marissa, discovers that the fetus Marissa is carrying has Down's syndrome. They have to decide whether to continue with the pregnancy when that means they may lose their family-run business and possibly their marriage. This leads to a debate about the moral permissibility of abortion in general, and in the couple's case, in particular.

C-Section by Choice: A woman requests a Caesarean section for non-medical reasons. Her physician refuses, but she finds another who is willing to grant her request, even though vaginal delivery is recommended in her case. This leads to a debate about the moral permissibility of Caesarean section for non-medical reasons. What, in general, are the moral obligations of parents to avoid needless risks to themselves, their children, and others?

Two-Tier Health Care: The case of two young hockey players who both need MRIs motivates a discussion on the justice of allowing expensive, privately funded MRIs in addition to the public health care system's provision of MRIs. Under what conditions, if any, is a two-tier health care system just?

Microallocation of Scarce Resources: A small-town emergency department must cope with a horrible car accident. There are not enough staff members and resources to treat all the patients who need care. This prompts a debate on the morally justified rules for triaging patients in emergency situations.

Alternative Medications and Professional Relationships: A man who received a diagnosis of cancer rejects the standard medical therapy and opts for a scientifically unproven alternative therapy. He finds a doctor who is willing to administer this unproven therapy, even though she thinks the standard therapy is a better option. This leads to a debate over how much discretion physicians should have to administer unproven therapies.

Debating Health Care Ethics also includes a number of **pedagogical tools**:

- **Up for Discussion questions** encourage readers to participate in the debate in various ways.
- **Definition boxes** demystify some concepts.
- **Background** and **Theory boxes** connect the discussion to everything from current events to great thinkers of the past.
- **Technique boxes** point out helpful strategies for presenting and critically examining arguments.
- **Key terms** are **bolded** in each chapter and are defined in an end-of-text **Glossary**.

RECOMMENDATIONS FOR USING THIS TEXTBOOK

There are various pathways through this book that an instructor may wish to consider. We recommend that all introductory students read the first chapter to gain some acquaintance with techniques of argument. Ideally, students will then work through the second chapter on ethical theories, and the third chapter where each author's approach to ethics is explained, prior to turning to the debate chapters 4 to 10. The debate chapters are self-contained and can be read in any order. In a one-semester course, however, especially for students in health professions not used to ethical theory, it may be advisable to initially skip over chapter 2. As questions arise, the instructor in such a course may wish to use chapter 2 as a reference text for students wanting more detail concerning theory.

The debate format of the book lends itself to novel and productive exercises. For example, when assigning a topic in health care ethics, instructors may ask students to write their own debates, using the text as a model. For many students, beginning with a conversation rather than formal prose also has the advantage of being less intimidating and more productive of ideas. It helps students produce, in an elementary form, the positions, arguments, objections, and replies that can form the basis of a more formal academic paper. This sort of exercise also avoids the copying and pasting of poorly understood passages from the Internet or other sources. After the instructor returns comments to students on their debates, the instructor may want to ask students to turn their debates into polished position papers.

Another sort of assignment that has worked well when using this material in medical ethics courses is to have students answer specific questions about the drama and debate. For example, on the issue of abortion, the instructor may ask the following questions:

1. Do you think it was morally permissible for Don and Marissa to obtain an abortion? Why or why not?
2. Consider an objection to your reasoning.
3. Explain why that objection fails.
4. Consider an argument discussed in the text that you think fails, even though it leads to a similar (or even the same) conclusion as your favoured argument.
5. Explain why that argument fails.
6. Explain what you take to be the strongest argument for the opposite conclusion to yours.
7. Explain why you think that argument is unsound.
8. What was your view about the permissibility of Marissa's abortion immediately after reading the drama, before reading the debate? At that point, what reasons did you have for your view? Has your view or have the reasons for your view changed, and if so, why?

The advantage of using these focused questions is that it requires students to state their own views and arguments, think critically about their own arguments, consider other arguments and why they think those arguments fail, and reflect about how their views and reasons have changed as a result of debate. It is also a relatively straightforward matter to have students transform their answers to these questions into a polished academic paper.

ACKNOWLEDGEMENTS

I am most grateful to my wife, Cara, for her patience, understanding, and support. Our children, Cashel and Reese, deserve special thanks too for their patience, but also for their curiosity and insight, which provide constant reminders of the excitement and value of philosophy. Finally, I would like to thank my colleagues and co-authors, Doran and Warren, for their hard work, perseverance, and friendship. —*Patrick Findler*

I want to thank Patrick and Warren for their tireless work on this project. The book could not have been written without them. They have my respect and admiration both as first-rate philosophers and, more importantly, as fine human beings. On a more personal note, I am most grateful to my best friend and wife, Julie, for her love, wisdom, constant support, and encouragement. I want to thank my children, Mischa, Andy, Kayti, and Elie, for their love and encouragement, for their good company, and for demonstrating that the future is bright and full of hope. Last, but never least, I am indebted to my mom and dad, Debby and Barry Smolkin, for their constant love and support. —*Doran Smolkin*

Thanks to Kwantlen Polytechnic University for an educational leave during which I prepared a website that turned out, with Doran and Patrick's efforts, to be a precursor to our book. I am grateful to my patient family who saw me through the years of debates, writing, and revision that led to this text. My students and colleagues, too, deserve thanks for their enthusiastic questioning of our positions. Of course, my co-authors deserve much gratitude for their persistence, dedication, and insight. I wrote the dramas and am grateful for Patrick and Doran's comments and those of my nursing students. I must also thank physicians and nurses who looked at these cases with an eye to verisimilitude. Their comments helped to bring the cases presented more in line with reality. Any lack of verisimilitude must, however, be laid at my doorstep. —*Warren Bourgeois*

Collaboration among three authors brings various challenges to a project. Invariably, disagreements surface, compromise is required, and each author ends up taking on certain roles and responsibilities. There are also great advantages in co-authoring a book. Different points of view make for more interesting reading, arguments are improved because of helpful suggestions made by one's co-authors, and the workload is shared. In our case, there is no doubt that our book is much stronger because it had three authors who each made different, though equally important, intellectual contributions.

We wish to thank Kwantlen Polytechnic University for several research grants that gave us much-needed time to do revisions. We are also grateful to the editorial team at Canadian Scholars for their encouragement and support.

Lastly, we owe a debt of gratitude to the following reviewers:

Eva Beattie, *St. Clair College*
Dale Beyerstein, *Langara College*
Leslie Burkholder, *University of British Columbia*
Carolyn Ells, *McGill University*
Ken Ferguson, *University of Ottawa*
Mazen M. Guirguis, *Kwantlen Polytechnic University*
Kenneth Kirkwood, *University of Western Ontario*
Arthur Schafer, *University of Manitoba*
Meredith Schwartz, *Ryerson University*
Karen Shirley, *Camosun College*
Jeremy Snyder, *Simon Fraser University*
Edrie Sobstyl, *Douglas College*
Duff R. Waring, *York University*
Brian Wetstein, *University of Guelph*

1 ARGUMENTS AND METHODOLOGY

INTRODUCTION

We should accept philosophical views in general, and moral views in particular, on the basis of the arguments offered in their support. It is therefore crucial to understand what an argument is, and how to evaluate an argument. In this chapter, we explain the kinds of arguments philosophers give, the features of good and bad arguments, and some common tools and methods that will aid in the evaluation of arguments.

LEARNING OBJECTIVES

After completing this chapter, you should be able to:

- Distinguish deductive from inductive arguments
- Define deductive validity and soundness
- Explain inductive strength and weakness
- Describe common fallacies when constructing and evaluating arguments
- Recognize the role of moral principles when constructing moral arguments
- Understand the nature and purpose of thought experiments
- Construct counterexamples to test philosophical analyses and claims

---

ARGUMENTS

What Is an Argument?

An **argument** is simply a set of claims; one of these is the conclusion, and the others are premises. The **conclusion** is the claim that one is trying to establish, and the **premises** are the reasons offered in support of the conclusion. To illustrate, consider the following example:

(1)   It is always wrong to kill an innocent person.
(2)   Abortion is the killing of an innocent person.
(3)   Therefore, abortion is wrong.

The conclusion of this argument is the claim that abortion is wrong. The other two claims are the premises or supporting reasons. Arguments must have at least one premise, but there is no upper limit to the number of premises an argument can have.

Sometimes the arguments given in support of a position are clearly and explicitly stated. Other times, however, the arguments may be buried in difficult and lengthy passages. In these cases, it will take work to spot the conclusion and supporting premises. Often, certain terms are present that can help you to piece together an author's argument. Philosophers call these terms **premise indicators** and **conclusion indicators**.

Premise indicators include the terms *for*, *because*, *since*, and *given that*. Here are two examples to illustrate how these terms are used in the context of an argument:

> *Because* active euthanasia involves the intentional killing of a person, it is always wrong.
> You should not deceive others, *for* this is disrespectful.
> *Since* abortion is murder, it is wrong.

The following terms are conclusion indicators: *therefore*, *thus*, *hence*, *so*, and *consequently*. Here are examples to show how some of these terms are used to signal the conclusion of an argument:

> Active euthanasia involves the intentional killing of a person; *therefore*, it is always wrong.
> Deceiving others is disrespectful, *so* you should not deceive others.
> Abortion is murder; *thus* it is wrong.

In some instances, arguments may be given without the use of premise or conclusion indicators. Determining the structure of an argument in such cases can be tricky. You have to ask yourself what *role* each sentence is playing in the passage. If a particular sentence expresses the point the author is trying to establish, then it is the author's conclusion. If a sentence is given as support for some other claim, then it is a premise. Still other sentences in the passage may not play a direct role in the argument, and these would be neither the premises nor the conclusion.

Upon finding a passage in a text that contains an argument, it is often helpful to rewrite it in what is known as **standard form**. In standard form, each premise is numbered and stated on its own line, and then the conclusion is stated last. Usually, the conclusion is separated from the premises by a horizontal line, with the premises above the line and the conclusion below it. To illustrate, consider the following argument:

Abortion is morally permissible, for it is morally permissible for women to make their own decisions when it comes to controlling their own bodies, and abortion is a decision that involves women and their own bodies.

We can rewrite the argument in standard form as follows:

(1) It is morally permissible for women to make their own decisions when it comes to controlling their own bodies.

(2) Abortion is a decision that involves a woman and her own body.

(3) Therefore, abortion is morally permissible.

There are numerous advantages in writing out an argument in standard form—not the least of which is that it makes the argument clearer and thus easier to evaluate.

Evaluating Arguments

The point of providing an argument in support of a view is typically to show that the view is correct and to persuade others to accept it.[1] Good arguments—ones we should accept—have two features. First, all of the premises are true. And second, the premises logically support the conclusion. Thus, when evaluating arguments, we need to ask two basic questions. First, are all of the premises true? Second, do the premises support the conclusion? If the answer to *both* of these questions is "yes," then the argument is a good one and we have good reason to accept its conclusion. If, however, the answer to *either* question (or both) is "no," then the argument is bad and we do not have good reason to accept its conclusion. Notice, then, that an argument might fail for one of two reasons: it might have a false premise, or it might have premises that do not support the conclusion. (Of course, an argument might have both of these problems.)

It is important to recognize that whether the premises are true and whether the premises support the conclusion are logically distinct issues. Consider the following example:

(1) All patients have cancer.

(2) All cancer patients have appendicitis.

(3) Therefore, all patients have appendicitis.

This, of course, is a bad argument. What makes it bad is not that the premises fail to support the conclusion. In this example, the premises very strongly support the conclusion. If the premises were true, the conclusion would have to be true.[2] The problem with this argument is that the premises are not true. Now consider an argument with the opposite problem:

(1) Some Canadians have cancer.
(2) Some Americans have arthritis.
(3) Therefore, a broken leg is painful.

This, too, is a bad argument. But what makes this argument bad is not that the premises are false. Rather, the problem with this argument is that the premises do not logically support the conclusion. Acceptance of the premises does not give us any reason to accept the conclusion. Even though the premises are true, the conclusion still *could be* false. It is important, then, not to assume that the conclusion of an argument is true simply because the premises are true. The premises must also logically support the conclusion.

Deductive Arguments: Validity and Soundness

A **deductive argument** is an argument where the truth of the premises is intended to *guarantee* the truth of the conclusion. For example, the following is likely offered as a deductive argument:

(1) It is seriously immoral to deprive an individual of a future of value.
(2) Abortion, in standard cases, deprives the fetus of a future of value.
(3) Therefore, in standard cases, abortion is seriously immoral.

When evaluating deductive arguments, there are certain technical terms that philosophers commonly use. In particular, philosophers use the terms *valid* and *sound* to refer to properties that deductive arguments can have or lack. A deductively valid argument (or, for simplicity's sake, a **valid argument**) is an argument with the following feature: It is *impossible* for all of the premises to be true and the conclusion false. Put a little differently, *if* all of the premises are true, the conclusion must be true. To illustrate, let's return to an example considered earlier:

(1) All patients have cancer.
(2) All cancer patients have appendicitis.
(3) Therefore, all patients have appendicitis.

Here's another example:

(1) No Canadian is an American.
(2) Justin Trudeau is a Canadian.
(3) Therefore, Justin Trudeau is not an American.

Notice that in each of these examples, *if* the premises were true, the conclusion would have to be true. The truth of the premises *logically guarantees* the truth of the conclusion. Hence, these are valid arguments.

It is very important to note that valid arguments need not have true premises. In saying that an argument is valid, we are not claiming that the premises are true. We are claiming, rather, that the premises, *if true*, guarantee that the conclusion

UP FOR DISCUSSION

Can a valid argument have false premises and a true conclusion? Explain your answer using an example.

is true. In other words, to say that an argument is valid is to say something about the *logical relationship* between the argument's premises and its conclusion: the relationship is such that if the premises are true, then the conclusion must be true. Deductive arguments that do not have this property are said to be **invalid**.

A **sound argument** is a valid argument with all true premises. A virtue of sound arguments is that they always have true conclusions.[3] Notice that this is guaranteed by the definition of a sound argument. Here is a simple example of a sound argument:

(1)   If mercy killing was illegal in Canada in 1993, then Robert Latimer broke the law when he committed the mercy killing of his daughter, Tracy.

(2)   Mercy killing was illegal in Canada in 1993.

(3)   Therefore, Robert Latimer broke the law when he committed the mercy killing of his daughter, Tracy.

This is a valid argument: if the premises are true, the conclusion must be true. The premises, moreover, are in fact true. Hence, this argument is sound.

An **unsound** argument is a deductive argument that is either invalid or has at least one false premise. Unsound arguments are therefore bad arguments. They are bad because if an argument is unsound, it has failed to establish the truth of its conclusion. Note, however, that this is not to say that the conclusions of unsound arguments must be false. To illustrate, here is an example of an unsound argument with a true conclusion:

(1)   Everyone who goes to a private clinic is terminally ill.

(2)   Some Canadians go to private clinics.

(3)   Therefore, some Canadians are terminally ill.

Here we have an unsound argument with a true conclusion. The argument is unsound because premise (1) is false. Thus, when we claim that an argument is unsound, we are not saying that its conclusion is false. Rather, we are saying that its conclusion should not be accepted on the basis of this argument. Either the argument is invalid, so the premises do not logically support the conclusion, or at least one premise is false, so the argument does not necessarily lead us to the truth.

Inductive Arguments

Not all arguments are intended to be deductive arguments. In some arguments, the premises, if true, may not be intended to *guarantee* the truth of the conclusion. Instead, the premises provided may be intended to demonstrate only that the conclusion is *probably* true. In that case, the argument is **inductive**. Here is an example of this kind of argument:

(1)   Most healthy pregnancies at 24 weeks result in successful births.
(2)   Tina has a healthy pregnancy at 24 weeks.
(3)   Therefore, Tina's pregnancy will result in a successful birth.

Now, the fact that healthy pregnancies at 24 weeks generally result in successful births does not guarantee or conclusively prove that Tina's pregnancy will result in a successful birth. That is, it is *possible* that the conclusion is false, even if the premises are true; however, if the premises of the argument are true, they certainly do provide some support for the conclusion. This support is not, however, the kind of support we talked about earlier when we looked at valid arguments. The premises just make the conclusion more probable.

When it comes to evaluating inductive arguments, philosophers do not use the terms *valid/invalid* and *sound/unsound*; instead, they speak of inductive arguments as being either **strong** or **weak**. A strong inductive argument is an argument that is not deductive, and where the premises, if true, make the conclusion probably true. The more support provided by the premises of an inductive argument, the stronger the argument. Here is an example of an inductively strong argument:

(1)   Dr. Badesh will see 100 flu sufferers this year.
(2)   Dr. Badesh has treated 99 flu sufferers this year with antibiotics.
(3)   Therefore, Dr. Badesh will treat all of the flu sufferers she sees this year with antibiotics.

This is a strong inductive argument, because if the premises are true, it is likely that the conclusion is true.[4]

An inductive argument is weak when the premises, if true, provide little support for the conclusion. Here is an example of an inductively weak argument:

(1)   Dr. Badesh will see 100 flu sufferers this year.
(2)   Dr. Badesh has treated 1 flu sufferer this year with antibiotics.
(3)   Therefore, Dr. Badesh will treat all of the flu sufferers she sees this year with antibiotics.

DEFINITION

Our definition of inductive strength closely follows that provided by Brian Skyrms in *Choice and Chance: An Introduction to Inductive Logic*, 4th ed. (Belmost, CA: Wadsworth Publishing, 1999; first published in 1967). Skyrms contends that "an argument is inductively strong if and only if it is improbable that its conclusion is false while its premises are true, and it is not deductively valid" (17).

Some philosophers, however, define inductive strength differently. Richard Feldman, for example, suggests that an argument is inductively strong if and only if: (i) it is cogent, (ii) the premises are true or at least justified, and (iii) the conclusion is not defeated by one's evidence. Feldman's notion of *cogency* appears to correspond to our (and Skyrms's) definition of inductive strength: an argument is cogent when it is not valid and when its premises make the conclusion probable.

Source: Richard Feldman, *Reason and Argument*, 2nd ed. (Upper Saddle River, NJ: Pearson, 1998).

What makes this an inductively weak argument, of course, is that the premises, if true, do not make the conclusion probable or likely to be true. In this instance, the argument commits the familiar error of generalizing from a single case. As the saying goes, one swallow does not make a summer. We should not infer conclusions from too little evidence.

Moral Arguments

What we call a **moral argument** is an argument in support of a **substantive moral claim**—that is, a claim about the moral status of acts, policies, persons, and so forth. The following, for instance, are examples of substantive moral claims: euthanasia is morally permissible; progressive taxation is unjust; an unrepentant serial murderer is evil. In the next chapter, we examine several influential normative ethical theories. One of the central aims of many of these theories, we shall see, is to provide correct, general principles that tell us what makes actions (policies, and so forth) right and wrong, and persons good and bad. As we'll now explain, these principles can play an important role in arguing for substantive moral conclusions.

Consider the following simple argument:

(1)   Active euthanasia minimizes overall suffering.
(2)   Therefore, active euthanasia is morally right.

Notice that this argument is invalid: the premise, if true, does not guarantee the truth of the conclusion. Although active euthanasia may well minimize overall suffering, it does not logically follow that it is right. But now consider the following moral principle:

Any act that minimizes overall suffering is morally right.

This principle tells us that minimizing overall suffering is a "right-making" feature of actions; any action that has this feature is morally right. With this principle in hand, we can now construct a deductively valid argument for our conclusion:

(1) *Any act that minimizes overall suffering is morally right.*
(2) Active euthanasia minimizes overall suffering.
(3) Therefore, active euthanasia is morally right.

Notice the structure of this argument. Premise (1) asserts a moral principle; it states that any act that has a certain property is morally right. Premise (2) asserts that a particular act has this right-making property. We can therefore validly conclude that the act in question is morally right.

Although we have been focusing on the role of moral principles in the construction of deductively valid moral arguments, it is worth noting that our comments about the interplay between moral principles and assertions that a given act has the relevant right- (or wrong-) making properties apply also in the case of inductive arguments. Consider, for example, the following argument:

(1) Usually, but not always, acts of dishonesty are wrong.
(2) By withholding relevant information, Dr. Badesh acted dishonestly toward her patient.
(3) Therefore, it was wrong for Dr. Badesh to withhold relevant information from her patient.

This argument is inductive. The premises, if true, are not intended to guarantee that the conclusion is true. Rather, the premises provided are intended only to show that the conclusion is probably true. Still, the omission of either premise would significantly weaken the argument.

 UP FOR DISCUSSION

Consider the following argument: Homosexuality is unnatural; therefore, homosexuality is wrong. What missing premise would make the argument inductively strong?

In summary, the general moral principles provided by normative ethical theories can play an important role in arguing for substantive moral claims. Moral principles commonly tell us what makes actions right or wrong (or persons good or bad). These principles, when combined with premises that assert that given acts (or persons) have the relevant properties, can be used to construct deductively valid or inductively strong arguments for substantive moral views. We critically examine the moral principles offered by leading normative ethical theories in the next chapter. First, however, we consider some useful methods for evaluating moral principles in particular, and philosophical claims in general. We also consider common fallacies to avoid when constructing and evaluating arguments.

PHILOSOPHICAL METHODOLOGY: COUNTEREXAMPLES AND THOUGHT EXPERIMENTS

We mentioned earlier that philosophical views should be accepted or rejected on the basis of the arguments offered in their support. If you disagree with an author's position on some issue, then you must believe that the author's argument for that view is unsound or weak. So you must believe either that the premises fail to adequately support the conclusion or that at least one premise is false. Let's now consider methods employed by philosophers to establish whether premises are true or false.

As noted in the previous section, moral arguments commonly involve a combination of both moral principles that specify right- or wrong-making properties and assertions that a given act has the relevant properties. Claims of the latter sort are often empirical—since they are often based on our *observations* that a given act has the relevant properties—and therefore can be shown to be true or false through ordinary observational methods. But observation alone will not suffice in the case of moral principles. So how might we try to demonstrate that a moral principle is true or false?

To evaluate or test moral principles, and philosophical claims and analyses in general, philosophers often employ *counterexamples* and *thought experiments*. A **counterexample** is just that—an example that counters a given claim or argument. A **thought experiment** is a kind of mental experiment one performs through an exercise of imagination. Thought experiments are a very useful way to generate counterexamples. To illustrate these methods, let's return to an argument discussed earlier:

(1) Any act that minimizes overall suffering is morally right.
(2) Active euthanasia minimizes overall suffering.
(3) Therefore, active euthanasia is morally right.

We noted earlier that this argument is valid. If you disagree with the conclusion, you must show that at least one of the premises of this argument is false.[5] The first premise expresses the moral principle that any act that minimizes overall suffering is morally right. But is that true? A good way to test this claim is to see whether we can find a counterexample to it. That is, we want to see whether we can find an instance of an act that minimizes overall suffering yet is not right. Engaging in a thought experiment will help us to discover possible counterexamples. The task here is to see if we can *imagine* a situation in which an act that minimizes overall suffering is not right. With a little thought, it seems that we can in fact imagine many such situations. The following paragraph presents one example.[6]

Suppose a teen from the neighbourhood knocks on my door one Saturday morning and offers to mow my lawn for $20. My lawn needs mowing, and I'm too busy to take care of it myself, so I agree. An hour later the teen knocks on my door again to collect her money. I inspect the lawn and see that she has done a very nice job. As I reach for my wallet to pay the teen, it occurs to me that I could minimize overall suffering by donating the $20 I promised to her to a local charity. Let's suppose that I'm right: breaking my promise to pay the teen and donating the money to a local charity re-

UP FOR DISCUSSION

Can you think of another counterexample to the claim that "any act that minimizes suffering is morally right"?

ally would minimize overall suffering. In that case, premise (1) implies that breaking my promise is the morally right thing to do. But our common-sense moral beliefs suggest that this is not the right thing to do. And so we seem to have a counterexample to premise (1); we have an example of an action that minimizes overall suffering, yet does not appear to be morally right.

This counterexample provides us with good reason for thinking that premise (1) is false, and that the above argument is therefore unsound. But remember, it doesn't follow from this that the conclusion of the argument—that active euthanasia is permissible—is false.

One might wonder why this counterexample provides good reason for thinking that the moral principle in question is false. After all, we seem to have done little more than show that the moral principle in question conflicts with what you and I happen to *believe* is the right thing to do in the example described. Perhaps, though, the principle is correct, and it is our belief about what's right that is mistaken. The more general question here is how the use of counterexamples can show that any moral principle or theory is false, if the counterexamples are simply based on our common-sense moral beliefs. There is a great deal to be said about this topic that we cannot address here. We shall have to limit ourselves to a brief discussion of the concept of **reflective equilibrium**. This will help to shed some light on the legitimacy of thought experiments and counterexamples when evaluating moral principles and theories.

Reflective equilibrium, in the context of moral philosophy, is the end point of a process of moral deliberation that involves going back and forth between moral principles and what they imply about specific cases. The ultimate goal of this process is to attain a state of coherence or consistency between the moral principles we accept and our considered moral beliefs. We have achieved reflective equilibrium when we have achieved this state of consistency. The basic process goes like this. If a principle or theory has implications that conflict with our moral beliefs, and we have a high degree of confidence in our moral beliefs, then we may reject or revise the principle until we find one that matches our beliefs; however, if a principle conflicts with our moral beliefs, but we lack confidence in these beliefs, then we may want to revise or reject our beliefs to achieve a state of consistency.

To illustrate, let's return to the principle considered above: *Any act that minimizes overall suffering is morally right*. We want to know whether this principle is correct and deserves our acceptance. So we then consider what this principle implies in specific cases. We saw earlier that this principle implies that it would be morally right to refuse to pay the teen who mowed your lawn and to give the money to a charity instead, for this would minimize overall suffering. Upon reflection, however, most of us believe that it would be wrong to give the money to the charity if that meant breaking the promise to pay the girl. That is our considered belief or judgment about this case. Since we have a high degree of confidence in this judgment—more confidence that this judgment is correct than that the principle is correct—we should revise or reject the principle in question and seek another that is consistent with our judgment. If we lacked confidence in this judgment, however, then we might want to seek consistency by revising or rejecting the judgment. The goal, again, is to attain a consistent fit between our moral principles and moral judgments about cases. And the fact that the moral principles we accept are in equilibrium with our considered moral judgments confers justification on both the principles and the beliefs.[7]

One final point about thought experiments is in order before we turn our attention to fallacies. Thought experiments often involve unusual and unrealistic situations, but it is important to see the relevance of these examples. The force of the counterexample described does not depend on whether the imagined example would ever actually happen, or whether it involves a situation in which we might actually find ourselves. The only constraint is that the imagined situation is one that is logically (or conceptually) possible. Notice that premise (1) asserts that *any* act that minimizes overall suffering is morally right. Given this, it is perfectly legitimate to test this claim by imagining situations that may or may not be very realistic. It is very important to bear this point in mind as you read the debates, for you'll sometimes encounter strange counterexamples and thought experiments that are used to test the authors' (and others') moral views.

COMMON FALLACIES

A **fallacy** is a mistake in reasoning. There are many different kinds of fallacies, but we focus here only on a few of the more common errors in reasoning.[8]

Circularity (a.k.a. Begging the Question)

A **circular argument** is one in which the truth of the conclusion is presupposed by one or more premises.[9] The most blatant form of circularity occurs when the conclusion you are arguing for appears as a premise in your argument. Consider, for instance, the following argument:

(1)   Abortion is wrong.

(2)   Therefore, abortion is wrong.

There are, however, less obvious cases of circularity, as illustrated by this example:

(1)   Abortion is murder.
(2)   Therefore, abortion is wrong.

This second example is simply a disguised version of the conclusion, for "murder" simply means "wrongful killing." To make this point explicit, the argument could be more clearly expressed as follows:

(1)   Abortion is wrong.
(2)   Abortion is killing.
(3)   Therefore, abortion is wrong.

The circle in the argument is now apparent. The problem with the circle is that we would not accept the premises of this argument unless we already accepted the conclusion. So if you are in doubt whether abortion is wrong, this argument will do little to persuade you that it is wrong. Although circular arguments are generally uninformative and unpersuasive, notice that they are valid and may be sound.

THEORY

It is rather difficult to state the problem of circularity in precise terms, because all valid arguments are circular in the sense that the conclusion is logically "contained" in the premises. Yet we certainly don't want to say that all valid arguments are fallacious. So why is circularity a problem in some cases, but not others? To answer this question, it may help to consider a common reason for giving an argument. The point is often to convince others that your conclusion is correct. It will not help to convince others that your conclusion is correct, however, if you appeal to the conclusion to help establish it. Circularity is a problem, then, when the conclusion you are arguing for appears as one of your premises, or is offered as a reason for accepting one of your premises, and you intend to convince someone of the conclusion.

 UP FOR DISCUSSION

Is the following argument guilty of circularity? Explain your answer.

(1)   The Bible is the inerrant word of God.
(2)   The Bible says that God exists.
(3)   Therefore, God exists.

False Dilemma

Presenting fewer options than are actually available when arguing for a view is known as the **false dilemma** fallacy. For instance, in defending the current Canadian health care system, one might fallaciously argue the following: we can have our current health care system or the US model, and we certainly don't want the US system of health care. But clearly this argument is guilty of containing a false dilemma. There are, in fact, other options besides our current model of health care and the American model, and so it would be a mistake to conclude our system was best merely because we prefer it to the American system.

Equivocation

There are a host of fallacies involving the manipulation of language in order to attempt to support a conclusion. We will consider two of the more common of these, beginning with the fallacy of **equivocation**.

An example of the fallacy of equivocation is the following:

(1)   Laws imply lawgivers.
(2)   There are laws in nature.
(3)   Therefore, there must be a supernatural lawgiver.[10]

This argument commits the fallacy of equivocation, and so is invalid. The word *law* is ambiguous. It can mean legislation enacted by a lawgiver, or it can mean regularities that occur in nature. The term *law* is used in the first sense in premise (1) but in the second sense in premise (2). Once this is noted, we can rewrite the argument without the ambiguous term, and the fallacy of equivocation becomes apparent.

(1)   Legislation implies a lawgiver.
(2)   There are regularities in nature.
(3)   Therefore, there must be a supernatural lawgiver.

Now that the premises are clarified, we see that even if they are true, they fail to establish the conclusion. As critical thinkers who are searching for the truth, we need to try to spot equivocation. And we need to try to avoid falling into the trap of committing this mistake when developing our own arguments.

Appeal to Emotion

Another fallacy involving the misuse of language is the **appeal to emotion** in order to argue for some claim. Claiming that euthanasia and abortion ought to be opposed because they're butchering would be an instance of using inflammatory language in order to make one's point. Of course, such claims not only beg the question, but they also are often advanced so as to get the reader or listener to accept the conclusion without having to think carefully about the issues involved.

Straw Man

The **straw man** fallacy is the fallacy of misrepresenting your opponent's argument so that it is easily shown to be unsound or weak. The fallacy is so named because a straw man argument is easily blown down. Suppose, for instance, that a philosopher offers the following argument in support of euthanasia:

(1)   If competent, seriously disabled adults express a preference to die, then they should be permitted to die.
(2)   Some competent, seriously disabled adults do in fact express a preference to die.
(3)   Therefore, some competent, seriously disabled adults should be permitted to die.

Now, suppose a critic objects as follows: "My opponent is claiming that we should euthanize all disabled persons, since all disabled persons desire to die. But it is not true that all disabled people want to die. So my opponent's argument is clearly unsound." This critic would be guilty of the straw man fallacy, since she has misrepresented her opponent's view to make it easier to refute. Her opponent's actual position is much more subtle and less easily refuted than the argument attributed to him.

Ad Hominem

Ad hominem is a Latin expression that means "against the man." One commits the **ad hominem** fallacy when one tries to refute an argument by attacking the one who offered the argument. For example, suppose that a leader of an evangelical church presented the following argument in support of his "pro-life" position on abortion:

(1)   All human lives are sacred.
(2)   Fetuses are human.
(3)   Therefore, fetuses' lives are sacred.

Now, imagine that a critic objects as follows: "We can safely reject this argument, since it is being advocated by a religious extremist who believes all sorts of crazy things!"

This critic would be guilty of committing the ad hominem fallacy, since he attempts to refute his opponent's argument by attacking his opponent. The only way to show that an argument fails is to show that there is a problem with the argument itself.

CONCLUSION

There are, of course, many other fallacies that we cannot explain here. What counts as a fallacy depends, moreover, on the context in which an argument is offered and the intentions of the person offering it. A full discussion would be very complex. The general point is that moral philosophy—indeed, philosophy in general—is first and foremost a matter of searching for the truth through the careful use of reason. We want to discover the truth by fairly and carefully considering the arguments on all sides of an issue. Doing philosophy therefore requires a sense of fairness, as well as a sharp, critical, and open mind. We want to arrive at the truth, but we should accept a claim as true only if we are reasonably confident that it is supported by a good argument.

REVIEW QUESTIONS

1. What are the two features of a good argument?
2. What is a valid argument?
3. Construct your own example of a valid argument.
4. What is a sound argument?
5. What is an inductive argument?
6. What makes an inductive argument strong?
7. What is a moral argument?
8. What is a counterexample?
9. Describe an example that counters the following claim: Killing human beings is always wrong.
10. What is reflective equilibrium?
11. Explain the fallacy of circularity.
12. Explain the straw man fallacy.
13. Explain the fallacy of equivocation.
14. Explain the fallacy of appeal to emotion.
15. Explain the ad hominem fallacy.
16. Explain the false dilemma fallacy.

NOTES

1.   Arguments can, of course, have different purposes. For example, in science, arguments can be used to deduce predictions from general principles and observations.

2.   Arguments that have this feature are said to be *valid*. We discuss the concept of validity in the following section.

3.   Notice, however, that not all sound arguments are informative or useful. Circular arguments, for instance, may be sound, but not informative or useful. Here's an example of a sound circular argument: Cancer is sometimes fatal. Therefore, cancer is sometimes fatal.

4.   When we say this is a strong argument, we do so against typical background assumptions like these: Dr. Badesh is not likely to suddenly change her treatment preferences, and one case of the flu is much like the others. Of course, there might be an unexpected difference in case number 100, but the very fact that a difference is unexpected attests to our thinking the argument is strong. The argument could be much stronger if we made all the background assumptions explicit.

5.   One could attack this argument by criticizing either premise (1) or (2). Since our present concern is to explain how to test philosophical claims in general, and moral principles in particular, we focus our attention on criticizing premise (1), and the moral principle that it asserts. Premise (2) does not assert a moral claim. It simply says that active euthanasia minimizes overall suffering. Whether this is in fact true is an empirical matter and can be evaluated through ordinary empirical methods.

6.   This example is based on an objection raised by Will Kymlicka in his *Contemporary Political Philosophy: An Introduction,* 2nd ed. (Oxford: Oxford University Press, 2006), 24.

7.   The method of testing moral principles against our considered beliefs is one that is both common and widely accepted among moral philosophers. We recognize, however, that there is some controversy about this method and about "coherence" accounts of justification, but discussion of this controversy is well beyond the scope of this book. For an excellent discussion of reflective equilibrium, see the *Stanford Encyclopedia of Philosophy,* http://plato.stanford.edu/entries/reflective-equilibrium/.

8.   For a more thorough discussion of fallacies, see the entry on fallacies in the *Internet Encyclopedia of Philosophy,* http://www.iep.utm.edu/f/fallacy.htm.

9.   An argument like "It is raining; therefore, it is raining" is clearly circular. Note that it nonetheless fits our earlier definition of an argument: "An argument is simply a set of claims; one of these is the conclusion, and any other claims are premises." There is no requirement in the definition that the premises all be distinct from the conclusion. In fact, circular arguments, though rarely useful, are nonetheless valid, for it is not possible for their premises to be true while the conclusion is false.

10. This example, and others, can be found on the Texas State University Department of Philosophy website: https://www.txstate.edu/philosophy/resources/fallacy-definitions/Equivocation.html.

2 PHILOSOPHICAL ETHICS: AN INTRODUCTION

INTRODUCTION

This book explores some key issues in health care ethics. Health care ethics is a topic within the broader field of normative ethics. Normative ethics is concerned, in large part, with general theoretical questions such as what makes acts morally right or wrong, what states of affairs are desirable or undesirable, what constitutes a good life for the person who leads it, which character traits are virtuous and which are vicious, and, most generally, how one ought to live. Philosophers have developed a number of normative ethical theories in an effort to address these questions. The principal goal of this chapter is to introduce you to some of the most important and influential ethical theories and to explain their major strengths and weaknesses. A grasp of these ethical theories is helpful, if not essential, for thinking about moral problems that arise in health care.

LEARNING OBJECTIVES

After completing this chapter, you should be able to:

- Distinguish between metaethics, normative ethics, and descriptive ethics
- Explain ethical relativism and its problems
- Define classical act utilitarianism, explain objections to it, and utilitarian responses to those objections
- Describe Kant's distinction between an action's having moral worth and an action's being morally right
- Understand and apply the universal law version and the humanity version of Kant's categorical imperative
- Outline the main strengths and weaknesses of Kant's moral theory
- Describe W. D. Ross's distinction between *prima facie* duties and duties, all things considered
- Explain Ross's moral theory, and describe its strengths and weaknesses
- Define what justifies moral rules according to social contract theory
- Explain why John Rawls's theory of justice is called *justice as fairness*

- Outline the strengths and weaknesses of Rawls's theory, and of social contract theories in general
- Recognize how virtue ethics differs from other approaches to ethics
- Describe Aristotle's concept of moral virtue and his doctrine of the mean
- Identify the strengths and weaknesses of virtue ethics
- Explain various feminist approaches to ethics
- Point out the strengths and weaknesses of the ethics of care

THREE TYPES OF ETHICAL INQUIRY

We begin by explaining **normative ethics** and distinguishing it from **descriptive ethics** and **metaethics**.[1] As suggested above, normative ethics addresses general theoretical questions about what sorts of things matter, morally speaking. When considering whether an act is right or wrong, for example, should we look only at its consequences? Or are other things important—for example, a person's motives? But normative ethics is also concerned with practical or applied issues. Here the concern is to try to resolve concrete moral problems, such as whether mercy killing is sometimes morally permissible, whether cloning is immoral, and what obligations people have to non-human animals and the environment. What is distinctive about normative ethics is that it is *prescriptive*: it is concerned with what ought to be, not with what is the case. Thus, to say that **health care ethics** is an area of inquiry within normative ethics, or more narrowly, within **practical ethics,** is to say that it is concerned with how one ought to act, the character traits one ought to develop, the policies that ought to be adopted, and so forth, when dealing with ethical problems that arise in and around the practice of health care.[2]

It is helpful to distinguish normative ethics from descriptive ethics. Descriptive ethics is concerned with the examination of a given population's beliefs about a particular moral issue. For example, we might ask, "What percentage of the Canadian population believes that abortion is sometimes morally acceptable?" Descriptive ethics seeks to describe what is the case; for instance, it seeks to describe what people actually believe about particular moral issues. Descriptive ethics also is concerned with questions of why people believe what they believe about ethics, and how they come to hold their particular moral beliefs and attitudes. Comparisons between different cultures' moral beliefs, and questions of what people in the past have believed about various ethical issues, also belong to descriptive ethics. So, while descriptive ethics is a rich and interesting area of inquiry, it is, for the most part, an area that properly belongs to the social sciences: careful empirical investigation is the key to doing descriptive ethics well.

But since normative ethics is essentially prescriptive, it differs importantly from descriptive ethics. Thus, for example, in doing health care ethics we want to know what Canadians (or people, in general) *should* think about the moral acceptability of abortion, and we are much less concerned about what people happen to think. Here there is the recognition that people's actual moral beliefs and society's laws, policies, and professional ethical codes can be mistaken (recall that prevailing moral beliefs, and many of society's laws and policies, used to favour whites over non-whites, men over women, and so forth), and we attempt to move toward moral beliefs, laws, policies, and ethical codes that are justified.[3]

While descriptive ethics requires careful empirical study, the key to doing normative ethics well is good reasoning.[4] That is, normative ethics is a matter of rational investigation. To be sure, this requires an awareness of the relevant facts, but it also requires the defence of various moral principles and careful argumentation from these moral principles and the relevant facts to conclusions about what ought to be done.

One of the most important steps in arguing for one's position in normative ethics is to begin by clearly defining the key concepts one is investigating. For instance, if we want to determine when, if ever, abortion is morally permissible, we should first determine what "abortion" involves. For instance, is it an abortion if one removes the premature fetus to save the pregnant woman's life, knowing that the premature fetus will die as a result? And is it an abortion if one prevents a fertilized ovum from implanting in the uterus (say by using an intrauterine device, or the so-called "morning-after pill"), or is this just a form of contraception? And what about the nearly 50 percent of fertilized eggs that end up being discarded in IVF clinics—should we view the destruction of these unused fertilized eggs as abortions?[5] Obviously, defining the concept one is debating can be a tricky matter, but it is terribly important to get it as clear as one can so that one knows exactly what one is investigating.

Also, when thinking about problems in normative ethics, it is very important to clarify relevant facts. For instance, on the topic of abortion, we will presumably need to know such things as when does pregnancy begin; when are fetuses able to survive if born; when, if ever, are fetuses conscious; and, in general, what changes go on throughout pregnancy as the fetus develops? We will also want to know the effects of pregnancy on a woman; for example, what health risks does she face in pregnancy, what health risks arise from abortion, what percentage of pregnancies are not consensual, what are the consequences to families and society of having unwanted children, and what effects would there be on women's lives if access to abortion was heavily regulated or even banned?

Finally, once key terms are defined and the relevant facts identified, the next step is to consider whether the act in question is supported (or opposed) by moral principles or moral considerations that we are willing to accept after careful reflection. For instance, we might propose the moral principle that a person should be free to do what she chooses provided that she does not violate others' rights, and provided that she is competent to make her own decisions. We might then argue that abortion can be freely chosen by competent persons without violating anyone's rights, and, therefore, abortion is morally acceptable in these situations. Alternatively, we might put forward the moral principle that it is morally wrong to intentionally kill innocent human beings, and since abortion involves intentionally killing innocent human beings, it is morally wrong. We then need to examine each of these arguments, and any others that can be brought to bear on this topic, to see whether they are (deductively) sound. (Arguments that are not deductive should be checked for inductive strength and for the truth of the premises.) There is no mechanical method for determining whether a given argument is sound or strong; instead, we have to carefully examine each premise (both the factual claims and the moral principles) and consider whether it is true or vulnerable to criticism. We also need to consider the logical structure of the argument to determine whether the premises, taken together, adequately support the conclusion. If a flaw can be identified either in one (or more) of the premises or in the logic of the argument, then we ought to reject the argument as rationally unpersuasive.

The process of developing, examining, and revising arguments is at the heart of normative ethics, health care ethics, and, indeed, all substantive areas of philosophy—it requires creativity, a sharp critical mind, and a sense of fairness. The goal is to find the best arguments on a particular topic and to understand why rival arguments fail. On occasion, on truly difficult issues, one may be unable to tell which argument is best—they may all appear problematic, or there may be opposing arguments that look equally good. In such cases, the appropriate thing to do is to admit that one does not know what to think. Even in difficult cases such as these, the investigation itself can be fruitful: for, at a minimum, one will better understand the debate around a moral issue—the arguments for and against, their strengths and their weaknesses—and why the issue is so difficult.

Finally, normative ethics should also be distinguished from metaethics. Metaethics concerns the rational investigation into the nature of morality. Here, the focus is on questions *about* morality, rather than questions *within* morality, such as "Are moral judgments capable of being true or false?" and "What are the meanings of moral terms?" For instance, one might ask, "What does it mean to say that something is morally wrong or that something is morally right?" Is this merely a report about the speaker's feelings, or an expression of emotion, or is it a statement that can be objectively true or false?[6] Metaethics is a rich area of philosophical research; however, because this is a book on health care ethics, not metaethics, we won't be able to explore these issues in depth here.[7]

One of the main purposes of this book, then, is to suggest a number of solutions to some problems that arise in health care ethics by reasoning about them. This will involve defining key terms; clarifying relevant facts; identifying, explaining, and defending relevant moral principles and values; and then drawing conclusions about these moral problems. In reading this book, you will see how arguments are formed, criticized, reformulated, and debated again. You will see how there can be progress in ethical debate, and how informed and intelligent disagreement sometimes remains. We hope that you will join our debates, reflect on the merits of the arguments presented here, and develop your own arguments for your views on these issues. Thus, in addition to attempting to shed light on some difficult problems in health care ethics, this text aims to improve your critical reasoning skills and to prompt you to develop your own arguments on these topics. We believe that such a process is intellectually exciting and rewarding. Thus, we also hope that in reading this book you will see how challenging these problems are and how stimulating it can be to think philosophically about these problems.

SKEPTICAL CONCERNS: ETHICAL RELATIVISM

Before we explore questions in health care ethics, and normative ethics generally, it is important to address and allay some of the skepticism about the entire enterprise of moral philosophy. There is a long and important minority point of view in the history of philosophy that claims there is no **objective truth** in ethics. Instead, it is suggested that right and wrong are simply relative to a given individual or group. For instance, some may suggest that right and wrong are merely culturally shared attitudes, or that right and wrong are just a way for an individual to communicate her particular preferences or feelings about an issue—for example, if a person says something is wrong, it just means she does not like it, and if she says something is right, it just means she likes it. Although each of the above views represents a slightly different understanding of the nature of morality, they share in common a general skepticism about morality: specifically, they deny that there can be objective truths in ethics. That is, they deny the existence of ethical claims that are true independently of whether some particular group or individual wants, believes, or feels that they are true. Let's call this basket of views **moral** or **ethical relativism**.[8]

Because this is not a text in metaethics, we cannot do justice to the issues raised by ethical relativism; however, a serious difficulty with this point of view is worth mentioning, namely, that there are dramatic costs to believing in ethical relativism. One such cost is that ethical relativism conflicts with the widely held common-sense belief that individuals or groups can be mistaken in their moral judgments. Most of us believe that some of our past moral judgments have been mistaken. Likewise, it seems clear that some previous prevailing moral beliefs (and practices) in our culture have also been wrong. And, if we are honest with ourselves, most of us would admit that some of our present moral views, and some of our culture's present prevailing moral views, could also be wrong; however, if one is an ethical relativist, it is impossible to believe these things. This is because in order to believe in the fallibility of one's own or one's culture's moral views, one would have to believe what the relativist denies, namely, that there is some standard of right and wrong that is not based on what the individual or culture happens to think. Once it is pointed out that ethical relativism implies that an individual's or group's moral views can never be mistaken, ethical relativism loses much of its appeal, for few are prepared to say that their own moral views, much less the moral views of their culture, are incapable of error. For ease of reference, let's calls this *the problem of moral infallibility*.

Moreover, because the relativist denies that there are standards of right and wrong that are independent of what individuals or cultures happen to think, the relativist is in the uncomfortable position of being unable to view one person's or group's moral views as objectively better than another's. The individual relativist must be willing to say something like, "Gandhi and Hitler had different moral views, but neither Gandhi's nor Hitler's moral views were objectively better or worse than the other's." Similarly, the cultural relativist must be willing to say that Nazi Germany had its moral views regarding the proper treatment of Jews, Canada has its moral views regarding the proper treatment of Jews, and neither Nazi Germany's nor Canada's moral views in this matter are objectively better or worse. But given that few people really believe that, objectively speaking, Hitler's moral views were as good as Gandhi's or Nazi Germany's were as good as Canada's, few should be willing to accept ethical relativism. For ease of reference, we may call this *the problem of moral equivalency.*

These concerns with ethical relativism directly apply to issues in health care ethics, for there is a long history in medicine of doing dreadful things. For example, consider the Tuskegee syphilis experiments carried on in the United States by the US Public Health Service for 40 years:

> The Public Health Service, working with the Tuskegee Institute, began the study in 1932. Nearly 400 poor black men with syphilis from Macon County, Ala., were enrolled in the study. They were never told they had syphilis, nor were they ever treated for it. According to the Centers for Disease Control, the men were told they were being treated for "bad blood," a local term used to describe several illnesses, including syphilis, anemia and fatigue. For participating in the study, the men were given free medical exams, free meals, and free burial insurance.
>
> At the start of the study, there was no proven treatment for syphilis. But even after penicillin became a standard cure for the disease in 1947, the medicine was withheld from the men. The Tuskegee scientists wanted to continue to study how the disease spreads and kills. The experiment lasted four decades, until public health workers leaked the story to the media. By then, dozens of the men had died, and many wives and children had been infected.[9]

Now, on the one hand, if one were truly a relativist about ethical matters, one would be in the odd position of saying that if the culture of 1930s, 1940s, and 1950s approved of such experiments, and if the experimenters felt that what they were doing was right, then they in fact did nothing wrong when they did it. On the other hand, if one thinks that these experimenters were doing something extremely immoral, say, because they violated the basic human rights of the participants, or because they deliberately caused great suffering to the innocent without their consent, or because they caused great distrust of the medical establishment, or because they exploited the most vulnerable in society, then it appears that one has straightforward reasons for criticizing such experiments. But it is hard to see how one can appeal to such reasons and believe that these experimenters were wronging these patients unless one thinks that there are objective moral standards.

Given these evident problems with ethical relativism, one might wonder why anyone would be tempted to embrace it in the first place. We will consider two of the principal arguments that have led people to embrace ethical relativism. One argument is motivated by a desire to be tolerant of other cultures' values and ways of life, and to avoid the kind of cultural imperialism and ethnocentrism that has characterized so much of European and North American history. Notice this, however: this motivation for ethical relativism stems from the belief that cultural imperialism is wrong and that respect for cultural differences is right. But if that is the case, then those who argue in this manner are being **inconsistent**. They are simultaneously saying (1) that there is no objective right or wrong in ethics, *and* (2) that cultural imperialism is objectively wrong and respect for differences is objectively right. It is clear that something has gone seriously wrong with this line of thought. Indeed, if one wants to defend the belief that cultural imperialism is morally wrong, it seems that one is best served by embracing **ethical objectivism** rather than by opposing it.[10]

Another argument that has led some to embrace ethical relativism is a general puzzlement about how ethical claims could possibly be objectively true. Many argue that, unlike the claim that tables and chairs exist, or that water boils at 100 degrees Celsius, moral claims are not subject to empirical verification. Instead, they say that moral claims seem closer to judgments of taste or preferences. (For, surely, if someone says something is wrong, they'd prefer it not to be done.) And it is quite reasonable to regard judgments of taste as mere expressions or reports of personal preferences. Thus, one might wonder how moral claims could be objectively true or false.

It is certainly true that judgments about right and wrong seem very different from empirically verifiable judgments such as "the earth is not flat." But it may be a mistake to immediately conclude from this that moral judgments must be expressions or reports of mere preferences or feelings. After all, certain propositions like "There is no greatest number" may not be empirically verifiable, but that does not lead us to conclude that this statement is not objectively true. Thus, it seems that there are ways for judgments to be known to be true or false even if they are not empirically verifiable. Further still, it seems far-fetched to say that moral judgments are similar to reports or expressions of feelings or preferences. Statements like "Vanilla is better than chocolate" seem very different in kind from statements like "Abortion is wrong." For one thing, we tend to think that the former statement needs no justification, while the latter statement requires defence. And indeed, that might be, in part, the sense in which moral judgments are objective—they require rational justification.

NORMATIVE ETHICAL THEORY

A principal concern of normative ethics is its focus on the development and defence of normative ethical theories, which include general moral principles (or approaches) that can be used to determine such things as what acts are morally right or wrong, what rules are morally justified and unjustified, and what character traits are virtuous and vicious. While there is no consensus about which normative ethical theory is correct, there are certain leading candidates that have been particularly influential. The following sections present an explanation and preliminary critical examination of each of these leading theories. We explain each theory and then present some of the most important objections to it. Sometimes, possible replies to these objections are suggested. A very important point to keep in mind is that this overview is intended as an *introduction* to the topic of normative ethical theory. Its aim is to build your critical understanding of normative ethical theories and to help you see their various strengths and weaknesses, while at the same time providing you with some background information that can help inform your thinking about the cases in health care ethics explored later in the text. Our aim is not to tell you what to think, nor is it to pronounce final judgments on any ethical theory. In other words, our aim is to present the beginnings of a conversation, not the final word.

In chapter 3, each author will present and defend his favoured approach to ethics. This will give you an indication of how ethical theories continue to be developed and defended. In subsequent chapters, as we take up particular issues in health care ethics, you may find the approach of one author or another particularly helpful; however, you may also find it helpful to appeal to some of the other ethical theories discussed below.

CLASSICAL ACT UTILITARIANISM

Perhaps the most influential normative ethical theory of the last 150 years is what is sometimes referred to as **classical act utilitarianism**.[11] Utilitarianism takes many forms, but in its classical formulation, as articulated by Jeremy Bentham and John Stuart Mill, it may be defined as the view that right actions, laws, and policies promote the greatest net amount of pleasure, or the least net amount of pain, where everyone's pleasures and pains receive equal consideration.[12] It is helpful to see that utilitarianism is composed of three distinct ideas:

- **Consequentialism:** The right act is entirely determined by its consequences; the right act promotes the most net good or the least net bad.[13]
- **Hedonism:** The sole intrinsic good is pleasure and the sole intrinsic bad is pain.
- **Equal consideration:** No one's good is to be counted as more important than anyone else's.

Putting these three ideas together we get, of course, utilitarianism. Right acts promote the most net good (pleasure) and the least net bad (pain), where everyone's pleasure and pain is given equal consideration.

To better understand this theory, it will be helpful to make a few points about each of these aspects of utilitarianism. Consequentialism is perhaps utilitarianism's most distinctive component. It is the idea that *only* consequences matter in the evaluation of the rightness or wrongness of actions, and that the right act, in any given circumstance, is the **optimific** act—the one that does the *most net good*, or the *least net bad*. Thus, for instance, if one has to decide whether or not active euthanasia is morally right, the only relevant issue is whether or not it will (all things considered) do more net good (or less net bad) than any other alternative. If active euthanasia will in some case do more net good (or less net bad) than any other alternative, then it is what ought to be done; however, if some alternative, say palliative care, would in some circumstance do more net good than active euthanasia, then, in that situation, palliative care would be right and active euthanasia would be wrong. So, in theory at least, this aspect of utilitarianism is strikingly simple: consequences are the sole determinant of right action, and an act that fails to produce the best net consequences is the wrong thing to do.

A second thing to note about the consequentialist aspect of utilitarianism is that it is a **situational ethic**; that is, whether an act is right or wrong depends on the particular situation. Unlike an ethical theory that claims, for instance, that active euthanasia is always wrong, utilitarianism looks at the specific situation to determine whether the act is required or forbidden. If, in a particular case, active euthanasia will do the most net good, then in that case it is morally required. If, in another situation, active euthanasia won't do the most net good—say, because it will spread fear in the community, or because the person would have recovered—then in that case it is morally forbidden. Thus, unlike supporters of some other ethical theories, the utilitarian holds that what is right or wrong depends on the situation.

A third thing to note about utilitarianism, stemming largely from its acceptance of consequentialism, is its radical implications. That is, it is a theory that frequently challenges common-sense moral beliefs and tries to revise them—to make them more rational and humane. Again, the case of active euthanasia will illustrate this point nicely. A principal belief found in many cultures is that it is always wrong to intentionally kill (innocent) human beings. For many, this seems to be a bedrock moral rule, and it seems to imply that active euthanasia is always morally wrong since it involves the intentional killing of an innocent human being. But utilitarianism invites us to consider *why* this rule is so important.

Presumably, a major justification for this rule against killing innocent human beings is that it promotes good consequences. By having such a rule, we are able to live, and to live without fear of murder—and that promotes much pleasure and avoids much pain for all of us. That is why the rule against killing innocents is a good rule; however, the utilitarian then points out, there are (rare) situations where killing innocents may actually produce the best consequences—for instance, in cases where the person is suffering terribly and has no hope for recovery, where he begs for death and is joined in that plea by his family who can no longer stand to see him suffer. In such a case, producing the most good may well require that the person be painlessly killed. If that is so, the utilitarian will encourage us to revise our traditional moral beliefs about the wrongness of killing, and to allow for killing innocents in some special circumstances. Thus, it is fair to describe utilitarianism as a radical theory, insofar as it often challenges traditional moral beliefs.

Another ingredient of utilitarianism is its view of what is to count as a good outcome. Classical utilitarians are hedonists: they view pleasure as the sole *intrinsic* good (and pain as the sole *intrinsic* bad). Other things—like health, income, freedom, and friends—can be good as a means insofar as they tend to lead to pleasure and to diminish pain, but they are not good in themselves. These things are **instrumentally good**, while pleasure is **intrinsically good**—it is valuable for its own sake. As hedonists are likely to argue, people vary greatly in their sources of pleasure—some like dancing, others like singing, others like reading, and so forth—but all people agree that what they want, ultimately, is to avoid pain and to get pleasure.[14] Further, people can explain why they like to sing or to dance or to read—it gives them pleasure; but they cannot explain why they want pleasure or want to avoid pain—they just do, since it is an ultimate end.[15] For these utilitarians, then, good consequences are understood as consequences that produce more net pleasure than pain, and right acts produce the greatest net amount of pleasure or the least net amount of pain for all concerned.[16]

Lastly, utilitarians believe that everyone's good (pleasure) counts and that it counts as much as everyone else's: the well-being of men and women, whites and non-whites, citizens and non-citizens, and so forth, is equally important. Thus, against a history of moral exclusiveness, utilitarians embrace the idea of impartiality. In assessing the morality of actions, one is to count the effects of one's actions on others as equally important as the effects of one's actions on oneself and on one's loved ones. Thus, for example, according to utilitarianism, it would be wrong to do an act that promoted a little bit of good (pleasure) for oneself or for one's friend if an alternative action would promote a greater amount of good (pleasure) for someone else.[17]

Having said that utilitarians accept equal consideration, it is important to clarify that equal consideration does not mean equal treatment. To see the distinction between equal treatment and equal consideration, imagine an emergency room situation where a triage nurse must decide who to treat first—here each person's interests must be equally considered, and the nurse should choose in such a way as to produce the most net good or least net bad. This will likely result in someone who is not critically ill waiting longer for care than someone else who is critically ill, since (typically) this will do the most net good. Although the people in the emergency room are treated unequally (some are waiting for care longer than others), the utilitarian requirement of equal consideration is satisfied. What a utilitarian would object to is counting the net pleasures and pains of some as more important (more deserving of consideration) than the net pleasures and pains of others; for example, if you were to view the pain of a family member as deserving greater attention than the pain of a stranger.

In conclusion, utilitarians claim that the right thing to do in any situation is to promote the most net good or the least net bad. Good is defined as pleasure and bad is defined as pain. And everyone's pleasure and pain matters and matters equally. Therefore, one is to do the action that would maximize net pleasure or minimize net pain for all concerned.

Objections to Utilitarianism

Despite the attractiveness of this theory, many philosophers find utilitarianism to be unacceptable. Some reject utilitarianism because of its consequentialist approach to moral problems; others reject the classical theory's acceptance of hedonism; while still others reject utilitarianism because of its insistence on strict impartiality.[18] In what follows, some important objections to each part of the theory are explained.

Against Consequentialism

Perhaps the most common, and powerful, objection to utilitarianism is the idea that it is too simple. While it can plausibly be maintained that producing good consequences and preventing bad consequences is one morally significant factor, it is hard to believe that it is the *only* morally relevant consideration. Many believe, for instance, that the moral rightness or wrongness of an act also depends on such things as whether or not the act is truthful or deceitful, a case of promise keeping or promise breaking, a case of violating someone's rights or respecting those rights. For example, it is a widely shared common-sense moral belief that it is at least sometimes wrong to violate an innocent person's rights, even if that will produce the best consequences.

To illustrate, suppose a person is dying and refuses to be an organ donor, even though her organs are needed to save another person's life. Suppose also that, after much discussion, the nurse caring for the patient tells her to sign a form stating her refusal to be an organ donor. In fact, though, the form is really an authorization *for* organ donation. The patient signs the form, falsely believing it is protecting her wish not to donate her organs. The patient then dies, the needed organs are harvested, and a transplant takes place that saves the life of someone else who otherwise would have died. Everything is done with great care, and no one ever finds out about the clever deceit. In this case, the best consequences were produced—a person who would otherwise have died is saved, and no one, not even the organ donor, suffers any pain as a result. Yet, it seems quite clear to most of us that the nurse did the wrong thing in deceiving the patient. If this is our reaction, then it looks as though utilitarianism sometimes gives the intuitively unacceptable answer. Utilitarianism says the nurse did the right thing, but common sense strongly suggests otherwise.[19]

Another common criticism of utilitarianism's reliance on consequentialism concerns our frequent inability to know the long-term consequences of our actions. Utilitarianism claims that the right act produces the most good, but, the critic urges, often we do not know what act will produce the most good; therefore, utilitarianism often will not be useful. Take, for instance, whether Canada should permit private health care to exist alongside a public system.[20] Some suggest that such a system will do more net good than bad because it will help to alleviate delays in the public system thereby increasing net well-being; others argue that a private system will just erode the public system and, thus, not produce the most net good. The seemingly simple utilitarian idea that we should do the act that will produce the greatest net good turns out to be a view that is strikingly difficult to apply, given the complexities of the real world. Now, strictly speaking, this objection does not show that utilitarianism is false, but it does show that the theory is very difficult to apply in these sorts of complicated, real-life cases.

Against Hedonism

Another criticism of utilitarianism focuses not on its principle of right action (consequentialism), but rather on its view of good results. As explained above, early utilitarians tended to be hedonists. Hedonism is the view that the sole intrinsic good is pleasure and the sole intrinsic bad is pain. Thus, the right thing to do according to these utilitarians is the act that produces the most net pleasure or the least net pain. But many argue that hedonism is a flawed theory of the good. This is because *it seems that pleasure is not always intrinsically good, and that some things are intrinsically good besides pleasure.*

Pleasures that we may not want to count as intrinsically good and worth promoting would presumably include pleasures obtained by violating the rights of others, or pleasures that a virtuous person would not find to be good. Think of a peeping Tom who gets pleasure from secretly spying on young boys in a locker room, or the pleasures that a sadist might experience when watching a newscast about a group of people who died in a tsunami. Arguably, we would not want to call these pleasures good, or claim that the pleasures the peeping Tom and the sadist experience help to justify their actions.

Further, we might regard other things as intrinsically good besides pleasure. Autonomy, important knowledge, beauty, creativity, and meaningful relationships often produce pleasure for an individual and for others, but even if they do not, we might want to say that a life is still good for having these things. To see this, you might imagine two lives with equal amounts of pleasure and pain: suppose the first life involves being lobotomized, and then given a daily dose of medication that results in one feeling great pleasure and very little pain throughout one's day; and suppose the second life also involves great pleasure and very little pain, though these pleasures come from a life of meaningful work, loving relationships, and enjoyable travels. Hedonism would imply that these are equally good lives for the ones that lead them, but surely the second life is the much more desirable life. But if that is right, then—contrary to hedonism—pleasure cannot be the sole intrinsic good.

To see that pleasure is not the only intrinsic good, it might help to consider a thought experiment made famous by Robert Nozick.[21] Consider *the experience machine*: scientists have developed a machine that can give people the experience of anything they desire. The way it works is that the patient lies down on a bed or sits in a chair and is given a drug that immediately makes the patient forget that they are about to go into an experience machine. Doctors then hook the patient's brain up to a computer that has the ability to simulate any experience or feeling the patient desires. If the patient wants to be skiing, or going out for a romantic evening, or winning the lottery, or doing well on a philosophy test, the machine lets the patient experience all these things. As a result, the patient is pleased, maximally so. The machine can even cause the patient to experience frustration, if later that will lead to super-intense pleasures.

Now, suppose a person could enter this machine for their entire life. (No need to worry about the patient's body—they could be kept alive indefinitely by inserting a feeding tube.) Suppose, by hypothesis, that life in such a machine would be much more pleasurable than the life any other person has ever lived. It would follow, according to hedonism, that the person who lived their life in an experience machine was living the best life ever. But, the critic argues, such a life is not best, and so hedonism must be false. Although this life contains a great amount of pleasure, it is severely lacking in other goods—for instance, it is a life full of false beliefs and inactivity, and utterly devoid of meaningful relationships and accomplishments. While the experience machine thought experiment does not reveal what is important in a good life, it does demonstrate that a good life consists of more than merely having a lot of pleasurable experiences. Other things are important, too. And if this is right, then traditional utilitarians, who are committed to the view that the right act produces the most good for all concerned, need to revise their theory of what is to count as good. Hedonism, the idea that pleasure (and the absence of pain) is the sole intrinsic good, seems false.

Problems with Equal Consideration

Finally, critics often reject utilitarianism because of two related factors: (1) it is unable to recognize the importance of special relationships, and (2) it is too demanding. In our daily life, we often put our own interests and the interests of our friends and family ahead of the greater interests of strangers. For instance, often we choose to stay home and read a book to our children, or to go out for dinner and a movie with our friends or loved ones, or to help out a friend who is in need. Indeed, it seems that being a good spouse, parent, sibling, or friend requires that we show special concern for those people who stand in those relationships to us. But, if utilitarianism is correct, and we are supposed to treat everyone's good with equal concern, then it seems that it would be morally wrong to do these kinds of things. We could no longer justify helping a friend who is in need simply because he is our friend; instead, we would have to do whichever act promoted the most net good with everyone's interests given equal weight.

In addition to making it seemingly impossible to have special relationships, it seems that utilitarianism is too demanding in another sense. Many of us enjoy things like going to the movies, or to the theatre, or to concerts or sporting events. In addition, many of us hope to buy a nice car and a comfortable home, and to take the occasional luxury vacation. But, if utilitarianism is correct, all of this would be seriously immoral. Going to a concert, for instance, will likely produce a certain amount of pleasure for you, but surely more good could be accomplished in the world if, instead, you gave the money to UNICEF or some other worthy cause, and then donated your time to volunteer at a local charity. Indeed, since going to concerts or out for dinner will never, or almost never, produce the most net good, it will always, or almost always, be morally wrong to do these things. Generalizing this point, given the tremendous amount of suffering in the world, it seems that it would be wrong according to utilitarianism to acquire any luxury goods, or to take any fancy vacations, or even to take the extra time to just hang out with friends and family, since these choices would not maximize utility.

But such an implication strikes many people as absurd. They believe that morality requires that you do not violate other people's rights, so you should refrain from things like stealing, lying, and doing acts of violence, and that sometimes you should help others who are in need, but that you are not morally required always to treat everyone's interests as if they are as important as your own. To think otherwise is to make it impossible for a person to lead a normal life. Thus, while an earlier objection to utilitarianism's commitment to consequentialism was that it requires us to do things that intuitively seem to be wrong (like lie, violate rights, and break promises in order to promote the greater good), this objection points to the concern that utilitarianism is *too demanding*. It seems to require that we sacrifice too much of our own lives in order to satisfy some of the unmet needs of others.

Utilitarian Responses

Faced with such objections, many are convinced that utilitarianism is hopelessly flawed, and that a different normative ethical theory is needed. But some continue to defend utilitarianism. Confronted with these objections, the utilitarian has several replies available.

Most, although not all, contemporary utilitarians acknowledge that hedonism is flawed. Instead, they appeal to a different theory of the good. Here is a brief indication of what non-hedonistic utilitarianism may look like. Some may argue that what is ultimately good is the satisfaction of people's preferences, and so the right thing to do is to maximize net preference satisfaction for all concerned.[22] Others argue that what is good is the satisfaction of "informed preferences"—preferences, for example, that one would have if one were free of cognitive impairments and prejudices, and knew all relevant information—and so the right thing to do is to maximize the net satisfaction of informed preferences for all concerned.[23] Still other utilitarians opt for a list of objective intrinsic goods—say, autonomy, knowledge, beauty, friendship, pleasure—and say that right acts best promote these goods.[24] What these views share is the perception that hedonism is a flawed account of the good; instead, they opt for another account of good consequences.[25]

While utilitarians commonly abandon hedonism in the face of serious criticism, their replies to the objections against consequentialism and to the doctrine of equal consideration tend to be more varied.

One common utilitarian response is to say that many of the objections are based on highly fanciful situations that would never occur in real life. When this is realized, they argue, people do not find utilitarianism to be at odds with moral common sense. For instance, in real life, violating people's rights, as in the organ donor case, will not in the long run have the best net consequences. The reason for this is that the nurse who tricked the patient will likely get caught and will be punished. Further, the nurse's act will then cause great suffering to countless others who worry that their dying wishes will not be respected. Further still, many will no longer offer to give their organs because they will distrust the system. As a result, even more people will not get the organs they need. Thus, despite initial appearances, utilitarianism would not support deceiving patients to obtain their organs.

Similarly, a utilitarian may argue that the critic exaggerates the objection that utilitarianism is too demanding. Utilitarianism may not, in fact, require that you give every moment of your day to helping others, that you choose a career that is best for humanity, and that you never take a weekend off, since such a life would not in the end do the most net good. Realistically, most people who tried to lead such a life would exhaust themselves and crumble psychologically; as a result, in the end they would not be particularly useful to anyone and would themselves be unhappy. Instead, it might be argued that the best way for most people to maximize the good is to choose a fulfilling career, to foster meaningful relationships, to get enough sleep and take the occasional vacation, and to take some time to help others (probably more than we customarily do). Thus, the utilitarian would argue that utilitarianism is not at odds (or is not too much at odds) with moral common sense and is quite compatible with leading a "normal" life, for that is the best way for most of us to maximize good results in the world.

It is unclear, however, how persuasive these utilitarian responses are to the theory's critics. Perhaps the utilitarian is correct to point out that *almost* always the most good will come from keeping promises, respecting rights, and being honest. But surely there are some real-life cases where violating rights and the like are at odds with common-sense morality and yet will do the most good. Thus, it seems somewhat of an exaggeration to say that utilitarianism is never at odds with common-sense moral judgments. Likewise, it seems highly doubtful that living a lifestyle of conventional North American prosperity will produce the greatest net good. Many, for instance, think nothing of buying an expensive new car or a new wardrobe or going to see a professional sports match, but it is extremely unlikely that such acts would do as much net good as volunteering at a homeless shelter, donating money to help people in impoverished countries, and so forth. An honest assessment of utilitarianism therefore suggests that it is sometimes at odds with common-sense moral attitudes—it *does* allow for some rights violations, and it *is* very demanding.

In the light of this, other utilitarians acknowledge that their theory is sometimes at odds with common-sense moral beliefs, although perhaps not as often as critics suggest. They admit, for instance, that utilitarianism sometimes requires rights violations, lying, promise breaking, and so forth, to produce the best result. Further, these utilitarians acknowledge that utilitarianism may sometimes prove to be extremely demanding, prohibiting the accumulation of luxuries and the privileging of family interests over the general good;[26] however, they argue that these implications are not flaws in the theory. Rather, they insist that, on reflection, their theory is preferable to common-sense moral beliefs. After all, common-sense morality has been terribly mistaken in the past. For instance, the keeping of slaves and the live vivisection of non-human animals were, for centuries, widely viewed as acceptable. So, we should not be too anxious if utilitarianism finds fault in some of our current moral beliefs. Rather than trust our prevailing mores, these utilitarians suggest that it is more reasonable to believe that what is morally right is to act in ways that maximize the good or minimize the bad for all concerned.[27]

RULE UTILITARIANISM

One further utilitarian reply to these criticisms should be mentioned. Utilitarians may concede that their theory is at odds with common-sense moral beliefs—such as respect for moral rights—and that it should be modified to make it more acceptable. One such modification is known as **rule utilitarianism**.[28] Rule utilitarianism says:

- The right thing to do is to follow the best rule.
- The best rule is defined as the one that, if consistently followed, will produce the greatest amount of net good (well-being) for all concerned.

Thus, if given a choice between following a rule that says "respect people's rights" or "violate people's rights," it is clear that the former rule if consistently followed will have better consequences than consistently following the rule to violate people's rights. Thus, the former rule is best, and according to rule utilitarianism, the right thing to do would be to follow that rule and always respect people's rights. Thus, unlike the act utilitarian, who, for example, would seem to support lying to the organ donor to save a life, the rule utilitarian would presumably view such a deception as morally wrong, since the rule, if always followed, would have very bad consequences. Put differently, while traditional (act) utilitarianism requires that one perform the optimific *action* in any particular situation, the rule utilitarian requires one to follow the optimific *rule*, even if doing so on that particular occasion won't produce the best consequences.

In response to the objection that utilitarianism is too demanding, rule utilitarians may concede that insisting on a rule that says to always produce the best consequences would likely be counterproductive, resulting in burnout or leading people to routinely ignore moral rules. Instead, they might reasonably suggest that the set of rules that would actually produce the most good, given the way human beings are, is one that is considerably less demanding—insisting on respecting people's rights, encouraging people to help others, and allowing people (to a degree) to show special concern for family and friends. Still, it is quite likely that rule utilitarianism would require considerable sacrifices on the part of individuals, for it seems likely that a rule that allowed people to acquire luxury goods and to take luxury vacations, instead of helping others who suffered from lack of food, shelter, and basic medical care, would not be the best rule from the point of view of maximizing the good. Instead, a far better rule might be one that required people to forgo their luxuries when doing so could greatly help the needy. Given this, it is fair to say that rule utilitarianism will still be rather demanding. It is certainly arguable, however, whether this should count as a reason against the theory, for it is unclear why a normative ethical theory should not be demanding.

Despite these arguments in its favour, rule utilitarianism faces a serious problem. Rule utilitarianism may still not be able to give a coherent response to the objection that focuses on people's rights. Here the problem becomes apparent when we ask the rule utilitarian how to determine what constitutes the best rule. Above, we considered only two possibilities: adopt a rule of violating people's rights or adopt a rule of respecting people's rights. Given these two options, it was only reasonable to think that the rule of respecting people's rights would lead to the best results and so is the best rule. But there is clearly a third rule we could adopt: respect people's rights, unless violating them is necessary to do a greater good. Now it seems that this third rule, if consistently followed, would have the best consequences. It would respect people's rights when that led to the greatest good, and it would violate people's rights (only) when *that* led to the greatest good—it is the rule, in short, that will always lead to the greatest good, if it is consistently followed. Thus, the critic argues, this rule is the one that ought to be adopted according to rule utilitarianism.

But, of course, this rule is really just another way of stating traditional act utilitarianism! On reflection, then, the critic argues that rule utilitarianism, if treated seriously, merely collapses into act utilitarianism. The rule that will lead to the best consequences if consistently followed is simply the rule that says to do whatever is necessary to produce the greatest good for all concerned—but that, as we just claimed, is just another way of stating act utilitarianism.[29]

In response to this objection, rule utilitarians may argue that the rules that one is to choose between must be more general than a "rule" that merely says "follow the rule unless it is better not to do so." For, they may argue, a "rule" that is so easily disregarded would be no rule at all. Instead, rules must be more absolute, more exceptionless, than the objection supposes; however, if rule utilitarians insist that one ought to follow some rule like "never lie" even when a lie would produce better net results, then it seems that the position suffers from "irrational rule worship." Why should one agree to act in accordance with some optimal rule if one could occasionally break that rule and produce even more good? To say that such rule breaking would be wrong even if it did more good seems irrational.[30]

NON-CONSEQUENTIALISM AND DEONTOLOGY

Unlike utilitarians, many philosophers think that the rightness of an act is not solely determined by the goodness of its consequences. Such philosophers are called **non-consequentialists**. Some non-consequentialists are **deontologists**. Deontologists see morality as a matter of doing one's (moral) duty.[31] Many non-consequentialists (and deontologists) think that the consequences of an act are one determinant of the rightness of an action, but not the only determinant. Others think that the consequences of an act are simply irrelevant to the rightness or wrongness of an act. The latter view is famously held by the deontologist Immanuel Kant.[32]

KANT'S ETHICS

Kant argues that we are to evaluate the morality of an action by focusing on the agent's intentions rather than the results of the actions. More precisely, it is helpful to think of Kant's ethical theory as falling into two parts. First, Kant develops a view of when actions have "moral worth." Second, he defends a set of principles that determine whether one's acts are morally permissible (or morally wrong).

The Idea of Moral Worth

Kant observed that people act on the basis of two different sorts of reasons, which he called **hypothetical imperatives** and **categorical imperatives.** Both types of imperatives can be expressed in terms of "oughts." Hypothetical imperatives state what one ought to do given the presence of a particular desire or goal. Categorical imperatives state what one ought to do regardless of one's desires. Hypothetical imperatives are commonplace—for instance, "If I am thirsty, I ought to drink" or "If you want to do well in this course, you ought to read the book carefully, attend class meetings, and study hard." There is nothing special or mysterious about hypothetical imperatives. As rational beings, we rely on them all the time. That is, we set goals for ourselves and then determine the most effective ways to accomplish those goals.

As rational beings, however, we are also capable of following categorical imperatives. Categorical imperatives take the following form: "Do *x*" or "Don't do *x*," where the idea is that you must do or not do some act, regardless of your desires, goals, or other inclinations. Examples of such imperatives would be "Tell the truth," "Keep one's promises," "Don't steal," "Don't cheat," "Don't harm others," and so forth. Kant calls these categorical imperatives the *imperatives (commands) of morality*. These imperatives are said to apply to all of us, and we ought to follow them regardless of whether they further our desires. Thus, as a rational being, you are capable of acting according to hypothetical and categorical imperatives; that is, you can act in a way that furthers the goals you happen to have, and you can act according to commands (moral duties) that are not related to any particular goals that you may have.

Now, there is nothing necessarily wrong with acting on the basis of a hypothetical imperative, but Kant maintains that acts based on a hypothetical imperative have no moral worth; however, if one does an act out of respect for morality—out of respect for a categorical imperative—then one is said to have a **good will**, and so one's act has *moral worth*. Thus, the person who gives to charity because she wants to get a tax deduction may be behaving rationally and presumably is doing the right thing, but nevertheless her act has no moral worth. Alternatively, if a person donates to a charity *because it is the right thing to do*, then not only is she doing the right act, but her act also has moral worth. For Kant, then, in order to have a good will, and for one's act to have moral worth, one must do the right act for the right reasons: namely, out of respect for morality. By contrast, if a person does an act not out of respect for morality, but because it furthers one of her own desires, then she may be doing nothing wrong, but her act has no moral worth.

The idea of moral worth is an extremely tricky one and gives rise to many questions. For instance, if a person donates to charity simply because she feels sorry for the needy and sympathizes with their plight, does her act have moral worth? Kant's answer is, surprisingly, "no." Such an act is still based on a hypothetical imperative—*If I feel sorry for someone, I ought to give that person charity*—and while such an act is certainly not morally wrong, it has no moral worth.

What about someone who gives to charity for several reasons—she wants a tax deduction, she feels sympathy for the poor, and she believes it is the right thing to do? The answer here is unclear. Some believe that Kant would say that such an act still has moral worth as long as respect for moral duty was a sufficient condition to motivate the person to do the charitable act. Others read Kant differently. They believe that such an act would not have moral worth because it was "polluted" by the presence of hypothetical imperatives. While it must be admitted that Kant is far from clear on this point, the former interpretation is the one we will adopt, since it seems to be both a reasonable interpretation of Kant's writings and it is the more *charitable* interpretation.[33]

The Categorical Imperative

By this point, you may wonder where these categorical imperatives come from. In other words, how does one determine what is and what is not a categorical imperative (a rule of morality)? This brings us to the second part of Kant's theory. Kant is famous for giving what he calls *the* **categorical imperative**, a test for determining whether a particular action is morally permissible or morally wrong. Indeed, Kant gives several different versions of the categorical imperative test. Two of his most influential versions will be examined here.

The Universal Law Formulation of the Categorical Imperative

One test that Kant gives to determine whether or not an action violates a moral rule is known as the **universal law version of the categorical imperative**. It says, "*Act only on those maxims that you can, at the same time, will as a universal law.*" In order to understand this principle, it is necessary to define its key terms. Specifically, we will need to clarify the terms **maxim, universal law**, and *will*. By the term *maxim*, Kant means the principle behind one's action. Thus, in the case of the forged organ donation, the nurse's *action* is to give the patient a pen and paper, but the nurse's maxim is to act on the principle "When needed, I will deceive my patient into donating her organs."

A *universal law* is a principle that states that everyone follows this maxim all the time, as if it were a law of nature. Thus, in the organ donor example, the universal law would be "When needed, everyone will always deceive patients into donating their organs."

Finally, before we can understand the test, we need to clarify the concept of being able to *will*. By this, Kant means two different things.[34] First, one is sometimes not able to will a maxim as a universal law because the practice would be self-defeating or self-contradictory if it were practiced by everyone all the time. Kant calls this **a contradiction in conception**, and he maintains that if the maxim of one's actions yields a contradiction in conception when it is universalized, then the action violates a **perfect duty** and is therefore strictly forbidden. A perfect duty is one that must never be violated. At other times, Kant admits that one can conceive of a maxim as a universal law, but still not be able to will it because a contradiction will arise between the universal law and what a person will (later) want—Kant called this **a contradiction in will**. Kant claims that to act on principles that can be conceived but not consistently willed as universal law is to violate an **imperfect duty**—a duty that one must sometimes follow, but which need not be followed all the time.

So, if we look at the organ transplant case, we will need to know if we can will the universal law "*When needed, everyone will deceive patients into donating their organs.*" Now it seems that the answer is that such a universal law would yield a contradiction in conception, since if everyone, when necessary, deceived their patients into donating their organs, then such deception would be self-defeating—patients would simply not be deceived by such tricks. (In other words, it makes no sense to say everyone will tell a lie in situation *x*, since a lie would no longer work if everyone lied in that situation!) Thus, because the nurse's maxim cannot be conceived as a universal law, the universal law test tells us that it is morally wrong for the nurse to lie to the patient. It violates a perfect duty.

Let's now tweak the example slightly and consider what the universal law test says about the patient who chose not to give up her organs. Let's suppose her maxim to be as follows: *"I will keep my organs even when I have no use for them and others need them."* We then universalize this maxim: *"No one will ever give up their organs to others even when others need them for survival and they are no longer needed by the donor."* Obviously, there could be a world where no one donated organs to anyone—such a world has existed for most of human history—but could one always *will* this as a universal law? Apparently not, since one day you may be in need of an organ donor (or some other kind of bene-factor), and then a contradiction will arise between the universal law of never donating organs (or more generally never helping those in need) and what you now want—an organ (or some other necessary good). Because there is a contradiction in will, it follows, in Kant's view, that there is an imperfect duty to donate one's organs (or at least to help others). What this entails is not exactly clear. Perhaps it means that all of us ought to donate some of our organs, although we are not obligated to donate all of our organs. More likely, it just means that we ought to help the needy at least sometimes, and not ignore their vital needs entirely.

By now it should be apparent that Kant's universal law test is extremely sophisti-cated and rather difficult to understand. It is sophisticated because this apparently simple statement—*to act only on maxims that can be willed as universal law*—purports to tell one not only whether one's act is morally permissible or a violation of moral duty, but also what kind of duty one is transgressing by one's act. This is truly an impressive accom-plishment, especially if the test works! But, before we turn to possible difficulties with the test, it may be helpful to explain the basic insight that is informing Kant's reasoning when he proposes this test. It seems to be the common-sense idea that *when one acts im-morally, one does something that one does not (or cannot) want everyone to do.* The mugger, who mugs, does not want everyone to mug. The shoplifter, who shoplifts, does not want everyone to shoplift. The promise breaker does not want everyone to break promises. Instead, the wrongdoer seeks to make an exception for himself—he wants to act in one way, while he wants others to act differently. But Kant's profound insight is that morality needs to be applied universally, or consistently: one should act only on principles that one can consistently will others to follow.

In turn, this point leads to another one of Kant's central claims: to act immorally is to somehow act in a manner that is contradictory. Kant's claim here is *not* that an act is im-moral because it leads to bad consequences—he is no utilitarian. Rather, his claim is that to act immorally is to behave irrationally. The reason for this is that, in acting immorally, one acts on maxims that cannot rationally (i.e., consistently) stand as universal laws.

Lastly, to simplify the universal law test, it may be helpful to think of it as a three-step procedure.

Step 1: Identify the maxim (principle) behind the action.

Step 2: Universalize the maxim, i.e., transform the maxim into a universal law (everyone acts on that principle, all the time).

Step 3: Consider whether the universalized maxim can be consistently willed.

    a.   If it can be consistently *willed*, then the act is morally permissible.

    b.   If it cannot be consistently willed, then determine why it cannot be consistently willed. If the maxim cannot even be *consistently thought of* as existing as a universal law, then the act violates a perfect duty and is morally forbidden. But if the universalized maxim can be consistently thought of as existing as a universal law but it cannot be *consistently willed*, then the act violates an imperfect duty—one that should not be ignored entirely but does not always have to be practiced.

Before we move on to another key Kantian principle, it may be helpful to illustrate one more time how the universal law test can be applied. This time, let's take one of Kant's own examples—a case of knowingly making someone a false promise.[35] Kant imagines that someone who is in need of money considers asking someone for a loan, even though he knows he will not be able to repay it. Here the maxim of the act is (Step 1) "When I need money, I will ask to borrow some money, promising to repay the loan, even though I know I won't be able to do so." Next, we need to universalize this maxim as (Step 2) "Whenever anyone needs money, that person will ask to borrow some money, promising to repay the loan, even though the borrower knows that they won't be able to do so." Kant then points out (Step 3) that such a universal law cannot be consistently conceived, and necessarily contradicts itself, for no one could make promises in a world where they were never kept. Thus, the universal law test tells us that knowingly making a false promise violates a perfect duty, and it is always morally wrong to do.

The Humanity Version of the Categorical Imperative

Kant also developed another equally influential and important principle to test whether one is acting on maxims that are morally permissible. This principle, known as the **humanity version of the categorical imperative**, states that *one must treat humanity, whether in one's own person or that of another, always as an end and never merely as a means.* Once again, in order to understand Kant's test, certain key terms need to be clarified. Specifically, the terms **humanity**, **end**, and **means** need to be explicated. In order to do this, it is helpful to recall the earlier notion of categorical and hypothetical imperatives. Kant thought that **rational beings** are special insofar as they can follow hypothetical and categorical imperatives. That is, rational beings can freely set goals for themselves and then determine the various means to accomplish those goals (hypothetical imperatives). Rational beings can also recognize and choose to follow (or not to follow) moral rules (categorical imperatives). In this sense, rational beings differ from what Kant calls

things. A *thing* can be defined as "not a rational being": things are not capable of following hypothetical and categorical imperatives. Thus, according to Kant's definition, you are a rational being, but a chair, a cactus, and a cat are things (remember, rational beings are capable of following moral rules—cats are not, Kant assumes).

When it comes to rational beings, it should be noted that Kant says that people differ greatly in their chosen goals. You may choose to exercise regularly, read for fun, and pursue a career in journalism; someone else may prefer playing and performing music. But what all rational beings value is their **rational nature**—that is, their ability to make their own decisions and set their own goals. (Even if you want others to make all your decisions, you still want to make the decision to let others decide for you, and it is the same if you are suicidal—you still value the ability to decide to commit suicide!) Thus, Kant thought that while we may differ greatly in the ends in life that we choose, we, as rational beings, all necessarily value the ability to make our own decisions.

With this explained, we can return to the key terms in Kant's humanity test. By *humanity*, Kant means "rational being." By *end*, Kant means "rational being," and by *mere means* he means "thing." Thus we can rewrite the humanity test as follows:

> *Act so you treat ~~humanity~~ every rational being, whether in your own person or that of another, always as ~~an end~~ a rational being, and never ~~merely~~ as a ~~means~~ thing.*

This means you must always treat beings who are capable of making their own decisions as beings who are capable of making their own decisions, and not as if they were things that are incapable of making their own decisions.

Some examples will help to illustrate Kant's humanity test. In the case of the deceived organ donor, the nurse certainly does not respect the patient's ability to decide what should be done with her organs; instead, the nurse disrespects this ability by manipulating her into signing the consent form. Or consider the case of rape. A rapist clearly treats his victim as a mere thing—that is, as someone who is incapable of making her own decisions. Instead, he forces his will upon another rational being, disregarding her ability to make her own decisions, and thereby dehumanizing her. Finally, consider the importance that contemporary ethicists place on obtaining informed consent prior to a medical intervention. This nicely illustrates the Kantian idea that people are rational beings who deserve to be respected by being given the information (or at least access to the information) that lets them make their own decisions.

At the heart of the humanity test is the conviction that to behave immorally is to dehumanize. To behave immorally is to treat someone who is deserving of respect merely as though they were a thing to be used.

Moreover, like the universal law test, the humanity test is able to distinguish between acts that violate perfect duties and acts that violate imperfect duties. Treating someone as a means *only* (as a thing) is strictly forbidden, a violation of a perfect duty. For instance, to lie or steal is to treat someone as a means only, and so these acts are violations of perfect duties. Failing *fully* to respect a person as a rational being is a violation of an imperfect duty. For instance, suppose my car battery is dead and I ask you for a boost, and you refuse to help me out even though you are able to do so. In such a case your refusal to help does not treat me as a means only—I am still free to ask someone else for a boost or to call a tow truck—but your refusal to help me does not fully respect me as a rational being, either. For, if you fully respected me as a rational being, you would have assisted me in my (morally permissible) goal of getting my car started. In general, according to Kant, there is an imperfect duty to help others, a duty that he thinks follows from the imperative to respect rational beings.

Now, interestingly, despite the very different appearances of the universal law test and the humanity test, Kant claims that they are equivalent—that is, they will always give the same answer about the moral permissibility or impermissibility of a given action. It is also fair to say that both tests have proven to be enormously influential—guiding people's thinking both within and beyond professional philosophical circles. Thus, it is quite common to hear the basic insight behind the humanity test. People sometimes say, "He used me *as a means!*" Or someone may condemn an act on the grounds that "the ends don't justify the means." Likewise, echoes of the universal law test are found in such common expressions as "Don't keep things that don't belong to you, since you would not want others to do that if they found something of yours." Similarly, someone might complain to a litterer, "How would you like it if everyone did that?" These expressions give testimony to the currency of what are, at least in part, Kantian notions about the nature of morality.[36]

Objections to the Universal Law and Humanity Tests

Despite the power of Kant's ideas, both his universal law test and his humanity test face serious challenges. One problem with the universal law test concerns the difficulty of identifying the principle behind one's actions (one's maxim). Kant's test instructs us first to identify the principle (or maxim) behind a person's action and then see if it can be willed as a universal law. But the problem is that the same act can be described by more than one principle (or maxim). Consider the act of giving the patient an organ donor consent form when the patient believes it is a form authorizing the refusal to donate her organs. This act can be described as falling under the maxim, "I will deceive the patient," but it also could be described as falling under the maxim, "I will procure an organ for a dying patient from someone who will no longer need her organs." Now, it seems that the former description of the action cannot be universalized, but the latter description of the action can be universalized. If so, this would mean that the same act can be both morally wrong and morally permissible depending on how its maxim is described. But this is highly problematic, for it now seems that those who are careful to describe their acts according to the "right" maxims can do more or less whatever they want.

Here is another problem with the universal law test. It seems too strict. There may well be morally permissible actions that the test views as wrong. For example, imagine a couple who decides to remain childless so that they can spend more time on important personal projects. (We needn't suppose they are selfish; we can suppose that one of their important projects is helping poor children around the world.) Now, there does not appear to be anything morally wrong with the couple's decision to remain childless, but the universal law test appears to claim otherwise. Here the couple's maxim is "We will not have children, so that we may spend more time on important personal projects." Next, as a universal law, the maxim says, "No one will have children, so that everyone may spend time on important personal projects." But, clearly, this universal law is self-contradictory. For if no one ever had children, then no one would ever exist, and if no one ever existed then the decision not to have children could not be made. Thus, the universal law test appears to tell us that it would be wrong for people to remain childless so as to be able to pursue important life projects. But contrary to this test, such a decision seems not to be wrong at all. The universal law test, therefore, sometimes gives the wrong answers; specifically, it views some morally permissible acts as morally impermissible.[37]

Finally, the universal law test seems to run into trouble because it appears to judge certain actions as morally permissible when they are clearly morally wrong. As an example, Russ Shafer-Landau gives the case of a lawn fanatic who (after issuing a warning) will shoot anyone dead who chooses to walk on his lawn. Clearly, such behaviour is morally wrong! But it may pass the universal law test, for the fanatic may very well be willing to accept it as a universal law that anyone who (after being warned) chooses to walk on other people's lawns will be shot. Here again, it seems like the universal law test gives the wrong answers; this time because it views morally impermissible acts as morally permissible.[38]

The humanity test also faces a number of problems. First, it does not seem to be a principle that covers all of our moral obligations. Specifically, it tells us how we are to treat rational beings, but it is silent on the question of our moral obligations to non-rational beings. Indeed, the test suggests that non-rational beings are merely things that can be used for any purpose that a rational being chooses, provided our actions do not dehumanize a fellow rational being. But that seems highly problematic. Most people think that it is morally wrong, for instance, to torture a non-human animal, and that this wrong consists primarily in the fact that one is needlessly harming the animal. But a Kantian cannot do justice to this moral intuition. A Kantian could say that it is wrong to torture a non-human animal if that animal belongs to (or is the pet of) another rational being, because that would disrespect the property rights of that other rational being.

For instance, if someone lights your puppy on fire for fun, a Kantian could say that this is wrong because *your* rights are violated, but a Kantian cannot recognize that anything wrong is done to the dog. Likewise, a Kantian will be hard pressed to satisfactorily explain why it is wrong for you to torture your own dog. Certainly, the main reason it is wrong to torture your dog is that it hurts your dog, but a Kantian cannot recognize this as a morally relevant reason, since he views dogs merely as things. Indeed, a Kantian would have to say that it is not wrong for you to torture your dog, or that if it is wrong it is only because it is likely to corrupt your character and make you more likely to injure a rational being in the future. But this seems to miss the principal wrong involved in harming the animal—namely, that it is wrong to make an animal suffer and it is wrong to act against its basic interests for no good reason.

It also worth observing that it is not only non-human animals that come out poorly on Kant's humanity test: the test also has problems explaining why we have direct moral obligations to non-rational humans, such as those who are significantly mentally challenged. The humanity test is (only) concerned with protecting the dignity of rational beings; it is the fact that we can freely choose goals for ourselves, and freely choose to follow moral rules, that marks rational beings out as possessors of dignity and deserving of respect. What, then, does it say of our obligations to non-rational human beings? Surely, we think they warrant respect and special concern, and we do not accept the idea that they are mere things to be used for our purposes. It is extremely difficult, however, to see how the humanity test can do justice to these important moral beliefs.

Lastly, one other problem with the humanity test is worth considering. The claim that one may *never* treat a rational being merely as a means seems problematic. For sometimes, the only way to prevent serious harm to rational beings is by treating a rational being merely as a means. To see this, consider Kant's own infamous case of the inquiring murderer.[39] Suppose a person comes knocking on your door, looking for your friend, because he wants to kill her. The inquiring murderer asks you where your friend is hiding. Your friend is hiding in your house, and you have to decide what you should tell the inquiring murderer. If you lie, you will be treating a rational being—the inquiring murderer—merely as a means. If you tell him the truth, he will be free to make his own decisions, and you will have treated him as an end. Now, the humanity test says that you must *always* treat rational beings as an end and *never* merely as a means. Thus, it seems clear that in Kant's view you must not lie to the inquiring murderer, even if that is the only way to save your friend. (Indeed, Kant explicitly states that lying to the inquiring murderer would be wrong in this case.) But surely that is mistaken.

There seems to be something irrational in Kant's insistence that we never treat rational beings merely as means. For if rational beings possess dignity and ought to be respected, then (the critic argues) it seems to follow that one should be prepared to treat rational beings as mere means if that is necessary to prevent even worse violations of rational nature. Thus, in the case of the inquiring murderer, it seems permissible, even required, to lie to the inquiring murderer, since that protects a rational being (the friend) from being destroyed, while, comparatively speaking, it only slightly devalues the rational nature of the inquiring murderer (he has been deceived, but his rational nature has not been destroyed). And surely, if rational nature is so important, we should prefer lesser violations to greater violations of rational nature.

Thus, like other moral theories, Kant's ethics faces numerous significant challenges. And yet, Kant's basic ideas—that we should act only on principles that could be applied to everyone alike and that we ought to treat rational beings with respect—have undeniable appeal. Beyond that, in the field of health care ethics, Kant's ethical insights, particularly the emphasis on respect for individual autonomy and the dignity of persons, continue to make their mark. It is therefore not surprising that many philosophers continue to defend at least part of Kant's ethical theory.[40]

PLURALISTIC DEONTOLOGY

Thus far, we have seen that two very different ethical theories, utilitarianism and Kant's deontological view, possess impressive insights into the nature of morality. Most people recognize the importance of promoting good outcomes and avoiding bad outcomes, that we should act only on principles that we are willing to apply to everyone in similar circumstances, and that we should not go around treating people as mere things. Nevertheless, it has also been argued that these two theories are in a sense too simple. Against the utilitarian, it seems that there is more to an act's being right than whether or not it promotes the best consequences—factors like promise-keeping, justice, and obligations based on special relationships seem important, too. Against the Kantian, it seems that moral rules need to allow for some flexibility. The objections discussed above suggest that our duties to keep promises, not lie to others, and never to harm the innocent are not absolute. In some cases, at least where much more good could come from lying, for example, it seems morally permissible or even morally required to lie. Thus, we would not want to say that people who told lies in order to hide Jews in their homes during the German occupation of Holland did something morally forbidden.

Many therefore argue that we need a moral theory that recognizes a variety of moral duties and also recognizes that these duties can sometimes be overridden by other duties. W. D. Ross attempts to develop just such a theory.[41] Ross is a *pluralist*; he does not think there is a single basic moral rule that explains all of our moral obligations. Instead, Ross argues that there are many general moral rules that generate the many different duties we have. Thus, for example, we have duties to tell the truth, to keep our promises, to help others, and so on. He calls these ***prima facie* duties**. The usual translation of the Latin phrase *prima facie* is "on the face of it," but in this context, *prima facie* duties should be understood as *conditional* duties. A conditional or *prima facie* duty can then be contrasted with duties that remain for us *when all things are considered*.

To illustrate, we have a *prima facie* duty to tell the truth. We also have a *prima facie* duty to prevent harm to others. Now, suppose you find yourself in a situation where these duties conflict, such as in the case of the inquiring murderer. In this situation, you can prevent the murder of your friend only by telling a lie to the would-be murderer. It seems clear, as we suggested above, that the moral reasons in favour of saving your friend are much weightier than the moral reasons that support telling the truth. If this is correct, then Ross would claim that the *prima facie* duty to tell the truth is overridden in this case by another *prima facie* duty—namely, the duty to prevent harm. In this situation, your **duty, all things considered** (that is, the duty you should act on), is to prevent serious harm to your friend.

An important feature of *prima facie* duties is that they are not absolute; they can be outweighed or overridden in various circumstances by other duties. When a *prima facie* duty is outweighed by another duty, the *prima facie* duty does not disappear. You still have a moral reason to tell the truth to the person who wants to murder your friend, for example, but there are weightier reasons in favour of protecting your friend. And since *prima facie* duties do not disappear in situations when they are outweighed, Ross suggests that we should feel a certain level of regret (or at least discomfort) for having violated a *prima facie* duty.

At this point, you might be asking yourself two questions: First, how does one know that something is a *prima facie* duty? Second, how does one know which duty is more pressing or weightier in a particular situation? That is, how do we know what our duties are, all things considered? Ross gives two very different answers to these questions. His response to the first question is this. *Prima facie* duties are known through what Ross calls **rational intuition**. Just as one "sees" that 2 + 3 = 5, or that triangles have three sides, one just "sees" the truth of such general principles as "repay debts," "keep promises," "tell the truth," "help others," "don't harm others," and so on. The suggestion here is that our *prima facie* duties, like basic principles of mathematics and geometry, are *self-evident*. That is to say, they require no proof, and are not the result of rational argument or inference, but instead can be seen to be correct just by reflection.

When it comes to how we determine our duties, all things considered, Ross's answer is very different. They are not self-evident, so there is none of the certainty that one finds when apprehending the general (i.e., *prima facie*) principles of duty. Instead, all one can do is to study the situation as carefully as one can, paying special attention to which *prima facie* obligations are at play, and then make a judgment about which duty is most pressing in that situation. Here, one can follow general rules, like the rule that normally the duty not to harm is stronger than the duty to help, or that the duty to keep promises is usually stronger than the duty to give to a charity. But these rules are only general guidelines and may not apply to every case. In the end, Ross says, in judging what duty ought to be followed, one takes a moral risk.

Thus, for instance, consider a case where you need to decide whether to keep your appointments at work or to stay home to care for your sick child. Here it is clear that you have a duty to keep your appointments and a duty to care for your child. Let's suppose that these are the only relevant duties at play. You might try to resolve the conflict by finding someone else to care for your child or by rescheduling your appointments. But if that is not possible, then you must try to determine which duty is the more important in this situation, and then follow that duty. The duty that is more pressing—say it is staying home with your child—then becomes the duty, all things considered, in that situation. Of course, Ross notes, your judgment about which duty is the more pressing could turn out to be wrong—this is what he sees as the moral risk. You may have misunderstood the factors at play, or you may have misjudged the relative strengths of these factors. For example, if you decided to keep your appointments rather than to stay home with your sick child, and if it turned out that the meetings were not that important and your child was sicker than you thought, then you may well have judged incorrectly about which duty was more important in that situation.

We can now understand why Ross's theory is often referred to as both **intuitionism** and **pluralistic deontology**. It is called "intuitionism" because Ross claims that the general principles of duty are self-evidently true (known through rational intuition). And his view is known as "pluralistic deontology" because he recognizes that morality is a matter of balancing many competing duties.

Difficulties with Ross's Theory

It is fair to say that many philosophers find Ross's pluralistic moral theory quite attractive, since it avoids the single-mindedness of utilitarianism (rightness is solely a function of producing the best consequences) and the absolutism of Kant's ethics (there are *no exceptions at all* to the duty never to treat others merely as means). Nevertheless, critics of Ross's theory rightly raise several important objections.

First, many doubt that there can be self-evident moral principles that are analogous to the basic principles of mathematics and geometry. This is in part because it seems inconceivable that someone who has the concept of triangles can deny that triangles have three sides, but it does not seem inconceivable that someone can have the concept of the duty of beneficence, and yet deny that one has a *prima facie* duty to be beneficent.[42]

In response, Ross may claim that our *prima facie* duties are analogous to basic principles of mathematics and geometry only in the sense that we do not (or need not) infer these truths from other, more basic, principles. Rather, he may contend that both *prima facie* duties and basic truths of mathematics and geometry can be seen to be correct by anyone of sufficient mental maturity. Someone who cannot see that there is a reason to repay a debt is morally defective, just as someone who cannot see that the longest side of a triangle is opposite its largest angle is geometrically impaired. It is unclear, however, whether this response will satisfy Ross's critics, since at least some of his critics regard a faculty of moral intuition as something completely mysterious.[43]

Another objection to Ross's theory is that it gives too little guidance when it comes to determining our duties, all things considered. An important point of a normative ethical theory, one might argue, is to be action-guiding, that is, to give people a clear mechanism for determining how one ought to act. But Ross's theory is lacking at this point. He says, in effect, that one should identify the various *prima facie* duties in a particular situation and then *do the best one can* to decide which is most important. But many will find this to be too little guidance. Not only that, but such a procedure could simply lead people to embrace their pre-existing prejudices about right conduct. One could well imagine, for instance, two people following Ross's advice and coming to opposite conclusions. There is a *prima facie* duty to tell the truth and a *prima facie* duty not to harm others. When faced with a choice of telling someone the truth or harming that person, one person might conclude that telling the truth is more important here, while another might conclude that not harming that person is more pressing. On Ross's theory, we would have no way of telling whose view is correct. If his ethical theory cannot help us see which course of conduct is morally right in a particular situation, then it is not a very useful theory.

In response to this objection, Ross argues that any attempt to provide a formula to solve moral problems will be overly simplistic and will ultimately result in giving wrong answers to some moral problems. Instead, we have to accept that morality is messy, and that all we can do is be sensitive to the situations we find ourselves in, be aware of the *prima facie* duties involved, and then make the best judgment we can about which duty is most pressing in that circumstance.[44]

Before concluding our overview of pluralistic deontology, we should note that a version of this general approach, called **principlism**, has been very influential in biomedical ethics. Tom Beauchamp and James Childress noted that rival ethical theories disagree on the ultimate basis of morality, but they can agree that certain principles can be used to guide ethical deliberations. These principles include respect for autonomy, benevolence, and justice.[45] So, when thinking about some ethical question in health care, we should consider factors such as: will autonomy be respected or violated, will the people affected by the decision be benefitted or harmed, and, finally, will there be any violations of justice in the allocation of health care? In easy cases, the actions performed will be consistent with respect for autonomy, beneficence, and justice. In more difficult cases, these principles may conflict, as when the most beneficent act will be one that conflicts with patient autonomy, or when beneficence in terms of providing a health care treatment (say a needed organ) may conflict with justice (e.g., someone else's prior claim to that organ). And, like Ross, according to this principlist approach, there will be no formal mechanism for prioritizing these principles when they conflict; rather, sensitivity to the particulars of the case, and judgment about which principle is most pressing, will need to guide decision-making. Principlism differs from Ross's ethics mainly in that Ross accepts a greater number of principles than do principlists like Beauchamp and Childress, and principlists avoid intuition as a justification for their favoured principles. Instead, the whole question of justification is left open.

SOCIAL CONTRACT THEORY

Social contract theory suggests yet another way of understanding the nature of morality and of determining which acts and policies are morally right and wrong, and why. Social contractarians differ in the details of their theory, but they share the fundamental belief that justified moral rules are the ones that rational individuals would agree to for their own benefit. For example, contractarians would argue that a rule against murder is justified because, if rational, we would each agree to this rule, since each of us benefits from it. In what follows, two versions of social contract theory are presented: the classic statement of the theory, defended by Thomas Hobbes, and a contemporary version of the theory, defended by John Rawls.

HOBBES'S SOCIAL CONTRACT THEORY

A classic defence of social contract theory is given by the 17th-century British philosopher Thomas Hobbes.[46] Hobbes, as a contractarian, thinks that moral rules are those that rational individuals agree to for their mutual benefit. To make his case, and to explain the nature of morality, Hobbes begins by asking what life would be like in a **state of nature**, that is, a time and place where there is no organized society and there are no recognized social rules, where everyone is free to do as they please.

What would life be like in a state of nature? You might think it would be a time of great peace, with no wars or conflicts over property, where people live as free, independent individuals in harmony with nature. But this is not Hobbes's view. Instead, he suggests that life in a state of nature would be dreadful, a state of war of everyone against everyone else, where people would live in constant fear of being assaulted and killed, and where life would be, as Hobbes put it, "solitary, poor, nasty, brutish, and short."[47]

You may suspect that Hobbes thinks that people are naturally evil, and that is why he believes the state of nature would be a state of war. But this is not the case. Instead, he makes the more modest assumption that people are primarily self-interested—typically caring more for their own well-being than the well-being of others—and they want to live and to have a better life. Next, he assumes that people need the same basic things: food, shelter, water, and so forth. Unfortunately, in a state of nature there is scarcity of the things needed. Food and shelter, for instance, are relatively scarce, given that they are needed by everyone, and yet there is no society to produce them. Finally, he assumes that people in the state of nature are roughly equal in power. That is, while some may be stronger or more rational than others, none is so strong or so rational that they can dominate for long over everyone else. Since people desire to live and lack the things needed for survival, they are going to be driven to fight for what they need. The result will be a war of everyone against everyone, where people live in continual fear of violent death.

Because life in the state of nature is so dreadful, and because people desire to live and to have a better life, they will eventually be driven to propose various "articles of peace." These articles of peace are moral rules—limitations on one's freedom—that each person accepts for their own benefit. For instance, it would be rational for everyone to agree to seek peace so far as others are willing to seek peace, to keep agreements with each other provided others are willing to do so, to not harm others provided others are willing not to harm them, and perhaps to even come to each other's aid, provided that too is agreed upon by others.[48] Thus, we can see that the rules of morality emerge as a tool that allows people to escape the misery of the state of nature and to obtain the benefits of social living. In short, moral rules are justified because they are in each person's self-interest: they are the rules that would be agreed upon by everyone so that all can live together and have a better life.

Now, it is important to realize that these rules of morality are supposed to be justified even if the state of nature did not actually exist, and even if they were not the product of an actual agreement. The social contractarian's point is that we all benefit from social living and by avoiding a state of nature, and the moral rules are justified because they are the rules needed for us to live together and to avoid this state of nature.

With this in mind, we can see why certain rules—those not needed for social living—would not be supported by social contract theory. For instance, on the one hand, rules prohibiting prostitution, same-sex relationships, or voluntary euthanasia would likely not be supported according to Hobbes's theory, since we could allow for such behaviour without threatening to fall back into a state of nature. On the other hand, rules that protect life and property do seem justified because they are needed for social living and to keep us out of the state of nature.

Hobbes's social contract theory has several attractive features. It does a good job of explaining and justifying some moral rules: justified moral rules are limited to those that everyone will agree to so as to enable people to live together in society. It also can explain why some of our most important moral rules are justified: rules against murder and violence, and rules that require keeping one's promises and telling the truth are all justified. They all appear to be rules needed for social living. Further, it can explain convincingly why practices like racial and sexual discrimination are morally wrong: people in the state of nature would certainly not agree to rules that said that they will get fewer rights and privileges than others.

Objections to Hobbes's Social Contract Theory

Nevertheless, Hobbes's social contract theory faces numerous objections. First, it seems unable to satisfactorily explain all of morality. For instance, we recognize obligations not to be cruel to non-human animals, to respect and try to promote the interests of those humans who are born seriously mentally and physically disabled, and to provide for distant future generations. Yet, social contract theory has a difficult time explaining the existence of such obligations. For, surely, self-interested humans could come together to form a society that benefits themselves without recognizing any of these moral obligations.

This objection seems to reveal a deeper problem with social contract theory. It views moral obligations as being justified because it is in each individual's interest to agree to them. But morality seems to be the kind of thing that it is not always in a person's interest to agree to: one might not benefit from living in a society that recognizes a duty not to torture animals or a duty not to be callous to those born with mental disabilities. Nevertheless, it seems clear that one has a duty to not do these things.

Further, it seems that social contract theory gets things wrong when it views morality as the product of agreement. For this implies that if we were in a state of nature, where there were no moral agreements, then nothing would be moral or immoral, just or unjust. Indeed, Hobbes admits this point when he writes of the state of nature that "the notions of right and wrong, justice and injustice, have there no place."[49] But that seems difficult to believe. Most would think that rape and torture would be wrong even in a state of nature (perhaps because it treats people merely as means or causes needless suffering), and kindness to children or sharing one's food with the hungry would be virtuous even if there were no social agreements (perhaps because they manifest respect for others or promote well-being). Yet social contract theory cannot explain these judgments.

Faced with these objections, social contract theorists have a number of responses. One line of response could go like this. First, social contract theorists may remind us that their theory is able to account for many of our moral obligations in a clear and convincing manner. As a result, they may argue that we should be confident in the truth of their ethical theory. With this confidence in mind, they may then simply bite the bullet and deny the common-sense moral claims that animals are directly protected by morality, and that there can be morality (or immorality) prior to agreements. As far as non-rational humans are concerned, social contract theorists might suggest that they would, in fact, be protected directly by a contract between rational individuals. The reason for this is that rational individuals may realize that it is in their best interest to accept a rule protecting vulnerable, non-rational humans, since one day they may become vulnerable and non-rational. We will leave it for you to judge whether these responses are adequate, and to think about what other responses contractarians might have to the aforementioned challenges.

RAWLS'S SOCIAL CONTRACT THEORY: JUSTICE AS FAIRNESS

At any rate, even if some philosophers find Hobbes's social contract theory to be problematic, many accept some version of contract theory. For many, the guiding idea that moral principles are justified if they would be agreed upon by everyone is a compelling one. Indeed, in recent years, numerous philosophers have tried to refine and defend certain aspects of social contract theory. The most influential modern social contract theorist is John Rawls.[50] Rawls's theory, called **justice as fairness**, is not intended as a comprehensive ethical theory, but rather as a theory of justice, aimed only at the question of how the major social institutions ought to be regulated.[51] Rather than beginning with the conception of a state of nature, Rawls begins with what he calls the **original**

position. The original position is a hypothetical situation from which people are to choose the principles of justice to regulate the major social institutions. Like Hobbes, Rawls assumes that the people who are choosing the principles of justice are rational and primarily self-interested, and want to have a good life for themselves; however, unlike Hobbes, Rawls imagines that the people in the original position are behind a **veil of ignorance**. That is, he imagines them as not knowing any particular facts about themselves: for instance, they do not know their race, gender, class, natural abilities, religious convictions, specific values, goals in life, and so forth.

The purpose of the veil of ignorance is twofold. First, ignorance of one's personal situation will *facilitate agreement* between people in the original position. If one is self-interested and knows one is from a wealthy family, one will choose principles that favour the wealthy, while those from impoverished backgrounds will favour principles that benefit the poor. Atheists will insist on principles that are beneficial to atheists, while strongly religious persons will seek principles advantageous to their particular religion, and so on. In short, if self-interested people know their personal situations and values, it will be very difficult, if not impossible, to reach unanimous agreement on principles of justice.

Second, and more importantly, the point of the veil of ignorance is to ensure *fairness* in the choice of principles of justice. Since people in the original position lack all knowledge of their personal circumstances and attributes, they cannot tailor the principles of justice to benefit their own particular circumstances and views of the good life. Instead, people will be forced to choose fairly, or in an unbiased manner. Hence, we get the name of Rawls's theory—*justice as fairness.*

As parties in the original position do not know their particular conception of the good life nor have any particular information about themselves, Rawls believes that they will be extremely cautious in the choice of principles of justice. They will not, for instance, choose principles of justice that favour one race over another, since they may be in the racial group that is forced to form part of the underclass. Likewise, they will not choose a society that is radically inegalitarian when it comes to social opportunities and the distribution of wealth, since they do not know which economic group they will occupy. Thus, parties in the original position will adopt a choice strategy that Rawls calls **maximin**: *Choose in such a way so that you will be doing maximally well if you should turn out to be in the minimum (or worst off) position.* With this in mind, Rawls believes that rational, self-interested people behind a veil of ignorance will choose the following principles of justice:

1. The **principle of maximal equal basic liberties**: Each person is to have maximal equal basic liberties.
2a. The **principle of fair equality of opportunity**: Each person should have a meaningful opportunity to attain employment, education, and positions of power.
2b. The difference principle: There should be social and economic equality, unless inequality benefits everyone, especially those in the worst-off group.

According to Rawls, these principles are to be ranked in order of importance, with one being unable to relinquish, for instance, some basic liberties for the sake of greater wealth or greater opportunities.

Thus, Rawls believes that his two principles of justice are the result of a rational choice from an original position that is set up so as to be fair. Because the original position is fair, and because people would choose Rawls's two principles from the original position, it follows, Rawls argues, that the two principles of justice are themselves fair.

Rawls's theory of justice has been enormously influential in the areas of social and political philosophy. Feminists, for instance, have used Rawls's ideas to argue for justice within the family.[52] (Would people from behind a veil of ignorance agree that one sex would do most of the housework and child-rearing? Would they agree that those who stay home with the children so their partners can go out and work would receive no direct financial compensation for their decision?) Likewise, Rawls's ideas have been used to argue for justice in the distribution of health care. Not knowing in the original position if they were going to be healthy or unhealthy, or if they would be able to afford or not afford needed medical care, would lead people to make sure that everyone had access to health care, regardless of ability to pay. A system that allowed only the rich to get access to health care would almost certainly not be chosen by people in the original position, because of the risks people would run if it turned out that they were not healthy and not rich.[53]

Difficulties with Rawls's Social Contract Theory

Rawls's theory is widely recognized for its contribution to political and social philosophy. Nevertheless, it has its detractors. For one thing, as Rawls himself acknowledges, his theory of justice will not apply to all moral issues—rather, it is meant only to regulate major social institutions. What one owes to friends, what it is to lead a virtuous life, and how one ought to treat non-human animals are among the moral questions beyond the scope of his theory. (Of course, this is not really an *objection* to Rawls's theory, since he never intended his view to be comprehensive. The point, rather, is to note a limitation of the scope of his theory.)

Moreover, many have argued that Rawls's characterization of the original position is problematic. One concern is that while the original position is meant to be characterized as a fair situation from which one is to choose principles of justice, it is not a fair choice situation. For example, some claim that Rawls's characterization of the original position is biased against certain religious groups. Rawls assumes that people in the original position do not know whether they're religious. He also assumes that people in the original position want more **primary social goods** (liberty and rights, opportunities, income and wealth) rather than less. Rawls's motivation for these constraints on the principles of justice, as we have mentioned, is primarily to ensure fairness and a lack of bias. But the religious critic of Rawls's theory will say that these assumptions are actually biased against ultra-religious individuals and communities—the Amish or ultra-Orthodox Jews, for example. These individuals do not view their religion and its teachings as biasing conditions; rather, they view their religion and its teachings as the source of truth. Further, these religious groups likely do not value the so-called primary social goods of liberties, opportunities, and income and wealth. Instead, what they may value is obedience to their religion and to their traditions, and the right to be left alone. And they may well view liberties, opportunities, and income and wealth as either not primary social goods or as positively harmful societal options.

Another objection to Rawls's theory concerns his claim that parties in the original position will choose the *difference principle* (which promotes social and economic equality) to regulate social and economic issues. Rawls argues that parties in the original position will choose the difference principle because they will want to guard against the possibility of being in an intolerable situation should they find themselves to be in the worst-off economic group; however, one could agree with Rawls that those in the original position will want to avoid intolerable outcomes, and yet deny that they would choose the difference principle to distribute income and wealth in society. Instead, in addition to a principle of maximal equal basic liberty and a principle of fair equality of opportunity, one might choose a principle that guaranteed that those in the worst-off group did tolerably well. In other words, people in the original position might accept a principle that allowed for significant economic inequality provided that those in the worst-off group have their basic needs met and have the meaningful opportunity to advance to a higher social and economic class.[54] Such a principle would allow people to prosper greatly economically and socially, should they be lucky to be born with the requisite natural skills and fortunate social circumstances; it would reward those who were hard-working (and fortunate), enabling them to have a way to move from one class to another; and it would allow for protections should one find oneself in the worst-off group. Thus, it is at least unclear why the difference principle should be preferred to this less egalitarian principle of justice.

People on the political Left may also argue that Rawls's difference principle would not be chosen from behind a veil of ignorance; however, their argument would be that the difference principle is not sufficiently egalitarian. For the difference principle allows for *some* economic inequality—some people are allowed to have more income and wealth than others, provided that it maximally benefits those in the worst-off group. Thus, the difference principle is compatible with the formation of economic classes (though, it is likely that the degree of economic inequality would be much less than in most—probably all—industrial countries today). But the critic on the Left argues that people in the original position would not choose a principle that, by allowing the formation of economic classes, would under-represent the interests of the poor in forming the political leadership and setting the political agenda. Instead, in order to safeguard their political voice and other basic liberties, provided everyone's basic needs can be met, it might be most rational for parties in the original position to prefer a system that required social and economic equality. Such a society may not be as wealthy as a society regulated by the difference principle, but it would be a more just society, since it would allow for more effective realization of people's basic liberties.

Further, many think that the difference principle is to be rejected because it is unfair. The concern is that it requires that the state assist people in the worst-off economic group regardless of why they are in that group. According to the difference principle, a person who is in the worst-off economic group because of illness or some other unfortunate circumstance has no greater claim to economic assistance than someone who is in the worst-off group because of laziness or choice. And this seems patently unfair. It is unfair to tax the hard work of some to assist those who are in the worst-off economic group because of choice, yet this is precisely what the difference principle requires.

Something like this unfairness criticism of Rawls's theory can also be raised against attempts to apply his theory to questions in health care. Is it right for the veil of ignorance to exclude knowledge of whether or not a person takes care of herself, or whether she is reckless with her health? If so, does that not penalize those who take great efforts to eat healthfully, exercise regularly, drink moderately, and refrain from tobacco use? And does it not reward people who make poor health choices? If that is the case, then one might rightly wonder if such an approach truly is a fair approach to questions of just health care.

Lastly, a concern with Rawls's theory is that it does not clearly settle problems of social justice, since it is sometimes unclear what the parties in the original position would choose. For instance, would parties in the original position opt for a single-payer health care system that covered everyone equally, or would they favour a two-tier system—one that gave basic coverage to everyone, but also allowed the rich to purchase private health care to buy more exotic medical treatments? Would parties in the original position support research into the development of cures for extremely rare diseases, or would they favour an emphasis on preventing illness and developing treatments for more common diseases?

Thus, it seems that Rawls's theory faces numerous problems. This is not to suggest that it cannot deal with these problems, or that a modified contractarian position could not do better. These matters are complex and debates continue. It is fair to say that Rawls's theory is justly famous, for it gives us a fascinating way to think about just social institutions. The idea of evaluating social institutions from behind a veil of ignorance has widespread (if not universal) appeal, and it is an approach that has been adopted by many philosophers, even if they do not fully accept Rawls's principles of justice. Furthermore, Rawls and others have argued that even if the original position/contract argument is rejected, other reasons can be marshalled in support of his principles—reasons that can appeal to religious minorities and non-religious groups alike.[55] Even if Rawls's theory does not get things exactly right, it may get many things right, and, like all good philosophical theories, it points others in promising directions.

ARISTOTLE'S VIRTUE THEORY

The ethical theories we have explored thus far have focused on identifying criteria for morally right and wrong actions or on identifying just and unjust principles. **Virtue ethics** is commonly taken to represent a fundamentally different approach to ethics. Rather than focusing on right and wrong action or justified or unjustified principles, virtue ethics is said to focus on *moral character*. While this distinction is somewhat misleading—the consequentialist and deontological theories explored above are concerned with moral character, and virtue ethicists are interested in right and wrong action—it does seem to capture an important difference between virtue ethics and these other normative theories. Consider a case of telling the truth. The utilitarian would say this is right (if it is right) because it produced the best consequences. The Kantian would say it is right because it is in accordance with the injunction to treat others always as ends, and so on. The virtue ethicist will say it is right because it is a manifestation of the virtue *honesty*; it is the kind of thing an honest person would do.

The most influential virtue theorist is Aristotle.[56] According to Aristotle, the best life for a human being is a virtuous life—a life in which one exercises the virtues. A **virtue** is a character trait that disposes one to act and feel in a way that is appropriate. Thus, for instance, a person who possesses the virtue of compassion acts compassionately when circumstances call for it, takes pleasure in acting this way, and feels badly for others' misfortunes. (One does not have the virtue of compassion if one does the right act but feels nothing or feels pained while doing it.)

Aristotle adds that virtues are *positive* character traits, because they are necessary for the supreme good—***eudaimonia***. The term *eudaimonia* can be roughly translated as "flourishing" or "happiness." The suggestion, then, is that possession of the virtues is necessary for leading a flourishing or happy life as a human being. Aristotle recognizes that human beings are rational, social animals. In order to live successfully as rational, social animals, certain character traits are needed. For instance, in order to get along with others, one needs to be honest and trustworthy. These traits will benefit you in your life, since they facilitate co-operation with others. Likewise, a human being faces challenges in life and so will need courage to overcome these challenges. This will be true not only of people like soldiers, firefighters, and police officers, but of all people, since all people face challenges that require courage to overcome. Industriousness, understanding, self-control, beneficence, generosity, perseverance, and loyalty are virtues since these too seem to be important character traits to possess if one is to live well over a lifetime.

For the virtue theorist, then, the focus is not on formulating principles of right action (or rules) and then acting according to those principles. Instead, the focus is on developing a virtuous character. One becomes virtuous by doing virtuous acts, and by learning over time to take pleasure in those acts. We begin to acquire the virtues, Aristotle suggests, in much the same way that we acquire special skills like playing a musical instrument or a sport. Consider two contemporary examples: learning to play guitar or tennis well takes much practice and proper training. Similarly, learning to be virtuous (courageous, honest, and so forth) requires practice doing virtuous acts and being properly educated in the virtues; however, unlike some special skill (like playing the guitar well), merely doing the right actions does not mean that one has the moral virtues. One also must have the appropriate *feelings* when doing virtuous actions. For example, the virtuous person not only acts generously, but also *enjoys* acting generously.

According to Aristotle, part of understanding the virtues, and learning how to become virtuous, consists in recognizing that the virtues exist as a mean between two extremes—one of excess and the other of deficiency. This idea is known as the **doctrine of the mean**. For an explanation, consider the virtue of courage. This virtue is the mean between the extremes of cowardice (the deficiency) and rashness (the excess). A coward fails to stand up and fight the battles that ought to be fought. The person who is rash rushes to fight (physically, verbally, or emotionally) when fighting is not wise (as when one cannot win, or when one could win more easily by being diplomatic). The courageous person, by contrast, fights at the right time and in the right way. Another example is honesty. This virtue is the mean between the deficiency of being dishonest and the excess of being brutally honest. The dishonest person will conceal the truth when it ought to be told, while the blunt person will state the truth when it should not be told or in a way that is inappropriate for the situation. The honest person, however, will be honest in the right way and at the right time, conveying what needs to be said but in a manner that is appropriately tactful. (Think about issues like telling a patient she has cancer. It is usually thought that one needs to be honest here, where this means communicating the truth, but in a sensitive and caring manner.)

That the virtues are characterized as means between two extremes is significant for several reasons. First, it helps people identify what the virtues are. Second, it can help one in becoming virtuous. For Aristotle points out that each of us has certain tendencies to go to one extreme or another, and that we are therefore more likely to hit the mark of acting virtuously if we aim at the opposite extreme. Excessively shy people, for instance, should know that they tend toward being shy, and so should aim at being excessively friendly and outgoing. In this way, they are more likely to overcome their shyness and develop the virtue of sociality.[57] Finally, the doctrine of the mean is an interesting idea because it explains why it is difficult to be virtuous: a given virtue is always "surrounded" by specific vices, so it can be quite easy to slip into one of the vices, as opposed to hitting the mark of being virtuous.

Objections to Virtue Theory

There is much to recommend virtue theory. It is unclear, however, whether virtue theory is a comprehensive doctrine. Ethics concerns itself with more than matters of character; there are also questions, for instance, about how to design just institutions. What would be a fair tax code? How much tax money should go to public schools and how much to health care? How should governments allocate health care dollars? These are all important ethical questions insofar as they greatly influence people's well-being, autonomy, and opportunities; however, it is unclear whether virtue theory can contribute to these debates. Perhaps the virtue theorist could say, when it comes to issues like allocating health care dollars or structuring our tax code, that we should do what a virtuous person would do—but the worry is that this admonition is too vague to be helpful.

On a related point, it is often unclear how useful virtue theory can actually be when it comes to issues involving tough ethical choices for which we need answers.[58] For instance, there are many cases where it seems that different virtues recommend different courses of action. For instance, would a virtuous person who has young children get a divorce if she is unhappy in her marriage? Loyalty, compassion, and concern for her children may speak against divorce, but courage, authenticity, and honesty might speak in favour of divorce. The virtue theorist tells us to do what a virtuous person would do, or to follow the virtues, but this seems unhelpful in a case where different virtues seem to push in different directions. Indeed, the *same* virtue seemingly can point in opposite directions. In the case of the unhappy woman, courage may speak in favour of staying and trying to make the marriage better, but courage may say to leave and try to make a fresh start on her own. Thus, the instruction to be "courageous" appears unhelpful.

In response to these objections, the virtue theorist can plausibly say that hard cases are hard cases, and we should not expect an ethical theory to make hard choices easy. (Recall that Ross had a similar thing to say to similar objections to his theory.) Indeed, Aristotle famously, and some may say wisely, writes that we should not expect more precision from a subject than the subject allows.[59] Perhaps, then, we can expect precise answers to problems in mathematics, but we cannot always expect neat answers to moral questions. Nevertheless, it does seem fair to worry that an ethical theory loses some of its appeal if the theory is too murky and too frequently lacking in guidance. And this is the worry that many have with virtue theory.

Alternatively, the virtue theorist could try to overcome the murkiness objection by appealing to a decision procedure to decide what to do in cases of conflict. For instance, suppose a person asks you a question, and the truthful answer to that question would hurt that person's feelings. A virtue theorist could say that we have a conflict between honesty and compassion, and if more good comes out of being compassionate than being honest, then a virtuous person would opt for compassion. But then, notice that the virtue theorist appears to be resolving ethical problems by ultimately appealing to their consequences. And thus, the worry is that virtue theory just collapses into a kind of consequentialism. Alternatively, if the virtue theorist says it is more important to be honest than compassionate, since a virtuous person would not be disrespectful of others, and to deceive the person would be disrespectful, then it appears that the virtue theorist has collapsed the view into something very much like Kantianism.

Thus, it seems that a real challenge faces the virtue theorist. Either the virtue theorist's view is frequently murky and unhelpful, or else it can give clear guidance, but only by resorting to a theory of right action. If it is frequently murky and unhelpful, then ultimately virtue theory is not a useful procedure for resolving ethical issues. Alternatively, if it gives clear guidance about how to prioritize or interpret the virtues, then it risks disappearing as a distinctive ethical position—that is, it threatens to collapse into consequentialism, Kantianism, or some other principle of right action.

Of course, virtue theorists today are trying to work out answers to these and other challenges to their view. We have already suggested one response—that it is a mistake to look for precise answers to complex moral problems. Also, virtue theorists could perhaps deal with the objection that their theory has little to say about moral problems that do not clearly involve issues of moral character by giving up the attempt to present their theory as the solution to all moral issues. Just as Rawls limited the scope of his theory to questions of social justice, virtue theorists may want to limit their theory's scope to questions of moral character and individual action. At any rate, many believe that virtue theory is particularly well suited to deal with a wide variety of ethical issues in health care, since so often these issues involve questions of character. Important ethical issues, such as the virtues of the physician or nurse, the appropriate professional-patient relationship, and compassionate care for the dying are just a few of many possible examples.[60]

FEMINIST ETHICS

Arguably, **feminism** is not just one ethical theory but many distinct approaches. These approaches are, however, united by the view that women have been, and continue to be, oppressed. They seek to understand the nature of the oppression and to determine how best to overcome it. As Hilde Lindemann explains, feminism is "about power. Specifically, it is about the social pattern, widespread across cultures and history, that distributes power asymmetrically to favor men over women."[61] For example, in Western medicine, we have the historically gendered relationship between doctors (largely men) and nurses (largely women). In many religions, there are "men who are supposed to occupy positions of religious authority and women are supposed to run the church suppers."[62] In education, there are university professors and day care workers, where the prestige and economic rewards are unequal, and where the positions of privilege are male-dominated and the positions of subservience female-dominated. So, feminism is concerned with power—power of men over women—but it is also concerned with other sorts of power relations, such as race, class, and ethnicity. As Susan Sherwin explains, "feminist ethics is characterized by its commitment to the feminist agenda of eliminating the subordination of women—and other oppressed persons—in all of its manifestations."[63]

Some philosophers embrace one of the standard ethical theories discussed previously in this chapter and use it to explain and critique oppression. For instance, utilitarians have pointed to the great amount of needless suffering caused by patriarchy. Kantians can point to how many traditional practices (such as sexual violence and harassment and unequal pay for equal work) could not be consistently willed as universal laws, and fail to respect women's and other oppressed people's rational nature. Social contract theorists have used the idea of the veil of ignorance to uncover how society needs to be reorganized to protect the interests of all women, including work within the family. Virtue theorists can point to how the mistreatment of women is incompatible with being a virtuous person.[64]

Yet, many feminist philosophers are highly skeptical of traditional ethical approaches, suggesting that they are incomplete or even inherently flawed. Lindemann, for instance, criticizes traditional ethical approaches as incomplete: "their neglect of gender and other factors that determine who has power over whom means that those of us who want to think clearly and carefully about ethics have got our work cut out for us. We have to get a better understanding of the consequences for ethics of taking seriously the moral claims and perspectives of people who don't occupy positions of social privilege."[65] Sherwin goes even further than Lindemann and claims the leading ethical theories need to be rejected; in her words, they are "not only inadequate, but also morally wrong, because they promote behavior and relationships that are morally reprehensible."[66]

What is clear is that feminism is a rich and diverse movement, with distinct approaches within it. In what follows, we will give a basic introduction to some of its main ideas, as well as an overview of two types of feminist ethics: the ethics of care and status-oriented feminism.

THE ETHICS OF CARE

In 1982, psychologist Carol Gilligan began to question the accepted psychological theory of moral development. The accepted view, developed by Gilligan's colleague and former professor Lawrence Kohlberg, claimed that moral development progressed through six stages, beginning with strict obedience to established rules (stage 1), then to seeing moral reasoning as a matter of understanding and maintaining relationships and each person's point of view within those relationships (stage 3), to an appeal to abstract moral principles and norms of justice (stages 5 and 6). Gilligan, in her research, discovered that many women scored lower than many men when using Kohlberg's scale, with women more often landing at level 3, and men at levels 5 and 6. She noted that women tended to emphasize the specific details of the cases before them and instead of appealing to general moral principles to solve moral problems, they would try to understand each person's point of view, seek compromise, emphasize values like empathy and care, and try to do what they could to preserve existing relationships. But Gilligan did not conclude from this that women tended to be less morally developed than men; rather she questioned the impartiality of Kohlberg's theory of moral development. In her book *A Different Voice*, she argued that there are different sorts of moral reasoning—what she called an ethic of principle and an ethic of care—and that neither form of moral reasoning is more developed than the other.[67]

Impressed by Gilligan's theory of moral development, some philosophers developed a distinctive approach to morality known as the ethics of care. The ethics of care begins with the observation that there are different kinds of moral knowledge. There is moral knowledge that comes from the articulation and application of abstract principles, as evidenced by such theories as utilitarianism, Kantianism, and contractarianism. But there is also a kind of moral knowledge that comes from attending to the relationships one finds oneself in. Sensing and interpreting the needs and interests of self and others, and learning how to appropriately respond to those needs and interests, one might argue, is every bit as important as being able to universalize maxims. Yet, this second way of moral knowing and acting has largely been ignored in the male-dominated history of moral philosophy.[68] The ethics of care aims at rectifying this omission.

Rather than using principles to arrive at the solutions to moral problems, one needs to adopt a perspective of caring. Here the focus is on maintaining and improving one's relationships. For instance, if a relative is sick and in the hospital, a Kantian may reason that one ought to visit the sick relative because one could not will it as a universal law that one should not care for the needy. Alternatively, the utilitarian may recommend visiting the hospital because he sees it as an effective way to promote overall welfare. But these seem like the wrong kind of reasons for visiting one's ill relative in the hospital. Instead, the reason one ought to visit one's relative in the hospital is because one *cares* about one's relative and one's ongoing relationship with him, and so one wants to be sensitive to and attend to his needs. Similarly, if one thinks about the ideal physician, one would hope that the physician would act in accordance with principles like respect for autonomy, beneficence, and non-maleficence, but one would also hope for more than that: the ideal physician cares about her patients and is sensitive to each particular patient's needs, concerns, and values.[69]

The ethics of care has been applied to health care ethics in interesting and important ways. For instance, feminists seek to deepen our understanding of such core notions as autonomy and competence, insisting that we become more sensitive to the background circumstances that affect people's understandings and choices. When thinking about the issue of abortion, for example, traditional philosophical approaches have focused on the alleged conflict of rights between the pregnant woman and the fetus. But the ethics of care might address this issue by focusing on different questions, such as the following: What circumstances led the woman to become pregnant? What social supports are available to make it easier for women to not abort and to have the child? What would continuing the pregnancy mean for her other relationships? Or, to take a different example, consider a case where patient autonomy and competency are at issue when it comes to accepting or rejecting some life-prolonging therapy. The ethics of care would insist on much more than just a meeting with the physician to explain the medical situation and a psychiatric evaluation to ensure that the patient understands her options and the likely consequences of her decisions. The ethics of care would encourage the patient and those close to her, including family and friends, nurses and physicians, to work together (in a non-hierarchical manner) to find a solution that works best for all concerned. In short, the ethics of care rejects the idea of the individual as an isolated being and sees her embedded in a series of relationships. Further, the ethics of care seeks to discover ways to understand, nurture, and support these relationships.

Difficulties with the Ethics of Care

While the ethics of care does well to remind us that ethics is more than just a matter of acting on principle, it is not at all clear that this approach can stand on its own as a complete ethical theory. One concern about the ethics of care is that it is doubtful that all relationships require "attending to." Feminists are well aware that many relationships are exploitative or abusive. Often it seems best that these relationships be ended, and that the "needs" of the abusers *not* be attended to but eliminated. Similarly, Sandra Bartky makes the point that caring for someone can be immoral if that care helps support immoral behaviour outside of the relationship. Bartky gives the case of Teresa Stangl, wife of Fritz Stangl, Kommandant of Treblinka. Appalled by what she knew of her husband's work, she continued to lovingly care for him, "and stood behind her man."[70] In cases such as these, caring for others can come at the cost of one's own integrity and render one complicit in wrongdoing.

Another concern with the ethics of care is that one often finds that one is involved in several important relationships, but that it is not possible to simultaneously attend to all of them. For example, at any given time, one's children may need looking after, relationships at work may require that one try to reduce interpersonal conflicts, and an elderly parent may be ill and in need of one's presence. The claim that in such cases one needs to be attentive and caring toward one's relationships now becomes unhelpful, since there is no way that all of these relationships can be jointly and simultaneously looked after.

The previous two points suggest a similar problem. It seems that the ethics of care needs to appeal to principles to help a person decide what to do. For instance, principles are needed to explain which relationships require nurturing and which require ending, and which needs or interests within a loving and good relationship require attending to and which are illegitimate and should be resisted. Similarly, when conflicting demands from distinct relationships arise, it seems one needs principles to help one decide which relationship should take priority, or which needs ought to be attended to first, which will have to wait, and which will have to be left unattended to. In short, it seems, there is no easy escape from the need for principles.[71]

A further limitation of the ethics of care is that it seems to limit the realm of ethics to the realm of one's relationships. But there are ethical obligations that exist even in circumstances where relationships do not. For instance, it seems clear that (1) we cannot have relationships with people that do not exist and (2) we have ethical obligations to people living in distant future generations. But then it follows, (3) not all of our obligations are based on attending to relationships. (4) An ethics of care views all of morality as a matter of attending to relationships; therefore, (5) an ethics of care cannot be correct.[72]

Now, it is unlikely that a defender of an ethics of care will resist premise (1), since "the caring relationship requires engagement with another's will."[73] And, similarly, it seems clear to most of us that premise (2) is true—we have ethical obligations to people who will exist in the distant future (not to leave them an uninhabitable planet, for instance). Line (3) of the argument logically follows from premises (1) and (2), so line (3) must be accepted if lines (1) and (2) are accepted. This leaves premise (4). It seems that the most promising strategy for a defender of the ethics of care may be to abandon premise (4) and to claim that not all of morality can be explained by an ethics of care. Instead, it could be maintained that a core part of morality can be explained in terms of meeting the needs of the relationships one finds oneself in; however, this is not all of morality, as there are other ethical concerns that fall outside of one's relationships. And another normative theory needs to be invoked to deal with these ethical issues.

If the above is correct, then the ethics of care seems to provide an important insight into part of morality—part of the moral life involves the sensitive concern for the needs and interests of those one is in a relationship with. This will involve developing and prizing the sensibilities necessary for identifying others' needs and understanding how to properly care for them. Nevertheless, it seems that it would be a serious mistake to think that this is all of morality. An appeal to principle appears necessary to tell people how to respond to the demands of conflicting relationships, how to determine which relationships (or needs within a relationship) are no longer worth attending to, and how to respond to the variety of ethical issues that do not involve relationships.

Status-Oriented Feminist Approaches

Other feminists reject the ethic of care—dubbing it a feminine ethic—and embrace instead what Rosemarie Tong and Nancy Williams call a status-oriented approach to feminist ethics.[74] These feminists accept many of the insights of an ethics of care—the view that individuals are not isolated subjects but are immersed in networks of relationships, that traditional ethical theories have been blind to the importance of emotions, that context is key to good moral thinking, and that moral issues that arise in interpersonal relationships need to be elevated to more than just footnotes. But status-oriented feminists move beyond the ethics of care by focusing their attention squarely on the question of oppression—identifying it in all its forms and seeing how it needs to be overcome so that people can lead fully autonomous lives. As Tong explains, "Status-oriented feminist approaches to ethics tend to ask questions about power—that is, domination and subordination—before moving on to questions about *good* versus *evil*, *care* versus *justice*."[75] Similarly, Sherwin explains, the principal insight of feminist ethics is that "oppression, however it is practiced, is wrong."[76] For status-oriented feminists, the personal is the political. This means, in part, that ethical issues are approached by looking at the broader societal ramifications of actions and policies. Marilyn Frye suggests that for any systematic barrier we should ask, "Who constructs and maintains it? Whose interests are served by its existence? Is it part of a structure that tends to confine, reduce, and immobilize some group? Is the individual a member of the confined group?"[77]

To illustrate, consider the topic of abortion. Sherwin begins her analysis of abortion by asking how women get pregnant. She writes that given existing powers of sexual dominance, women have little control over their sexual lives—many women do not feel free to refuse a man's demands for intercourse. Further, no form of birth control is both fully effective and safe over the long term. Next, she emphasizes the fact that pregnancy takes place in a woman's body and has profound consequences for her body. It is the woman and not the fetus that is the central focus of her analysis. The fetus's status is relational, gaining value through the mother valuing it; it is not a person, for a person is a matter of being in relationships with others, and she claims this does not occur until after one is born. Finally, access to abortion is necessary for women to maintain control over their lives. Seeing as women are the primary child-rearers in our society, they need to be able to have the freedom to decide for themselves whether they can care for a child (or another child), for having a child dramatically affects their ability to govern their own lives in the future. Prohibiting abortions would work to impoverish women, trap them in relationships that are potentially dangerous to them and their children, and lead women to lose control over their own lives.[78]

So, status-oriented feminists remind us that ethical analysis needs to concern itself with the effects of social policies and behaviours on those that are oppressed. It also reminds us to be critical of the questions that we are asking. Are we neglecting issues that are of concern to those who are oppressed? At the same time, we must realize that feminists can reasonably disagree. Some feminists might see oppression where others don't. Take the issue of the moral status of non-human animals and the environment. As some ecofeminists have argued, do we need to oppose all hierarchical thinking and patterns of domination, including those of persons over non-persons and the environment?[79] Or should our concern be limited to ending the exploitation and domination of persons, or perhaps persons and sentient non-humans? In addition, it is not always clear how best to respond to oppression when it is seen. Should we accept as morally permissible the choices of individual women, or should we instead object to those choices as perpetuating oppression? For instance, some lesbian feminists argue for refusal to engage in heterosexual relationships as the most appropriate way to oppose the oppression of women by men, whereas Sherwin is not willing to go so far, accepting the permissibility of heterosexuality.[80] Others are willing to accept the use of assisted reproductive technology to help women have children who badly want them, whereas Sherwin is highly critical of such technologies.[81] Despite these challenges, status-oriented feminists do well to emphasize the fact of oppression and the need to overcome it. In fact, this may be, currently, the uniting theme among most feminists.[82]

CONCLUSION

As this chapter makes clear, normative ethical theory is a rich and complex area of philosophical inquiry. We have examined several different philosophies. Each of these theories contains compelling insights into the nature of right and wrong, and each of these theories faces objections. In the light of these objections, philosophers continue to develop and refine their theories. As in other areas of inquiry, disagreement persists over which theory is, on balance, best. In the following chapter, each author explains his favoured ethical theory. Specifically, you will see Doran defend a version of pluralistic deontology, Patrick defend a version of virtue theory, and Warren defend a version of social contract theory. These approaches will then guide each of us as we debate the ethical problems in health care that make up the remainder of the text. In addition to our favoured approaches, it is quite likely that readers will find it useful to appeal to the other ethical theories discussed in this chapter as different ethical issues in health care are considered.

REVIEW QUESTIONS

1. Explain the difference between normative ethics, descriptive ethics, and metaethics.
2. What is the difference between ethical relativism and ethical objectivism?
3. Define classical act utilitarianism and explain why it is said to be too simple.
4. Give an example of a situation in which utilitarianism conflicts with the protection of individual rights.
5. Does utilitarianism require equal treatment or equal consideration? Explain.
6. What is Kant's distinction between an action's having moral worth and an action's being morally right?
7. Use Kant's universal law version and humanity version of the categorical imperative test to explain why it is wrong for health care professionals to deceive their patients.
8. According to Ross, what is a *prima facie* duty, and how does it differ from a duty, all things considered?
9. According to social contract theory, what justifies a moral rule?
10. Explain why John Rawls's theory of justice is known as *justice as fairness*.
11. According to Aristotle, what is a moral virtue? Give an example of a moral virtue and explain Aristotle's view of how that virtue would be acquired.
12. What is the ethics of care? Explain two problems with an ethics of care.
13. What is the key insight of status-oriented feminists? Explain how status-oriented feminists would analyze cosmetic surgery. Do you agree or disagree with their analysis and why?

NOTES

1. Some philosophers distinguish between the meanings of the terms *ethics* and *morality*. However, for the sake of simplicity, we use these terms interchangeably.

2. Philosophers sometimes carve up the moral terrain differently than we have done here. For these philosophers, normative ethics is described as focusing only on the kinds of general theoretical questions outlined above, while practical or applied ethics is described as a separate area of inquiry that focuses on specific moral problems. We prefer to describe practical/applied ethics as a branch of normative ethics in order to emphasize the normative (prescriptive) focus of practical/applied ethics.

3. Of course, those who work in normative ethics may be concerned with descriptive matters like the content of established ethical codes of conduct, insofar as some may argue that people ought to act in accordance with these ethical codes. In these cases, however, what is being examined is the acceptability of the normative claim that people ought to follow established ethical codes.

4. For a more detailed discussion of sound philosophical reasoning, see chapter 1.

5. See Andrew Hough, "1.7 Million Human Embryos Created for IVF Thrown Away," *The Telegraph* (UK), December 31, 2012, https://www.telegraph.co.uk/news/health/news/9772233/1.7-million-human-embryos-created-for-IVF-thrown-away.html.

6. The notion of objectivity is notoriously difficult to define, and the term gets used in strikingly different ways. By saying that a statement is objectively true, we mean (roughly) that the statement is true independently of what people think or prefer about the statement. Thus, a statement like "The earth orbits around the sun" is objectively true, because it is true regardless of whether people happen to believe it or prefer it to be true. Likewise, to say that the moral claim "Putting people's lives at risk for no good reason is morally wrong" is objectively true is to say that it is true regardless of whether people think that it is true or prefer it to be true.

7. Readers interested in metaethics would do well to begin by consulting Geoff Sayre-McCord's excellent entry in the *Stanford Encyclopedia of Philosophy*, http://plato.stanford.edu/entries/metaethics/.

8. Sometimes philosophers refer to the view that right and wrong are based on the culture or have some other group basis as *ethical relativism*, and the view that right and wrong are based on the individual as *ethical subjectivism*. We will refer to both such views as *ethical relativism*. What they share in common is a skepticism about objective truths in ethics, and a belief that moral truths are *relative*—either to individuals or collections of individuals (cultures).

9. Alex Chadwick, "Remembering Tuskegee: Syphilis Study Still Provokes Disbelief, Sadness," *Morning Edition*, NPR, July 25, 2002, https://www.npr.org/templates/story/story.php?storyId=1147234 (no longer available).

10. This point is forcefully made by Bernard Williams, *Morality: An Introduction to Ethics* (New York: Harper Torchbooks, 1972).

11. For brevity's sake, *classical act utilitarianism* will be referred to simply as *utilitarianism*.

12. Although utilitarianism is intended to apply to the evaluation of actions, laws, and policies, for the sake of simplicity, we will refer to it as a theory of right action.

13. Some prefer to define *consequentialism* simply as the view that consequences are the sole determinant of whether an action is morally right or wrong. This would then leave room for different sorts of consequentialism. A *maximizing* consequentialist would claim that the right act produces *the most* net good; a *satisficing* consequentialist would claim that the right act produces *enough* net good; a *negative* consequentialist would claim that the right act avoids *negative* consequences, and so on. Given this taxonomy, utilitarians are maximizing consequentialists. For simplicity, though, we will follow fairly standard usage and refer to maximizing consequentialism as, simply, *consequentialism*.

14. Even the masochist seeks pleasure, though the means to this pleasure happens to be pain!

15. See John Stuart Mill, *Utilitarianism* (1861), ed. George Sher (Indianapolis: Hackett Publishing, 1979), ch. 2.

16. One way to think of hedonism is that it is a view of well-being. In other words, it is a view about what makes one's life better or worse for that person. According to hedonism, the life with the most well-being is the life that contains, on balance, the greatest amount of pleasure and the least pain. Once hedonism is understood as a theory of well-being, we can again see why utilitarianism is such a tempting idea: it views morality as the attempt to bring about the greatest net amount of well-being. Such an idea is, at least on its face, very compelling.

17. Another radical aspect of utilitarianism is how it regards non-human animals. Many moral theories view moral rules and moral protections as applying only to human beings, or only to rational beings. But utilitarianism takes into consideration the good of everyone affected by an action, and insofar as many non-human animals have a good of their own, utilitarians argue that their interests also need to be taken into account when evaluating whether an act is right or wrong. Thus, for instance, painful experiments on non-human animals raise profound moral concerns for utilitarians. That is not to say that all such experimentation is wrong (remember, it is not an absolutist ethical theory!), but rather that such experimentation needs to be justified by showing that it is necessary to promote the greatest good. If no such justification is possible, the experimentation is immoral, according to utilitarianism.

18. Of course, some philosophers think that utilitarianism—either in its initial formulation or suitably modified—can withstand these objections.

19. Notice here that a counterexample is being used to criticize consequentialism. Consequentialism is at odds with people's deeply held convictions about what is right, since it implies what moral common sense strongly denies—namely, that it is right for the nurse to lie to the dying patient in this case. Insofar as philosophers are searching for moral principles which can explain and justify our deeply held moral convictions, consequentialism appears to be in trouble.

20. We explore the topic of two-tier health care in chapter 8.

21. Robert Nozick, *Anarchy, State, and Utopia* (New York: Basic Books, 1974), 42–45.

22. For a defence of preference utilitarianism, see Peter Singer, *Practical Ethics,* 2nd ed. (Cambridge: Cambridge University Press, 1999).

23. James Griffin, *Well-Being: Its Meaning, Measurement, and Moral Importance* (Oxford: Oxford University Press, 1988), part 1.

24. For a defence of ideal or objective list utilitarianism, see David O. Brink, *Moral Realism and the Foundations of Ethics* (Cambridge: Cambridge University Press, 1989).

25. An excellent account of various theories of well-being can be found in Griffin, *Well-Being: Its Meaning, Measurement, and Moral Importance*. For a recent spirited defence of hedonism, see Fred Feldman, *Pleasure and the Good Life: Concerning the Nature, Varieties, and Plausibility of Hedonism* (New York: Oxford University Press, 2004).

26. See, for example, Peter Singer, "Famine, Affluence, and Morality," *Philosophy and Public Affairs* 1, no. 1 (1972): 229–43.

27. An excellent defence of utilitarianism against the "rights" objection and the "too-demanding" objection can be found in J. J. C. Smart's "An Outline of a System of Utilitarian Ethics" in J. J. C. Smart and Bernard Williams, *Utilitarianism: For and Against* (New York: Cambridge University Press, 1973). A more recent defence of consequentialism is Shelly Kagan's *The Limits of Morality* (Oxford: Oxford University Press, 1989).

28. See, for instance, Richard B. Brandt, *A Theory of the Good and the Right* (New York: Oxford University Press, 1979).

29. David Lyons, in *Forms and Limits of Utilitarianism* (Oxford: Oxford University Press, 1965), was perhaps the first to raise this objection to rule utilitarianism. See also part 1 of Smart and Williams's *Utilitarianism: For and Against* for a classic presentation of these objections to rule utilitarianism, and for a defence of act utilitarianism.

30. Whether rule utilitarians can, in the final analysis, respond satisfactorily to these and other concerns remains a matter of significant debate. Students interested in this topic might want to turn first to Brad Hooker's entry on rule consequentialism in the *Stanford Encyclopedia of Philosophy*, http://plato.stanford.edu/entries/consequentialism-rule. For a leading defence of rule consequentialism, see Brad Hooker, *Ideal Code, Real World: A Rule-Consequentialist Theory of Morality* (Oxford: Oxford University Press, 2000).

31. *Deontology* comes from the Greek word *deon*, which means "duty." As we will see later, not all non-consequentialists are deontologists. Some non-consequentialists, for example, view morality as a matter of living virtuously or of caring for others.

32. The following discussion of Kant's ethics is based on chapters 1 and 2 of his *Groundwork of the Metaphysics of Morals*, trans. Arnulf Zweig (New York: Oxford University Press, 2002). An extremely helpful commentary on Kant's ethics is H. J. Paton's classic work, *The Categorical Imperative: A Study in Kant's Moral Philosophy* (Philadelphia: University of Pennsylvania Press, 1948).

33. On this point, see Paton, *Categorical Imperative*, 56. When given a choice between more than one interpretation of an argument or view, philosophers should follow the **principle of charity**. That is, they should go with the interpretation that is most reasonable. Philosophers do this in part because to do otherwise would be to commit the **straw man fallacy**, and in part because philosophers should be searching for the truth, and so it is only reasonable to go with the strongest interpretation of an argument or view. This is one way in which philosophy differs from debate—there, the goal is to persuade by any rhetorical means possible, including the deliberate oversimplification of the opponent's position.

34. Kant's work is notoriously difficult to understand. Not surprisingly, then, there is a great deal of debate over how to interpret Kant's work. One such area of dispute is the nature of the contradiction, if any, in being unable to will a maxim as a universal law.

35. Kant, *Groundwork,* 233. The example of making a lying promise, or of lying in general, could easily be related to issues in health care ethics. Examples are giving a patient a false promise of confidentiality or telling a patient that their condition is treatable when in fact it is not.

36. Some might hear echoes of the golden rule—"Do unto others as you would have them do unto you"— when they hear Kant's Universal Law test. Notice, though, that the tests differ. For one thing, the golden rule mentions only how to treat others, while Kant's principle deals with duties both to others and to oneself. There are also certain difficulties with the application of the golden rule that do not apply to the universal law test. For example, according to the golden rule, it would be permissible for a person to break a promise if she did not mind other people breaking promises to her. But, according to a Kantian view, such a person would still be obligated to keep her promises, since the maxim of promise-breaking cannot be universalized without contradiction.

37. The previous two objections may be related, in the sense that if the Kantian could solve the first objection by explaining how to unambiguously identify the maxims of our actions, then perhaps the problem raised in the second objection could be avoided.

38. Russ Shafer-Landau, *The Fundamentals of Ethics*, 4th ed. (New York: Oxford University Press, 2018), 170.

39. See his "On a Supposed Right to Lie from Philanthropy," in *Practical Philosophy,* trans. Mary Gregor (Cambridge: Cambridge University Press, 1996), 605–16.

40. Important defences of Kant's ethics include the following works: Thomas E. Hill, *Commentary on the Groundwork* (New York: Oxford University Press, 2002); Christine Korsgaard, *Creating the Kingdom of Ends* (Cambridge: Cambridge University Press, 1996); Marcia Baron, *Kantian Ethics Almost without Apology* (Ithaca, NY: Cornell University Press, 1995); and Barbara Herman, *The Practice of Moral Judgment* (Cambridge: Harvard University Press, 1993).

41. W. D. Ross, *The Right and the Good* (Oxford: Oxford University Press, 2002); first published 1930.

42. The duty of beneficence is the duty to contribute to the well-being of others. According to Ross, the duty rests "on the mere fact that there are beings in the world whose condition we can make better in respect of virtue, or of intelligence, or of pleasure." See Ross, *Right and the Good,* 21.

43. For a powerful classic attack on the idea that moral truths can be known through moral intuition, see J. L. Mackie, *Inventing Right and Wrong* (London: Penguin, 1989).

44. For a contemporary defence of many of Ross's ideas, see Robert Audi, *The Good and the Right: A Theory of Intuition and Intrinsic Value* (Princeton, NJ: Princeton University Press, 2004).

45. Tom Beauchamp and James Childress, *Principles of BioMedical Ethics*, 7th ed. (Oxford: Oxford University Press, 2012).

46. Thomas Hobbes, *Leviathan*, Book 1, ch. 13.

47. Hobbes, *Leviathan*, Book 1, ch. 13, 9.

48. Hobbes also argues that in order to escape the state of nature and gain the benefits of social living, people need to agree to the existence of a government that has the power of enforcing

agreements and punishing wrongdoers. While Hobbes's insistence on the necessity of a government is crucial for understanding his political philosophy, it is not something that needs to be emphasized here.

49. Hobbes, *Leviathan*, Book 1, ch. 13.

50. John Rawls, *A Theory of Justice* (Cambridge, MA: Harvard University Press, 1971).

51. A comprehensive ethical theory is one that attempts to explain all of our moral obligations. An ethical theory that is not comprehensive aims at explaining a certain subset of our moral obligations. Rawls's theory is not comprehensive, since he attempts to use it only to arrive at an answer to the question "What is the just society?" He does not seek to solve moral questions that exist beyond this topic. Notice how this strategy avoids many of the objections raised against Hobbes's version of social contract theory.

52. Susan Moller Okin, *Justice, Gender and the Family* (New York: Basic Books, 1991).

53. See, for instance, Norman Daniels, "Equal Opportunities and Health Care," reprinted in *Ethical Issues in Modern Medicine: Contemporary Readings in Bioethics*, 7th ed., ed. Bonnie Steinbock, John D. Arras, and Alex John London (Boston: McGraw-Hill, 2009).

54. We might call the idea that people in the original position will want to ensure a tolerable outcome should they turn out to be in the worst-off group *tolemin*, in contrast to Rawls's idea of *maximin*.

55. John Rawls, *Political Liberalism* (New York: Columbia University Press, 1993).

56. See, especially, Aristotle's *Nicomachean Ethics*.

57. Thus, Aristotle speaks of the doctrine of the mean as being a mean relative to the individual. Just as it is true that all people should eat the proper amount of calories, but this will mean different things for an Olympic athlete than for a couch potato, so all people should be honest, but one would expect a different degree of honesty from a close friend than from a mere acquaintance.

58. Virtue theory is not alone in having to deal with the objection that it does not always give clear guidance. As we have seen, this is also a problem, for instance, for pluralistic deontology.

59. Aristotle, *Nicomachean Ethics* 1094, 24–25.

60. Important contemporary works in virtue theory include the following: Thomas Hurka, *Virtues, Vices and Morals* (New York: Oxford University Press, 2001); Rosalind Hursthouse, *On Virtue Ethics* (New York: Oxford University Press, 1999); and Philippa Foot, *Virtues and Vices and Other Essays in Moral Philosophy* (Berkeley: University of California Press, 1978).

61. Hilde Lindemann, *An Invitation to Feminist Ethics* (Boston: McGraw-Hill, 2006), 9.

62. Lindemann, *Invitation to Feminist Ethics*, 9.

63. Susan Sherwin, *No Longer Patient: Feminist Ethics and Health Care* (Philadelphia: Temple University Press, 1992), 54.

64. An excellent introduction to the variety of feminist theories is Rosemary Tong's *Feminine and Feminist Ethics* (Belmont, CA: Wadsworth, 1993). For a fascinating feminist application of Rawls's theory, see Susan Moller Okin, *Justice, Gender, and the Family* (New York: Basic Books, 1989).

65. Lindemann, *Invitation to Feminist Ethics*, 83.

66. Sherwin, *No Longer Patient*, 57.

67. Carol Gilligan, *In A Different Voice: Psychological Theory and Women's Development* (Cambridge, MA: Harvard University Press, 1982).

68. A noteworthy exception to this may be virtue theory, since, as we have seen, the virtues require not only right action, but also appropriate feelings.

69. See, for instance, Nel Noddings, *Caring: A Feminine Approach to Ethics and Moral Education*, 2nd ed. (Berkeley: University of California Press, 2003).

70. Sandra Lee Bartky, *Femininity and Domination: Studies in the Phenomenology of Oppression* (New York: Routledge, 1990), 113.

71. A defender of the ethics of care may respond to these objections by trying to argue that we can best determine how to balance conflicting needs in different relationships, and how to best deal with destructive relationships, in a contextual manner, without appealing to principle. The idea may be that we bring the parties involved together (wherever possible) to try to work out for themselves acceptable solutions for that particular difficulty.

72. Instead of the example of future generations, a similar point could be made with such examples as famine victims in a far-off land who need our aid, or people in our own society who are isolated and alone but in need of help. Surely we have moral obligations to assist these people in need, even though it would be a stretch to say that we were in any sort of relationship with these people.

73. Lindemann, *Invitation to Feminist Ethics*, 93.

74. Rosemarie Tong and Nancy Williams, "Feminist Ethics," *The Stanford Encyclopedia of Philosophy*, https://plato.stanford.edu/entries/feminism-ethics/.

75. Tong and Williams, "Feminist Ethics."

76. Sherwin, *No Longer Patient*, 54.

77. Marilyn Frye, *The Politics of Reality: Essays in Feminist Theory* (Freedom, CA: Crossing Press, 1983), 14.

78. Sherwin, *No Longer Patient*, ch. 5.

79. Karen Warren, *Ecofeminist Philosophy: A Western Perspective on What It Is and Why It Matters* (Lanham, MD: Rowman & Littlefield, 2000).

80. Sherwin, *No Longer Patient*, 31.

81. Sherwin, *No Longer Patient*, ch. 6.

82. If you are interested in pursuing these and related issues, you would do well to begin with Rosemarie Tong and Nancy Williams's entry "Feminist Ethics" in *The Stanford Encyclopedia of Philosophy.* You should also see Hilde Lindemann, *An Invitation to Feminist Ethics* (Boston: McGraw-Hill, 2006); Susan Sherwin, *No Longer Patient: Feminist Ethics and Health Care* (Philadelphia: Temple University Press, 1992); Marilyn Frye, *The Politics of Reality: Essays in Feminist Theory* (Freedom, CA: Crossing Press, 1983); Virginia Held, *Feminist Morality: Transforming Culture, Society, and Politics* (Chicago: University of Chicago Press, 1993); and Virginia Held, ed., *Justice and Care: Essential Readings in Feminist Ethics* (Boulder, CO: Westview, 1995).

3 OUR PHILOSOPHICAL APPROACHES

INTRODUCTION

In the previous chapter, we critically examined some of the most important and influential normative ethical theories. While Doran, Patrick, and Warren subscribe to theories which were explained in that chapter, each has his own particular way of understanding and interpreting his favoured approach. The purpose of this chapter is for each author to explain and give his reasons for supporting his preferred normative ethical theory. This will help you to understand how each author approaches the ethical problems that will be debated in the coming chapters.

LEARNING OBJECTIVES

After completing this chapter, you should be able to:

- Explain and apply Doran's pluralist approach to ethics
- Describe Doran's objections to utilitarianism, Kantianism, social contract theory, and virtue ethics
- Distinguish metaethics from normative ethics
- Explain and apply Patrick's virtue-based approach to ethics
- Identify important similarities between colour properties and moral properties, on Patrick's view
- Explain and apply Warren's social contract theory
- Describe Warren's version of the original position, including the veil of ignorance and the sympathy metarule

---

DORAN'S PLURALISTIC APPROACH TO ETHICS

Philosophers have developed a wide variety of **normative ethical theories**. As was explained in the previous chapter, a normative ethical theory consists of a set of principles which purport to tell one how one ought to lead one's life. For some normative ethical theories the focus is on defending principles of right action; for other theories, the concern is more with determining which character traits ought to be developed. But all normative ethical theories share the common concern of determining how we are to lead ethically good lives. Although I cannot fully defend this here, I believe that each leading ethical theory provides important insights into the ethical life. However, I also find that each leading ethical theory fails to provide a complete explanation of right and wrong. As a result, I believe the best way to approach ethical problems is by adopting a kind of **moral pluralism**. That is, there are a *variety* of principles that help determine whether an act is morally right or wrong. As I explain below, the thoughtful philosopher draws on the insights of the leading philosophical theories, determines which particular moral principles are relevant to a given moral problem, and then uses those considerations to reason about what ought to be done. Such an approach to ethics is messy and unsystematic. However, I believe that rigidly following one ethical approach is less likely to provide reasonable answers to the variety of moral problems that we encounter. In what follows, I very briefly explain some of the main reasons why I find the leading ethical theories to be false, and what, in the light of this, is the best way to proceed.[1]

Leading Ethical Theories and Their Problems

Act utilitarians argue that the consequences of an action are the key factor in determining whether an action is morally right or wrong. Indeed, they believe that the right act in any situation is the one that produces the *best* consequences. I believe utilitarians are right to insist that the consequences of an action are important; however, like many, I believe that utilitarians err in thinking that the *only* determinant of a right act is its consequences. For example, when thinking about whether to honour a contract, one thing one should consider is the consequences of violating one's word. But, it seems, another reason to honour a contract, independent of consequences, is that it is in itself morally important to keep one's word. Further against utilitarianism, it seems that it gives the intuitively incorrect answer in many cases. For instance, a person can be quite confident that he should pay the teen who mowed his lawn the $20 he promised, rather than, say, give the money to UNICEF, even though he may not be at all certain that paying the teen will produce the most good.[2] Promoting good consequences is a morally significant factor, but it seems that it is not the only morally relevant consideration.

Kantians, by contrast, maintain that there are certain moral duties that are absolute, and must never be acted against. Keeping promises, not lying, not stealing, and not assaulting others are all examples of absolute moral duties, according to Kant. Underlying this belief is the idea that it is wrong to act on principles that one cannot consistently will that everyone follow. For instance, breaking a contract is wrong since one cannot always will that everyone break contracts. Also, Kantians defend the existence of these absolute moral duties because they think that it is wrong to act on principles that treat people (rational beings) merely as means (things). Thus, for example, it is wrong to lie to someone because it is disrespectful—it treats the person as a thing rather than an end in himself. But, unlike the Kantian, I do not think that these moral duties are absolute nor do I think that such considerations entirely determine the rightness or wrongness of an act. Failing to tell the truth, for example, may be disrespectful, but sometimes it is morally permissible or even morally required to lie, such as when it is the only way to save someone from being murdered. Similarly, on some occasions, an act may be morally permissible even when it is based on principles that cannot be followed by everyone. For instance, Kant claims it is always morally wrong not to keep one's contracts, but if repaying a bank loan (keeping one's contract) would mean that a parent would not have enough money to buy medicine for her very sick child, then it seems morally permissible not to repay the loan. Respecting people's rational nature and acting on principles that can be applied universally are important moral factors, but it appears that they are not all that is morally relevant.

Social contract theory argues that moral rules are those that all rational people would agree to for their mutual benefit. Rules against stealing, murder, and mugging, for instance, are all justified because such rules would be chosen by everyone as a means of protecting their own self-interest. In contrast, limitations on free speech or on religious worship, for instance, are not necessarily mutually beneficial, and so would not be justified moral rules. Now, social contract theory does a nice job of explaining and justifying many core moral rules, but, nevertheless, I do not think that it explains all of morality. Social contract theory is notoriously weak, for example, in satisfactorily explaining our obligations to non-rational beings and entities, such as mentally incompetent humans, non-human animals, the natural environment, and future generations. Yet, it seems we do have direct moral obligations to at least some, if not all, of these things. However, it is very hard for contractarians to satisfactorily explain why there are such obligations.

Finally, I think **virtue** theory contains numerous profound insights into the nature of morality that are overlooked by other ethical theories. Rather than searching for criteria of right action, the focus of virtue theory is on such questions as "What is to be a good person?" and "What is it to live well?" Typically, virtue theorists argue that the character traits needed for being a good person and living well include the moral virtues: courage, honesty, industriousness, trustworthiness, compassion, loyalty, and other traits. While virtue theory provides an important approach to ethics, it too seems incomplete. Many critics think that it gives too little direction about how to act when the virtues conflict. For example, the virtues of honesty and compassion seem to frequently clash. The honest act may not be compassionate, while the compassionate act may not be honest. The virtue theorist's admonition "Be virtuous!" or "Do what a virtuous person would do!" is hardly helpful in such cases.

Moreover, the virtue theorist seems to miss the main reason an act is morally right or wrong. Consider, for example, animal abuse. Intuitively, the main reason it is wrong is not because it shows a lack of virtue on the part of the abuser, but because it causes needless suffering *to the animal*. It would be odd to say that animal abuse is wrong because it manifests a vicious character, since we think the animal abuser has a vicious character because he is doing something wrong. Indeed, I think that virtue theorists err when they conflate two distinct issues—what makes an act right or wrong and what makes a person morally good or bad. To see this, consider someone who performs an act that he reasonably thinks is beneficial, but which turns out to be harmful. Perhaps he donates to a charity because he wants to help famine victims; however, it turns out that the charity is a fraud, and the money actually supports the lavish and corrupt lifestyle of a con artist. In this case, it is clear that giving to the charity was *not* the right thing to do, although we may still want to view the person who donated as having a good character (as being charitable). But if this is correct, then right action cannot be understood simply in terms of virtuous character. What makes a person virtuous or vicious is one thing, and what makes an act right or wrong is another. If this is right, then again it seems that we have a moral theory that is of great interest—for assessment of a person's character *is* an important part of morality—but that still fails to capture all of morality.

Roughly analogous remarks apply to my analysis of an **ethics of care**. A complete moral theory ought to recognize the significance and importance of care and of attending to the needs of others. But an ethics of care seems to me to be incomplete in some important ways. That an act is caring may be a reason to perform the act, but other considerations also need to be taken into account, such as whether *other* obligations are more pressing. Also, it is not clear that one should, morally speaking, always care about caring. It seems morally permissible, for instance, not to care about the needs of an abusive partner or parent. But if these points are correct, then ethics is more than just a matter of caring.

Moral Pluralism

For the above reasons and others, I am in the rather uncomfortable position of appreciating both the insights and the difficulties of each of the leading ethical theories. Fortunately, I am not alone in this regard. Indeed, it seems that many philosophers working in ethics routinely appeal to the insights found in more than one ethical theory. Like these philosophers, when I approach a moral problem, I try to identify the moral reasons for or against the case: Will such an action have negative/positive consequences? Will such an action violate/respect someone's autonomy? Will such an action involve dishonesty/honesty, or the sacrifice/promotion of the agent's personal integrity? And so forth. I then try to weigh these varied considerations. In easy cases, these moral reasons all lean in the same direction. For example, murder is wrong since it tends to have harmful consequences, is disrespectful of rational nature, cannot be universalized, undermines social living, and for other reasons. Similarly, keeping one's promises is normally right, since it normally has good consequences, respects rational nature, can be universalized, facilitates social living, and involves personal integrity. These are the easy cases.

Our book is full of the hard cases—cases where respect for personal autonomy seems to conflict with the promotion of the best consequences, or with caring, or with respect for one's personal or professional integrity, and so on. Indeed, cases like these are interesting precisely because they are so difficult. My approach in these hard cases is to identify the moral reasons for and against, and to try to reach a determination about which moral reasons are most pressing in each case. In this regard, my work in ethics is most closely aligned with what is sometimes referred to as **pluralistic deontology**.

Following W. D. Ross, I'd say that morality consists in many conditional duties: to be honest, to promote good consequences, to repay debts, to not harm, to promote virtue, and so forth. In many cases, these conditional duties conflict. In cases of conflict, one must study the situation carefully and try to reach a considered judgment about which duties are most pressing in that situation. Whatever the strongest duties recommend in any situation constitutes the right thing to do in that situation.[3]

Here are some examples to make the point clearer. Recall the case of the homeowner who hires a teen to mow his lawn for $20. Upon completion of the task, the teen comes to collect his fee. The homeowner suddenly realizes that he could give this $20 to a charity like UNICEF or he could pay the teen what he promised. In this case, it seems quite clear that the duty to keep his promise is more important than the duty to help others. Thus, the right thing to do in this situation would be to pay the teen, and the reason is "he promised." In other situations, though, the duty to keep a promise may be outweighed by considerations of welfare. For instance, if forced to choose between keeping a promise to meet a student in my office at a certain time or to come to the aid of someone in mortal danger (say, another student who had just been hit by a truck and who needs my first aid skills in order to survive), then clearly my duty to help the needy would take priority in this situation over the duty to keep my promise, and it would be morally right (indeed, required) to help the needy student in this case.

Beyond the identification and weighing of competing duties in favour of and against a particular act, part of my approach to moral philosophy involves attempting to identify guiding principles to deal with cases that are similar in kind. For instance, I might try to defend the principle that says promises must be kept unless breaking them is necessary for preventing much greater harm or promoting much greater good. I would then test whether such a principle would give the right answer in a variety of situations. The more generalizable the principle, the greater the confidence I'd have that the principle is correct. If, however, it turns out that the principle is vulnerable to **counterexamples**, then I'd either have to modify the principle or scrap it entirely and search for another underlying rationale for our moral judgments in cases like these.

Finally, in addition to identifying general principles of right action that are able to yield reasonable answers in a variety of cases, I think it is important to be able to *explain* why the proposed principles are morally significant. Ideally, for instance, one should be able to say why it is normally right to keep promises even if doing so will not always do the most good, but why it is not always morally required to keep promises.

Thus, to summarize, when approaching a moral problem I consider the various morally relevant factors—such as consequences, virtue, care, universalizability, autonomy, and mutual benefit—weigh which factors are most pressing in this particular case, develop a principle that can handle other similar situations, and explain why this principle is reasonable independently of this particular case. If I can do this, I then become reasonably confident that I have reached the right answer about the particular moral problem in question.[4]

The approach is messy. In hard cases, the conclusions are often tentative. But I think that is a virtue of my approach, for hard cases are hard, real-life scenarios are messy and complicated, and we are fallible in our moral judgments. Any moral theory that glosses over the complexities of the moral life is likely to be unsatisfying. All we can do is to try to sort things out, get some clarity on the issue, and reach a conclusion that is sensitive to as many considerations as possible.

PATRICK'S VIRTUE-BASED APPROACH TO ETHICS

My approach to ethics is the product of an investigation of issues in both **metaethics** and normative ethics. Let me begin, then, by saying a few words about this distinction. It is not easy to provide a precise account of the difference between these two levels of moral inquiry, but the rough idea is this: Metaethical issues are "second-order" issues; that is to say, they are issues *about* morality. Normative ethical issues, in contrast, are "first-order" issues—that is, issues *within* morality. For instance, normative ethics is concerned with questions about which moral principles are correct, and which actions are right and wrong. Metaethics focuses on more abstract questions *about* normative ethics. The normative ethicist asks: Are physicians always morally required to tell their patients the truth? The metaethicist asks: What does it *mean* to say that an action is morally required? Other examples of metaethical issues include the following: Are moral claims (such as the claim that eating meat is morally wrong) **descriptive** or merely **prescriptive**? If they are descriptive, are any moral claims true? That is, are there any moral truths or facts? If there are moral truths or facts, are they **objective** or **subjective**? Do our true moral claims describe a moral reality that is objective in some important sense, or do they merely describe the moral attitudes of particular individuals or cultures? Metaethical theories provide answers to these and other important questions about the nature of morality. These theories are typically characterized as either realist or antirealist. **Moral realism** is the view that moral claims are (at least partly) descriptive, and that some of these descriptions are true. So moral realists hold that there are moral truths or facts. **Moral antirealism** denies that moral claims are descriptive at all, or accepts this but denies that any of the descriptions are true. So moral antirealists deny that there are any moral truths or facts. For reasons that I touch on below, I favour a realist theory of ethics.

Let's turn now to normative ethics. As mentioned above, normative ethics involves "first-order" issues—that is, issues *within* morality. These include questions about what sorts of things contribute to the rightness of actions and the goodness of persons. For instance, do consequences matter? If so, are consequences *all* that matter? Are people's motives also important? Among the most influential normative ethical theories are utilitarianism, deontological ethics, and virtue ethics. These theories generally aim to provide us with an account of the properties that make actions right (or wrong), and persons good (or bad).

The metaethical views one adopts put constraints on the normative views one can hold. For this reason, as I mentioned, my approach to ethics begins with an investigation of metaethical issues. As I explain below, this investigation lends support to a **secondary quality view** or, more specifically, **dispositional view of moral properties**. With this view in hand, I turn to normative ethics. I believe that virtue ethics provides a natural, and I think very plausible, way to fill in the details of the dispositional view. The end result is a realist version of virtue ethics: there are facts about what is right and wrong, and these facts are constituted, in part, by the judgments of virtuous persons.

Metaethics

Let's pretend, for the moment, that you and I have stepped outside of our normal moral practices and are observing what's going on "in" there. What will we see? Perhaps the first thing we'll notice is that people, in their day-to-day lives, make moral claims. People say things like the following: "Keeping one's promises is right," "Killing someone for no good reason is wrong," "Abortion is sometimes permissible," and so on. The **surface grammar** suggests that these and other ordinary moral claims are (partly) descriptive, like familiar sorts of non-moral claims. And like ordinary non-moral claims, our moral claims seem capable of being true or false. We also think of ourselves and others as having moral beliefs and, in some cases, moral knowledge. We claim to know, for instance, that it is morally wrong to sexually abuse children. And we often engage in moral arguments with others about questions we take to have correct answers. These considerations strongly support a view called **cognitivism**. This is the view that our moral claims describe the moral features of actions, persons, and other things we evaluate morally. Consequently, moral claims are the kind of thing that are true or false, and that we believe, know, assert, doubt, and deny.[5]

A host of other considerations support the view that morality is *objective* in an important sense. Morality is objective in at least the (minimal) sense that the rightness and wrongness of actions is independent of the personal attitudes and feelings we happen to have toward the actions. For instance, many people in the past believed that it was morally permissible to keep slaves. But the fact that these people happened to believe that slavery is permissible does not, according to ordinary moral thought, make it permissible. The thought is, rather, that these people had a mistaken view of the moral status of slavery. So we think that an action's being right or wrong is independent of whether you and I, in our ordinary circumstances, happen to think that it is right or wrong, or whether we happen to have a favourable attitude toward the action. In this sense, at least, morality is objective.[6]

The above two considerations suggest that moral claims are very much like familiar sorts of non-moral claims. Both are descriptive of a reality that is, in an important sense, independent of our feelings and attitudes. There is, however, a crucial difference between moral and many non-moral claims. Moral claims are prescriptive (or "normative"), whereas many non-moral claims are not. That is, moral claims give us reasons or motives for acting in certain ways;[7] familiar sorts of non-moral claims do not have this prescriptive force. For example, if you sincerely judge that it is wrong to eat meat, it seems you thereby have a reason or motive not to eat meat. The judgment, say, that your car's tires are black, however, does not automatically give you a reason or motive to act a certain way or adopt a certain attitude toward the car. These considerations help to support a view called **internalism**—the view that reasons or motives are in some sense internal to, or built into, the fact or judgment that an action is morally right (or wrong).

To sum up the discussion thus far, our ordinary moral claims are descriptive and, moreover, they describe a moral reality that is objective in an important sense. But, as we just saw, our moral claims are not merely descriptive; they are prescriptive or normative too. According to many philosophers, this prescriptive component is plausibly understood in terms of an internal connection between moral facts or judgments and our reasons or motives for action.

A common complaint of many metaethical theories is that they fail to capture one or more of the features described above. By construing moral properties as secondary qualities or, more specifically, dispositional properties, however, I believe we can accommodate the descriptive, objective, and prescriptive elements of morality.[8] The dispositional view I have in mind is analogous to a dispositional account of colours. A dispositional account of colours holds that an object's being red consists in the fact that it would appear red to "normal" observers under "normal" conditions. The dispositional account of moral properties I favour holds that an action's being right consists (roughly) in the fact that it would appear right to appropriate observers when they are under appropriate sorts of conditions. The phrase "appear right" is shorthand for a more complicated psychological state—one that involves the apprehension of a reason or motive for action.

Now, notice that according to this dispositional view, moral claims are descriptive. They describe the dispositional properties of actions (or persons). And these properties are objective in the sense that an action might be right, even though you and I do not think or feel that it is right; similarly, an action might be wrong, even though you and I think or feel that it is right. Mistakes of this sort happen when either the evaluators or the conditions of evaluation are not appropriate. The dispositional view also (arguably) captures the prescriptive or normative element of morality, since it implies that reasons or motives are "built into" moral properties or judgments.[9]

Normative Ethics

I suggested above that central metaethical considerations support the view that an action's being right consists in the fact that it would appear right to appropriate observers when they are under appropriate sorts of conditions. But who are the appropriate observers? And what are the appropriate conditions? As I explain below, the appropriate observers are those who are virtuous, and the appropriate conditions are ones in which virtuous persons have, and fully appreciate, all relevant information. The upshot of this is the view that an action's being right consists in the fact that it would appear right to virtuous persons if they had, and fully appreciated, all relevant information.

Let's begin with the question, What are the appropriate conditions? What we are looking for here is a specification of the ideal conditions for evaluating the moral status of actions, persons, and other things we evaluate morally. We often make mistakes in moral evaluations when we lack an important piece of information or have incorrect information. For instance, suppose I hear that someone named Smith killed someone named Jones. Then, at first blush, I might judge that Smith did something wrong. But suppose I later learn that Smith killed Jones in self-defence. In that case, I might see my earlier judgment as mistaken, owing to a lack of relevant information. So the ideal conditions of evaluation are ones where we have all relevant information.

I'm not sure this is enough, however. It seems we can and do arrive at mistaken moral judgments, not because we lack information, but because we fail to appreciate the significance of some information, or fail to see how the information we have fits together to generate an obligation. To illustrate, suppose we are morally obligated to stop eating meat and become vegetarian, but I fail to see this, even though I know that meat production causes significant animal suffering. My failure here might be due to a failure to take sufficient note of animal suffering, or perhaps to see how this suffering connects with other things I know to generate an obligation not to eat meat. Examples of this sort suggest that the appropriate conditions should require not just possession of all relevant information, but *full attention to,* or *appreciation of,* that information.

Let's now turn to the "appropriate persons" clause in the dispositional account I am proposing. Who are the appropriate persons? For reasons that I cannot fully defend here, I believe that the most plausible answer is that the appropriate persons are those who are morally good or virtuous.[10] Being virtuous in this sense consists in possessing particular virtues—for example, honesty, kindness, generosity, benevolence. Following Aristotle, I take these individual virtues to be deep and stable character traits that dispose those who possess them to act and feel in appropriate ways. Honest people, for instance, are disposed to act honestly, and to feel disapproval toward persons who are dishonest.

I believe that possession of virtue amounts, moreover, to possession of a certain kind of sensitivity or "perceptual capacity"—that is, a capacity to perceive the moral requirements situations impose on us. The rough idea here is this. We acquire virtue by acquiring certain sorts of concerns and feelings. These feelings and concerns enable us to clearly see the moral features of actions, persons, and so forth. Some simple examples will help to illustrate the idea I have in mind here. A sociopath might fail to see how his violent and abusive behaviour is wrong, because he is insensitive to the feelings and well-being of others. Similarly, a racist may fail to see how her discriminatory ways are insulting and disrespectful, because she lacks concern for the feelings of minorities. A good or virtuous person, however, has a concern for the feelings and well-being of others and therefore sees certain ways of treating others as morally better or worse, right or wrong. This is the rough idea, anyway.

Return now to the analogy between colour properties and moral properties. An object's being red consists in the fact that the object appears red to people with the right sort of perceptual equipment when they view the object in the right sort of light, under suitable conditions. Similarly, I am proposing, an action's being right consists in the fact that it appears right to people with the appropriate sorts of feelings and concerns—that is, virtuous people—when they have and appreciate all relevant information. And just as defects in our perceptual equipment can lead to colour blindness, defects in our moral character can lead to a kind of moral blindness.[11]

Some Objections and Responses

I would like to conclude by offering a brief defence of the view sketched above. I believe that perhaps the most attractive feature of this view is that it does a better job than other familiar metaethical views of accommodating and explaining the descriptive, objective, and prescriptive features of our moral discourse and practice. To repeat and expand on points made earlier, this view preserves the idea that moral claims are descriptive claims, just as their surface grammar suggests. It preserves the idea, moreover, that morality is objective, at least in the sense that what is right or wrong is not simply a matter of what you and I *happen* to think or feel. Finally, this view preserves the idea that there is an internal connection between moral properties or judgments and our reasons or motives. If one is virtuous, and one has and fully appreciates all relevant information, then one will have a reason or motive to do those acts that one perceives as right.[12]

Another supporting consideration is that this view is not vulnerable to the kinds of objections that pose a problem for utilitarian and Kantian theories.[13] On my virtue ethics perspective, consequences are not all that matter, as the utilitarian mistakenly argues. Nor, on my view, are moral rules absolute, as the Kantian claims. It is important to promote one's own good and the good of others. And it is also important to treat others with respect, to be kind, honest, generous, and loyal, and to practice other virtues. But all of these rules admit of exceptions.

I turn now to potential problems with the view. One common objection to dispositional accounts of colours is that they are **circular**, and some have argued that dispositional accounts of value properties suffer from the same problem. My simple response is this: Yes, the account is circular in a sense, for it holds that an action's being right consists (partly) in the fact that virtuous persons think it is right. But why is this circularity a problem? Is it supposed to be an **epistemic problem**? A **metaphysical problem**? Some other kind of problem? The alleged problem with circularity is, unfortunately, seldom explained. In any case, I believe that any circularity in my view is harmless, but showing this in detail would require a lengthy detour into the nature of properties and philosophical analyses. Since I can't take that detour here, I won't try.[14] However, let me say this: the circularity in my view is only at a surface level—an action's being right consists roughly in the fact that it would appear right to virtuous persons. But as I noted earlier, "appear right" is shorthand for a more complicated state involving the apprehension of a reason (or reasons) for action. At this point, the circle vanishes.

In the section explaining his favoured normative ethical theory, Doran raises several other common objections to virtue ethics which I would like to address. One of the alleged problems is that virtue ethics may provide little in the way of practical guidance, since it leads to conflicting rules or virtues. For instance, the virtuous person is one who is honest and kind. But suppose I ask my friend, who happens to be virtuous, what he thinks of my new jacket. Let's suppose that he hates it. Then, if he tells me the truth, I will be deeply hurt, and if he tells me a lie, he will be dishonest. So the virtues of honesty and kindness seem to conflict in this situation. The apparent problem, then, is that owing to these conflicts, virtue ethics provides little in the way of practical moral guidance.

One response to this objection is to find partners in crime. Conflicting virtues or rules is a potential problem not only for virtue ethics, but for any pluralistic view—that is, any view which asserts more than one moral rule. This is a frequently cited problem for contractarian and pluralistic deontological views, for instance. So, to the extent that this is a problem for virtue ethics, it is also a problem for many other moral theories, including the pluralistic approach Doran takes.

One way for pluralistic views to avoid conflicts is to provide a ranking of rules. Virtue ethics *can* similarly provide a ranking of the virtues. One might say, for instance, that honesty always trumps kindness. This ranking would then provide a way to resolve any conflicts among the virtues. I do not think, however, that this is a promising response to the objection. The problem is that there is no plausible ranking of the virtues that will hold true in all circumstances. In some situations, it is best to be honest, while in others it is best to be kind. Put otherwise, morality is not **codifiable**, as the point is sometimes put.[15] No matter how carefully we try to specify and rank moral virtues (or rules), we are bound to meet with exceptions. Notice that our experiences trying to reach correct moral decisions in hard cases help to prove this point. In these cases, no simple rule, or ranking of rules, seems to lead to the correct answer. Rather, finding the correct answer requires the capacity to see which facts are most salient in the situation. There is no shortcut to the acquisition of this capacity; it comes from experience and wisdom. In hard cases, virtues or rules conflict, and we should expect moral theories to reflect this feature of our moral lives. The fact that virtue ethics does not provide simple answers to difficult moral questions is not, then, a problem with the view; rather, it is a point in its favour.

Another objection to virtue ethics that Doran raises is that virtue ethics gives the incorrect account of the reason why actions are right and wrong. He notes that the main reason why it is wrong to abuse animals, for instance, is not that it manifests a vicious character or because, on my view, virtuous persons would see it as wrong. The reason why animal abuse is wrong is that it causes needless suffering to the animal. But this is a point that virtue ethicists can fully agree with. The objection, I believe, is based on a failure to distinguish between two different questions: What *is* rightness/wrongness? and What *makes* an action right/wrong?[16] My answer to the first question is that rightness and wrongness are dispositional properties. More specifically, and simplifying somewhat: for an action to be right just *is* for it to be such that it would appear right to virtuous persons. And for an action to be wrong just *is* for it to be such that it would appear wrong to virtuous persons. When we consider the question What *makes* an action right or wrong? we are asking (on my view) what makes an action such that it appears right or wrong to virtuous persons. Now, to return to Doran's example, what makes animal abuse wrong is just what he says—that it involves the infliction of needless suffering. This is what makes the action wrong; that is, this is what makes the action such that it appears wrong to virtuous persons. Once we distinguish between these two questions—What *is* rightness/wrongness? and What *makes* an action right/wrong?—I believe this objection evaporates.

A final objection that Doran raises is that virtue ethicists are themselves guilty of failing to draw an important distinction—in this case, the distinction between what makes an action right or wrong and what makes a person good or bad. The alleged failure to note this distinction is illustrated by considering well-meaning individuals who unwittingly act wrongly. In such cases, we may want to say that the individual did something wrong *and* that the individual is nonetheless morally good or virtuous. Doran provides a specific example to make the point: Consider someone who performs an act that he thinks is beneficial, but which turns out to be harmful. Perhaps he donates to a charity because he wants to help famine victims; however, it turns out that the charity is a fraud, and the money actually supports the lavish and corrupt lifestyle of a con artist. In this case, it is clear that giving to the charity was *not* the right thing to do, although we may still want to view the person who donated as having a good character (as being charitable).

Doran concludes that "if this is correct, then right action cannot be understood simply in terms of virtuous character." Perhaps this is a problem for some versions of virtue ethics; I'm not sure. But it is not a problem for my view. An action's being right or wrong, on my view, consists in the fact that it would appear right or wrong to *fully informed* virtuous persons. Since a fully informed virtuous person would know that the charity was a scam, then the act of giving to the charity would not appear as right to this person. So I have no difficulty saying that the action in question is not right. But can I also say that the person who gave to the charity has a good character, since he exemplifies the virtue of charity? Sure, there's nothing at all that prevents me from saying that the person is morally good (or virtuous, or praiseworthy) insofar as he was trying to be charitable. (I would add, however, that he might also be deserving of some blame, if he *should have known* that the charity is a scam.)

So, how will I, from my virtue ethics perspective, attempt to answer difficult moral questions, such as the ones we will investigate in this book? The first thing I will try to do is get a firm grip on the relevant facts in the situation. Then I will ask what the virtuous person would do in the situation. More specifically, however, I will be asking what the kind, considerate, honest (and so forth) thing to do is in the cases discussed. Of course, it will not always be easy to determine this. And even when I can, the various virtues will often conflict. In these cases, I will rely on whatever moral experience and wisdom I've managed to acquire at this point in my life to determine which facts are most salient in the case, and so which virtue(s) should prevail in the situation.

WARREN'S APPROACH TO ETHICS: PRACTICAL SOCIAL CONTRACT THEORY

The Main Contractarian Ideas for Warren's Purposes

I defend the particular moral views I take by showing how they would be acceptable to a bunch of selfish, ignorant people. That is only partly a joke, as you will see. I will consider what rules self-interested people would choose if they were ignorant of their advantages, allegiances, biases, and the other particular things about them that determine what rules they accept. My view is inspired by a longstanding tradition in philosophy. Plato, Hobbes, Locke, Rousseau, and Kant, among the most famous of philosophers in history, have all been associated with some form of social contract theory. The contemporary philosopher John Rawls is a huge influence on my thinking, although Rawls would disagree with many of my uses of contract theory. Social contract theory is often used to justify claims about what political system is just. My use of the ideas of contractarians, however, is to generate a method for debating any moral rules that are proposed. I do not confine attention to questions about the justice of institutions. My question is, rather, how to fairly choose rules that guide us in what we ought to do in all areas, personal, political, and others.

Think for a moment about people who make rules. Members of the Canadian Parliament, for example, make laws. They also make many regulations that affect members of Parliament. For example, they, unlike most of us, determine what kind of pension plan their members will have. Not surprisingly, they gave themselves an astoundingly good pension plan, much better than the one nurses have, for instance. Even after being moderated in response to public outcry, it is still exceptionally generous. Now, many have thought this unfair. We might say that nobody who was not a parliamentarian or hoping to be one would have set up the rules in such a way as to give such a lush pension plan to that group.

Now, this is a crucial idea: nobody would accept the plan unless he or she was sure to be a member of Parliament. Ignorance of advantages and disadvantages is the kind of ignorance I want to build into my test of rules. I will take my cue from the contractarians who make use of a kind of ignorance of one's own contingencies. Here is a brief explanation of contractarian theory and my use of it.

Contractarians ask us to follow the rules of the **ideal social contract**. We discover what these rules are by asking what rules people in the **original position** would choose. The original position is a hypothetical situation in which people are:

1. equally powerful (so nobody can force others to accept a rule);
2. equally intelligent (so nobody can trick others into accepting a rule);
3. self-interested (so no other moral theory enters social contract theory in a Trojan Horse);[17] and
4. ignorant of their own advantages and disadvantages, loyalties, biases, or anything else about themselves that would influence their choices of rules that would govern their behaviour. (Behind this **veil of ignorance**, participants cannot skew the rules in their own favour or in favour of their group.)

People are never really in the original position. It is just a useful fiction that we can use to figure out what rules are fair. We can ask, What rules would people in the original position want to apply to themselves in the real world? Given that people in the original position are self-interested, they will want to choose rules that will benefit themselves in the real world. However, in the original position, people do not know any personal facts about themselves, including where they will end up in the real world. This means that they will not be able to tailor the rules to suit their own particular circumstances. It also means that in the original position, people will choose rules that give everyone in the real world a chance to successfully pursue their own interests.

Another major restriction on people in the original position comes into play when they choose the rules that will govern people's behaviour in the real world. This is the **human-sympathy metarule**, *a rule about how to make other rules*. It says: *Choose rules that people with ordinary human sympathies could follow.* I construe "sympathy" very broadly to include most of the positive emotions we have toward one another. Vague as "sympathy" is, people in the original position would still be restricted significantly in the rules they could choose. They could not, for example, choose a rule like this: *Maximize human happiness.* That rule requires, for example, a mother to starve her own children so that she can feed many more children in Peru if she knows the consequences for human happiness would certainly be better that way. That is clearly over the top. This human-sympathy restriction prevents the theory from asking too much of people. Rules that are too hard to follow will be ignored by people in the real world, so people in the original position would not choose them. The rules people would generate in the original position would be usable moral rules in the real world—rules that real people could follow. They would not require us to be saints or superhuman ethical calculators.

Of course, where some kinds of sympathy lie can depend on one's culture, or family or other ties. If we were in the original position, we could not rely on that kind of sympathy. We would not, after all, know what ties might bind us. Instead, we would have to attend to feelings that are common to human beings the world over, like the strong attachment of most mothers to their own children.

It may be objected that we need to know our personal degree of sympathy and other characteristics in order to choose rules in the original position. Otherwise we might end up making rules that favour people with an uncommonly high degree of sympathy. The solution to this problem is one that we would have to use widely if we were in the original position. Not knowing how sympathetic we might be to others, we would be wise to choose the *mean between extremes*. We should make rules appropriate for people who have neither the sympathy of saints nor a total lack of sympathy but who have sympathy to a moderate degree. In general, we would be guided by moderation if we were in the original position. It would keep us from going too far from where our interests lie.

The Committee Metaphor

Now consider a fanciful metaphor to explain what it would be like to choose rules in the original position. This metaphor makes limited sense, but is intended not as a genuine possibility but only to reveal what we believe about fairness in terms of two concepts: the *original position* and the subordinate concept of a *veil of ignorance*. You will, I hope, find the metaphor useful for revealing your own beliefs about what is fair.

Suppose that a new anesthetic has been developed which makes people temporarily **amnesiac**. They retain their general intellectual and emotional abilities, but they forget who they are and where they are. They are also temporarily blind. They cannot feel their bodies except to the extent that they can speak coherently. These people, though rational, are behind a veil of ignorance about their own personal advantages and disadvantages in society. They do not know if they are crippled, average, or athletic in their bodily capacities. They do not know their positions in society, what sort of personalities they have, nor any other personal information, not even their genders or ages. They retain general knowledge about the human condition, but no particular religious or moral beliefs. This peculiar **amnestic anesthetic** is put to an interesting political use.

Under the auspices of the Hospital Ethics Committee, a subcommittee of volunteers takes this anesthetic in order to approximate the original position from which to write a charter of rights of patients and health care providers. They communicate with each other only indirectly through intermediaries. As much as possible, the veil of ignorance is thickened. They do not know whether they are patients, administrators, physicians, nurses, or janitors. The anesthetized committee members are told that they may have children and grandchildren they care deeply about who are mentally impaired or much more brilliant than they are. The volunteers have been chosen to be equally intelligent, rational people.

These volunteers, acting in their own self-interest, have insufficient information to be unfair. They cannot even favour their own generation. The rules they choose must be acceptable to an arbitrarily chosen person, for the volunteers do not know who they will turn out to be. They also realize that they must choose rules that people with ordinary human sympathies can follow.

The point of this odd metaphor of the volunteers is to explain what the original position is like. Asking what rules the volunteers on this subcommittee would choose is like asking what we would choose if we were in the original position. The rules people would choose in the original position are the justified moral rules. They would form the fair rules of the ideal social contract. They might be a great deal like the rules that some other moral theorists choose to tell us what our moral rights and duties are, but their justification is different. Whatever rules we come up with in any theory, if there is more than one rule and no rules are given priority over others, then we need to say what happens when rules conflict. Conflicts of rules are decided for my kind of contractarian by asking which rule would be given heavier weight in the original position if the choosers of rules were given the facts of the case but did not know their roles, if any, in the particular case.

Consider the case of a mentally fragile hospital patient, Zelda, who wants to know her diagnosis, and of her physician, Zeke, who thinks it will harm her to learn her diagnosis just now, although he knows that Zelda has a fatal illness. If you were in the original position you would not know if you were a patient like Zelda, a health care provider like Zeke, an administrator, a family member, or a person in some other role. You would have to select general rules to govern people's behaviour in such situations. These would be rules that you could live with no matter who you turned out to be in the real world. You would want honesty, in order to protect your own interests, but you would realize that brutal honesty might not be in your interest. While you would want the truth to be revealed, it might be allowed to emerge gradually with education and emotional support. You might try to write a rule of compassionate honesty into your social contract. Zeke would be required to educate his patients and break difficult news to them gradually and gently when possible.

If you were in the original position, you would want to protect your right to **autonomy**, your right to determine how your own life goes, by protecting your access to knowledge about yourself. You would know that few would look after your interests the way you would. At the same time, you would accept, in the original position, some limitations on autonomy that would be required to prevent you from getting too much choice when you could not handle it in the real world. If you are fragile, like Zelda, or if you are a child, you might want your autonomy in gentle doses.

One way to describe the balance to be achieved by those wishing to satisfy the requirements on the choosers of rules in the original position is to say it is a balance between protecting autonomy and **weak paternalism**. In other words, we are trying to balance protecting our ability to make choices for ourselves with allowing others to make choices for us that are intended to be in our own best interest. Those in the original position would accept certain slightly paternalistic rules the way we in the real world may accept seat belt legislation. This kind of legislation discourages us from temporary irrationality that would be contrary to our best interest. The freedom to drive without seat belts is not worth dying for. Some other more basic freedoms are worth dying for, and we want to make distinctions among the various types of freedom and the ways we should protect them. The choosers of rules in the original position would try to set the rules so as to protect their interests, primarily by ensuring respect for personal autonomy, but also by allowing for our protection against our own temporary irrationality. Any restriction on autonomy would have to be justified by an appeal to the protection of our interests.

The Video Game Metaphor

In another attempt to make the original position understandable, I am going to explain it in terms of an imaginary video game. Suppose you are playing a video game that you want badly to win—Sim Society. To win you must maximize the personal satisfaction of the character you control in an imaginary society and culture. You will do this through using opportunities for personal growth, wealth, health, and happiness. You do not, however, know in advance which of many characters you will control. The computer decides which one you get. Your character may turn out to be one with many advantages—wealth, beauty, family connections, a large inheritance, great intelligence, energy, strength, supportive social networks, and the like. Of course, your character might lack any or all of these advantages and might even be extremely disadvantaged. Some characters suffer from poverty, membership in a despised group, physical and/or mental disabilities, living with drug-addicted parents, and other disadvantages.

Before you are given your character, you are asked to choose some rules that the characters will play by as they pursue fulfillment. Your only motivation is to win, but you don't know which character you will get. Your task is just to choose rules that will give your character the best chance no matter who he or she turns out to be. In choosing rules this way, you are like the choosers of rules in the original position in social contract theory, behind a veil of ignorance about the particulars of their lives. The sort of rules you would choose would be fair rules.

Warren's Use of Social Contract Theory

Let me assume that you have a rough idea of how a social contract theorist uses the fiction of the original position to argue for the acceptance of rules in the real world. The way I use it is not, as some have, to argue that any particular set of rules is an **absolute moral truth**. I am content to use it as a way to generate debate and to argue for rules.

We cannot know for sure what rules people in the original position would accept. We do not have to know this. We only need to be able to give reasons for or against accepting particular rules. Contractarian thinking gives us a way of justifying principles but does not guarantee that we will come up with a justification on which we can all agree. All I expect is a basis for public debate. I seek merely *intersubjective*, not absolute, principles.

Cultural Relativism

One might object that the contractarian method of justifying rules is a part of the culture of the West and not something that is genuinely universal. That may be so, but this method gives us a degree of objectivity that is as close as we can get to the probably unattainable absolute and universal rules for which we long. The choosers of rules in the original position would not know their country, culture, or religion. Hence they would, in their own self-interest, choose rules that encourage tolerance of various cultures, so long as those cultures were not harmful to each other or their own adherents. A cultural rule that requires human sacrifice would be contrary to the rules chosen by people in the original position, but cultures that live and let live would not run afoul of the rules chosen in the original position. Some would, nonetheless, call my view **cultural imperialism**, but the poor person on the sacrificial altar would probably (though not necessarily) welcome this sort of interference. Be that as it may, this is the most culturally neutral moral theory I have seen.[18]

Ethics Regarding Non-Humans

Earlier in this chapter, Doran mentioned a serious criticism: "Social contract theory is notoriously weak, for example, in satisfactorily explaining our obligations to non-rational beings and entities, such as mentally incompetent humans, non-human animals, the natural environment, and future generations." I have wrestled with this problem in my book *Persons: What Philosophers Say about You,* and I refer you there for more details.[19]

I do not recognize obligations to the natural environment, but this is no problem. It is in the interest of people in the original position to accept rules that preserve the natural environment, since their interests will be tied to that environment in the real world. The more difficult questions for me have to do with our obligations to incompetent humans and non-human animals.

Since I do not think that being human is essential for being a person, I have less trouble with this than some contractarians. Intelligent non-humans are not automatically banned from the moral community. One thing that is morally relevant on my view is ability. I think that human beings and any other creatures that are capable of the kind of mental and emotional feats that most humans can perform must be given special consideration in our moral judgments. We have capacities, for example, for anticipation of the future that some creatures do not have. These give us special capacities for pleasure and pain quite different from those of other animals. We are free to make choices. This makes praise and blame reasonable for people, though not for most other animals. Making rules in the original position, we could take such things into account and realize that they are matters of degree. In that position we would recognize, for instance, varying degrees of responsibility corresponding to varying degrees of capacity to understand what we are doing and anticipate consequences. It would make sense to distinguish between those who are competent to make decisions and those who are not, and to give those who are competent more power and responsibility. Because choosers of rules would not know whether their children might be mentally at a great disadvantage in the real world, they would want protections for human beings who are mentally disadvantaged, but they would not want these human beings to be given power or responsibility that they cannot reasonably exercise. That would be in nobody's interest.

This still leaves the problem of rights of non-human animals, since the choosers of rules know they are not in that group. Their children too will be human, however minimal their mental abilities turn out to be in the real world. Remember, however, that I have a special restriction on the choosers, the sympathy metarule. The choosers of rules must give us rules that people with ordinary human sympathies can follow. Our sympathies for a person remain even after that person's mental abilities have drained away. Our strong sympathies for animals and those among the mentally disabled who never did have the capacity to make free, informed choices are also important. I have argued in *Persons* that rights of animals and disadvantaged human beings would be preserved by the choosers of rules in the original position because it would be in their interest to nurture the kind of sympathy that they might very well need for their children or, in the future, for themselves. We would give animals rights appropriate to beings that cannot bear responsibilities but that can feel pleasure and pain and have limited virtues. Unless our rules require their humane treatment, we encourage cruelty and risk that it will extend to us.

People manage to suppress sympathy for animals by keeping their suffering out of sight and out of mind. People who eat burgers would often go to great lengths to help a cow they found tangled in a barbed wire fence. In the original position, we would know that there is a danger that someone who could walk by the cow without a thought would also be able to suppress feelings for human beings. That is one reason why the rules would be set up to protect animals. Even if only a part (and I think the larger part) of the human population extends sympathy to animals and people in the same way, these rules protecting animals would be useful protection for interests of persons as seen from the original position. That is why fair rules would require us, for instance, to give up some of the cheap but inhumane food production methods on which agribusiness currently relies.

This does not mean that my theory supports fully the extreme animal rights movement. On a contractarian basis, animals can only gain rights via the interests of people.

These interests, however, can be quite broad. Even if we knew that people would soon be extinct on Earth, it might be in our interest to set up arrangements to prevent animal suffering after our extinction. It might make us feel better in the present to work for a future with less animal suffering. Admittedly, saying that animal suffering only has importance with respect to interests of persons makes me uncomfortable. It does, however, give an intuitively right answer when we look at decisions like whether to save persons at the expense of animals. My view has the effect of putting persons first but avoiding the inhumane treatment of animals and human non-persons.

It is important, as well, that our moral rules in the ideal social contract be consistent with ordinary human sympathy. The rules affecting animals will have to take into account the strong sympathy people frequently have for non-human animals.

Social Contract Theory beyond Ethics

Another way in which I depart greatly from contractarian tradition is to extend the contractarian method to metaphysics (the theory of reality) and to epistemology (the theory of knowledge). I believe that our claims about what is real and what we can know are value-laden. These would be subject to the same test as our moral principles. Indeed, the advantage of this way of proceeding is that we get a unified theory of knowledge, morality, and reality just as Plato wanted, but without claims about such things as Platonic Forms or other absolutes that are just too hard to believe.

An example of this way of proceeding can be seen in my approach to **rationality**, a concept that draws deeply on our metaphysical and epistemological ideas. Rationality is a much-contested concept. Many think they have a lock on absolute truths about what is reasonable, but it turns out that others are equally convinced of contrary views on the subject. These views are often highly coincident with the advantage of those who adopt them. Behind a veil of ignorance, people might not be so confident. I think we should ask ourselves what we would accept as the mark of the rational if we did not already know where our advantages lay. I would say that the rules we follow to determine if a belief, a choice, a goal, or a person is rational would have to be rules we could agree to if we were in the original position. It would not be in our interest to allow others to declare us irrational to further their own interests. We need a standard of rationality we can live with in the real world, especially where this is used to determine the competence of patients to decide on their treatment.

Warning

In general, I will continually appeal to the original position to defend not only my ethical positions but also my other philosophical positions in the coming debate. This may become annoying after a while, but that is my job. I am a philosopher.

CONCLUSION

Each author has now explained his favoured approach to ethics. Doran will apply a version of pluralistic deontology, Patrick will use his distinctive virtue ethics approach, and Warren will turn to his social contract theory to address the moral problems in health care that are explored in subsequent chapters. Remember to return to this chapter from time to time, if you are having difficulty remembering the details of any of their approaches.

REVIEW QUESTIONS

1. Explain why Doran's theory is called pluralistic deontology.
2. Why does Doran reject utilitarianism, Kantianism, social contract theory, and virtue ethics?
3. What steps does Doran think must be taken to resolve a particular moral problem?
4. What is the distinction between metaethics and normative ethics?
5. According to Patrick's version of virtue ethics, what does it mean to say that something is morally right or wrong?
6. In what ways does Patrick believe that colour properties and moral properties are analogous?
7. What is the original position? What is the veil of ignorance? What role do these concepts play in Warren's ethical theory?
8. Explain the sympathy metarule, and give an example to explain its use.
9. Consider a case of mercy killing—say it is the case of Tracy Latimer, where her father Robert deliberately ended Tracy's life so that she could avoid a life of horrible suffering. The details of this story can be found at https://www.thecanadianencyclopedia.ca/en/article/robert-latimer-case. How would Doran, Patrick, and Warren approach this difficult ethical issue?

NOTES

1. Chapter 2 contains a more detailed discussion of the strengths and weaknesses of some of the leading normative ethical theories.
2. The example is based on a similar case initially introduced by R. Sartorius and used by Will Kymlicka in his *Contemporary Political Philosophy*, 24.
3. Ross, *The Right and the Good*. While my approach to ethics is closest to Ross's theory, I do not necessarily accept Ross's claim that general moral principles are both self-evidently true and known through a faculty of moral intuition.
4. This is sometimes referred to as **reflective equilibrium**, a concept explained in somewhat greater detail in chapter 1. An excellent discussion of reflective equilibrium can be found in the *Stanford Encyclopedia of Philosophy*, http://plato.stanford.edu/entries/reflective-equilibrium/#3.2.

5. For the sake of simplicity, I ignore here potentially important distinctions among sentences, claims, and propositions.

6. The concept of *objectivity* is ambiguous. Readers should therefore be aware that different philosophers often mean different things when they speak of the objectivity of morality.

7. Because this is an introductory text, I am ignoring potentially important differences between *reasons* and *motives*. Put very roughly, the difference is that reasons are considerations that *justify* one's actions, whereas motives are considerations that *explain* one's actions.

8. My thinking about this issue was inspired by John McDowell's paper "Values and Secondary Qualities," which appears in Ted Honderich's book *Morality and Objectivity* (Boston: Routledge and Kegan Paul, 1985).

9. The claims I assert here obviously require much more defence, but providing a more adequate defence is well beyond the scope of this section.

10. The basic line of argument is that just as the redness of an object consists in the fact that it appears red *to those with a properly developed colour sensibility,* so the rightness of an action consists in the fact that it would appear right *to those with a properly developed moral sensibility.*

11. There are, of course, important differences between a dispositional account of colours and the dispositional account of moral properties that I propose here. One important difference, for instance, is that the appropriate observers in a dispositional account of colours can be specified *statistically.* However, a statistical specification of the appropriate observers is not plausible in a dispositional account of moral properties. I do not believe that this difference undermines the value of the analogy, although some may disagree.

12. This internal connection is admittedly rather loose. However, for reasons that I cannot defend here, I believe that any tighter internal connection is not plausible. But it is less plausible that there is no internal connection at all. David Lewis makes a similar point about his own view in "Dispositional Theories of Value," *Proceedings of the Aristotelian Society* suppl. vol. 63 (1989): 113–37.

13. These objections are discussed at length in chapter 2, where we critically examine the leading normative ethical theories.

14. For an interesting discussion of dispositional views and the problem of circularity, see Jeffrey C. King's "On the Possibility of Correct Apparently Circular Dispositional Analyses," *Philosophical Studies* 98 (2000): 257–78.

15. This point has been made, in various ways, by several virtue ethicists, including Aristotle and John McDowell.

16. This is a distinction that was intentionally ignored in the previous two chapters, given that it raises a number of complex issues. It is necessary to introduce the distinction here, however, in order for Patrick to respond to one of Doran's objections to virtue ethics.

17. The Trojan Horse was a hollow statue used to sneak soldiers into their enemy's city during a siege. Here it is being used to refer to a device for sneaking moral rules into the very procedure that is supposed to determine which moral rules are good ones.

18. More detail on relativism can be found in chapter 2's discussion of normative ethical theory.

19. Warren Bourgeois, *Persons: What Philosophers Say About You,* 2nd ed. (Waterloo, ON: Wilfrid Laurier University Press, 2003).

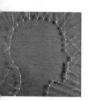

4   AUTONOMY AND THE RIGHT TO REFUSE TREATMENT

INTRODUCTION

Common-sense moral thinking strongly supports a principle of respect for **autonomy**. The rough idea here is that we ought to respect individuals' right to choose how to lead their lives. Within a medical context, this principle suggests that we ought to respect the right of patients—at least insofar as they are **competent**—to choose their own course of care. Respecting patient autonomy seems to imply, among other things, that we recognize a right to refuse medical care. These basic points are relatively uncontroversial. Controversy quickly emerges, however, when we attempt to get beyond the basics and specify more precisely what we mean when we speak of autonomy, competence, and the right to refuse medical care.

To help us think through these issues, we consider the case of Jonathan Edwards. Mr. Edwards was recently diagnosed with **multiple sclerosis** (MS). Because of his MS, he also suffers from **dysphagia,** a potentially very dangerous condition where one is prone to choke. He recently had a choking incident and has been admitted to the hospital for observation. His doctor prescribed a soft diet; however, Mr. Edwards is in denial about his condition (both his MS and the dysphagia), and he insists on eating solid foods. He is at times disoriented and confused, but at other times he seems to understand his doctor's warnings and just thinks they're overblown. Mr. Edwards is a very strong-willed individual and he is determined not to have his diet restricted, yet allowing him to eat solid foods would put him at a high risk of serious harm. After arguing with his physician over his diet, Mr. Edwards insists on being discharged from the hospital. His doctor and nurses are concerned that if he is allowed to leave the hospital he will return to his normal diet and will be risking grave harm to himself. A psychiatric assessment finds Mr. Edwards competent, but his eccentric and at times seemingly irrational behaviour leads some of the members of his health care team to believe otherwise.

By debating Mr. Edwards's case, we are able to explore the difficult issues of autonomy, competence, **informed** or **valid consent**, and the right to refuse care. Was

Mr. Edwards competent to make his health care decisions? Was Mr. Edwards's refusal of care valid? As you read through the drama and the debate, be mindful of such issues as when a competent person's liberty may be interfered with for that person's own good, and under what conditions a person should be permitted to make their own health care decisions. Focusing on these general questions may help you to develop a clear approach not only to the issue of whether Mr. Edwards was competent to make his health care decisions, and whether his health care team erred in releasing him when they did, but also to a wide variety of cases involving patient autonomy and the right to refuse medical care.

LEARNING OBJECTIVES

After completing this chapter, you should be able to:

- Define *autonomy*
- Explain what it means for a person to be competent (or incompetent)
- Distinguish soft paternalism from hard paternalism, and weak paternalism from strong paternalism
- Discuss Patrick's and Doran's view that greater paternalistic interferences were warranted in Mr. Edwards's case, even if he was competent to make his own health care decisions
- Discuss what is required for people to be competent to make their own health care decisions
- Distinguish informed consent or informed refusal from what Warren views as valid consent or valid refusal
- Understand the relationship between autonomy, competence, and valid consent or refusal
- Describe Warren's reasons for thinking that Mr. Edwards's health care team did not err in releasing him from the hospital when they did
- Explain Patrick's and Doran's reasons for thinking Mr. Edwards's health care team erred in releasing him from the hospital when they did

---

DRAMA

Please note: This case is based on various true stories, although names, places, and some uncontroversial elements of the case have been changed to preserve anonymity and confidentiality. Discussions of this and similar cases with health care professionals have also informed this fictional case. The drama merely raises issues. The philosophical arguments are to be found in the debate following the drama.

CHARACTERS

Jonathan Edwards: a patient with MS causing dysphagia

Brad Edwards: Jonathan's husband

Charles Nolet: a nurse assigned to Mr. Edwards's care and his friend of many years

Dr. Paula Paladin: the attending physician

Eva Kowolski: the head nurse

Jane Kruala: a social worker

Scene 1

A patient, Jonathan Edwards, is talking animatedly to nobody while his friend and nurse, Charles Nolet, observes him, unseen, from the door to the ward.

Jonathan: Nonsense! The idea! Me, with multiple sclerosis? Why, I'm as healthy as a horse. I'm sure my problems come from something much less exotic than MS. (*He spots Charles, who walks in with his arms out to his old friend.*) Oh! Goodness. (*Laughs*) You caught me rehearsing. How are you, my old friend?

Charles: Very well, Jonathan, but how are *you?*

Jonathan: Oh, never mind about me. Oh, it's so good to see you. Your mother said you were working here and I knew I'd be getting a visit.

Charles: More than that. I got myself assigned to your care. Nothing but the best for you.

Jonathan: Oh, lucky me. It is a good thing, since my doctor is trying to starve me to death. Brad brought me in a nice chop. Even if it is cold, it's better than that hideous gruel they expect me to put up with. I won't have it. It is utterly *nauseating.*

Charles: Let's see your chart. Ah, yes. Dr. Paladin ordered a soft diet. She thinks you're having trouble with your swallowing reflex. The **motility** test they gave you...

> **DEFINITION**
>
> **Multiple sclerosis** or **MS** is a disease in which the central nervous system is damaged by deterioration of a protective covering called the myelin sheath. It causes a variety of symptoms including weakness, lack of coordination, speech disturbances, vision problems and strange sensations. It can also cause dysphagia, i.e., difficulty in swallowing. MS can vary from mild to debilitating. The course of the disease is usually prolonged with remissions and relapses over years. The cause is unknown.
>
> *Source:* W. A. N. Dorland, *Dorland's Illustrated Medical Dictionary* (Philadelphia: Saunders, 1985), 1180.

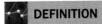

DEFINITION

Motility is the ability to move spontaneously. If this ability is lost in the parts of the body used to swallow, dysphagia results.

Jonathan: I swear, that young doctor hasn't a brain in her head. My chop was delicious, thank you, and I swallowed it all. Yes, I choked once upon a time, but who hasn't done that? No doctor is going to tell me what to do.

Charles: Well, I see you're just as stubborn as ever.

Jonathan: And I always will be. By the way, I'll need your help. I can get to the kitchen to get the little care packages my family leaves in the fridge, but I can't reach the food when it is pushed to the back. Pull it up to the front for me, will you? My things all have a little green ribbon taped on them. Oh, and one more thing, that chair that Brad has to sit in when he visits is so hard on his bad back. What possessed them to buy such ridiculous chairs? See if you can get something else, will you, Charles?

Charles: I'll see what I can do.

Jonathan: Much appreciated. I think I'll just nap now. The door isn't open, is it? There's a draft. We wouldn't want Nettles to get out.

Charles: Nettles?

Jonathan: Yes, my cat. Oh of course, you went away before Brambles died, poor old thing. Nettles can't hold a candle to Brambles, you know. Do see that the door is closed and ask Brad to open a tin for little Nettles, won't you?

Charles: I will.

Scene 2

Charles and Eva Kowolski, the head nurse, are discussing Mr. Edwards.

Eva: Well, there is a question of competence.

Charles: Oh, Mr. Edwards is okay. I've known him for years. He's always been a little bit *eccentric*, you know, but he's got all his marbles, all right.

Eva: Maybe knowing him for years clouds your objectivity about this patient just a little.

Charles: What do you mean?

Eva: He refused to get an MRI scan because he doesn't think he needs one and thinks it's a waste of tax dollars. He says he's perfectly healthy when he can barely get into his wheelchair. Charles, he talks to himself. He shouts and gesticulates at the empty air. He's forever pushing the call button to have us feed his imaginary cat or put it out or let it in. Alice in Wonderland was straighter.

Charles: He's always been like that. He built and ran a travel agency talking to himself all the while. He calls that talking to nobody "rehearsing." It's just a quirk.

Eva: Did he always have a Cheshire Cat?

Charles: Okay, he is a bit confused about being here or being at home sometimes. Nettles is a real cat, just not here.

Eva: Look, Charles, he's practically family to you. You said he helped finance your education as a nurse. Gratitude would make you want to give him the benefit of the doubt.

Charles: Of course I'm grateful. But that isn't the whole thing. You have to know him. He's always been so peculiar. People thought he was crazy before, and he was crazy like a fox. He's made millions being different, and he put a lot of that loot into this hospital. Maybe he is a little bit confused, but I owe it to him—we all owe it to him—not to write him off too soon. I swear, when I'm talking to him, he can be as sharp as a tack.

Eva: Your judgment may be clouded by your friendship. Seriously, think about the possibility of his choking. I think we should make sure Dr. Paladin's order for a soft diet is strictly followed.

Charles: I'll see what I can do, Eva.

Scene 3

A patient-care conference between Paula Paladin (physician), Eva Kowolski (head nurse), Jane Kruala (social worker), and Charles Nolet (nurse), concerning Mr. Edwards.

Paula: Have there been any incidents of choking since the first one that led us to do the motility test?

Eva: No, we've been lucky.

Paula: I don't want to depend on luck. Let's keep him on soft foods.

Jane: Mr. Edwards is in denial. Until he's convinced and his family is convinced that he really has MS and really has a problem with swallowing, we aren't going to get co-operation.

Paula: Well, Mr. Edwards is not competent to consent.

Charles: We can't say that. He does some quirky things, but he's right on top of it when we discuss his treatment.

Paula: So why doesn't he comply?

Charles: Because he doesn't agree that it is necessary. I've discussed the risks with him and he says he is willing to take those risks. He's been a big risk-taker all of his life.

Eva: Yeah, well, I don't want him aspirating on my watch.

Paula: A rational person wouldn't risk death for a lamb chop.

Charles: We all eat fast food, and that box of doughnuts Brad left for us disappeared pretty quick. We're slowly digging our graves with our teeth, and we know it. He's just making tougher choices. The threat of death is a little closer. We might not share his values, but anyway, he's one of the most rational people I know.

Paula: So what do the rest of you think? Is Mr. Edwards competent? Should we respect his autonomy?

Eva: I don't know. He seems too scattered to me.

Jane: Well, let's have the psychiatrist test him. If he really understands the consequences of his choices, then we should respect those choices.

Paula: Okay, but keep a close eye on him in the meantime. Be ready to suction him. Try to talk him into accepting the soft diet.

Eva: (*Laughs*) Nobody talks Jonathan Edwards into anything.

Charles: He's got a strong mind.

Eva: A strong will, anyhow.

Paula: Well, Charles, you're close to him. See if you can persuade him to be a little more co-operative.

Charles: I'll see what I can do.

Scene 4

Dr. Paula Paladin and Jonathan Edwards talk about Jonathan's second choking incident.

Paula: You don't seem to appreciate the situation. If Charles had not been right there to help you out, you could have suffered some serious long-term consequences.

Jonathan: Like what?

Paula: Brain damage from **hypoxia** or death, for instance.

Jonathan: What was that, dear? High what?

Paula: Hypoxia is not getting enough oxygen. When you can't breathe, you're in deep trouble.

> **DEFINITION**
>
> **Hypoxia** is a reduction of oxygen to tissue in spite of adequate blood circulation. If it is not remedied immediately, the brain is deprived of oxygen, causing damage.

Jonathan: Oxygen, my word. There's none in this stuffy little room, in any case. Of course, if we leave the window open, Nettles will get out. Now, don't roll your eyes, young lady. Nettles may be just a cat, but she's a dear little thing. Now, about this choking business, what this tells me is that I need somebody to stand by with one of those dreary little suction machines when I eat. Giving me baby food, my dear, is not an acceptable solution.

Paula: Mr. Edwards, we haven't the staff to watch over every patient who might choke and aspirate during every meal. For us to help you, you must listen to some of our advice.

Jonathan: I'm not sure I like your tone, doctor. The very independence of mind that seems to be such a problem at this institution has served me so well in life that I can afford to hire some twit to stand around with a tube in hand while I have my meals.

Paula: Speaking of tone, do you think that the people who have been caring for you deserve a little respect? Charles…

Jonathan: Oh, the nurses here have been wonderful. Don't put words in my mouth.

Paula: Words like "twit"?

Jonathan: What are you saying? I have never used such language.

Paula: Mr. Edwards, you seem rather unhappy with your care here.

Jonathan: What gives you that impression? Nettles and I are quite happy here, I assure you. I don't know where she has gotten to. Frisky little thing. Always off and about somewhere.

Paula: We were just speaking of your soft diet…

Jonathan: Out of the question, my dear.

Paula: And this latest choking incident of yours. I was saying that we couldn't provide staff to watch over you at every meal.

Jonathan: Then I will provide staff. It won't be hard to find someone to stand around with a tube in hand waiting to suction me if need be.

Paula: Your life depends on it. You need a trained nurse. This is not a task for an unskilled person.

Jonathan: Stuff and nonsense! There's nothing to it. My cleaning woman could do it.

Paula: Trained nurses know how to deal with quite a variety of complications that can arise as a result of choking and aspirating. Speedy responses are vital when you're not getting air.

Jonathan: As an employer, I am used to staff exaggerating their own importance. Suctioning me is a minor task. Don't you make much of it just to justify the high-priced help.

Paula: If you don't want our advice and care, then you can seek help elsewhere, but…

Jonathan: I shall. Thank you for your efforts. And really, dear, don't take it ill. It's not that I'm an ingrate. I'm sure you're all quite sincere and doing your best with a difficult old man, but I am accustomed to acting on my own opinions, isn't that right, Brad?

Paula: Your husband is not here at the moment, Mr. Edwards, nor is your cat in this hospital room.

Jonathan: Oh! Oh, yes, of course.

Paula: Why don't you rest? We'll talk tomorrow.

Jonathan: Excellent idea.

Scene 5

A patient-care conference with Eva, Jane, Paula, and Charles.

Eva: So Mr. Edwards is back, but he's not going to be a difficult patient this time. He still protests, but he is barely coherent and certainly incompetent.

Jane: What happened?

Paula: Predictably, he got into trouble at home under his husband's care, and by the time he got to Emerg he was hypoxic. **Dementia** has set in thoroughly now.

Charles: Jonathan's gone. Unfortunately, his body is still alive. He would have hated that. Poor Brad, he's finally going to take charge.

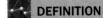

> **DEFINITION**
>
> **Dementia** is a loss of intellectual function, in this case from severe brain damage. Jonathan's intellect has been reduced to an infantile state.

Paula: It was all so maddeningly preventable. I don't think he was competent to book himself out and decide on his own care. I just could not get through to him.

Charles: Nobody ever could. He was a wonderful person but never did really listen to anyone. If he could look at the whole thing right now, he would just say, "Well, I made my choice and I was wrong. Win some, lose some."

Jane: Well, the psychiatrist said he was competent. We had to respect his autonomy.

Paula: Autonomy comes in degrees. It's wrong to treat it as all or nothing. You wouldn't have let him drive if he were drunk. Why should we have let him book himself out when he was in the initial stages of dementia? People ought not to be allowed to risk their lives when they are not on top of things. We should have gotten a second psychiatric opinion. Jonathan Edwards had some good years left.

Jane: Maybe so, but wouldn't it look different to you if you were in his shoes? Physicians themselves are always difficult patients because they want to take charge of their own care, just as Jonathan Edwards did.

Charles: I visited him at home and described to him in detail the dangers he was facing. He thanked me and said that he used to ride a motorcycle without a helmet to feel the wind in his hair. I'm not saying he was totally sharp at the end or able to keep the risks in mind, but if he had his old self back, he would still make the same decision.

Paula: I don't see that. He would have at least hired a home-care nurse if he really was sharp and appreciated the dangers. He was not suicidal. Come on, let's face it. We did the wrong thing. We should have fought harder to keep him. It's a damn good thing we're not bartenders or we'd all be in big trouble for giving him back his keys.

DEBATE

Identifying Relevant Facts

Patrick: Let's clarify some relevant facts before we begin our debate. How old was Mr. Edwards?

Warren: He was 62.

Patrick: What were his long-term prospects? Suppose Mr. Edwards had followed his doctor's orders: How long, and how well, would he have been expected to live?

Warren: MS patients may live long lives, but with limitations. These can be quite minor, but in Mr. Edwards's case, the dysphagia was dangerous, as we saw. Mr. Edwards's prognosis was poor given his lack of co-operation with Dr. Paladin's treatment plan.

Patrick: Where on the scale of harms from MS did Mr. Edwards fall?

Warren: If he followed his prescribed diet, Mr. Edwards was probably in the middle of the scale of harms from MS. He could have had a decent life, but he would've been low on energy.

Patrick: Okay. So he wasn't obviously doomed to a life of pain and suffering.

Warren: No, he had a chance, at least, of a good life.

Patrick: How about his mobility? I recall something about him having trouble getting in and out of a wheelchair.

Warren: Yes, it was something like having the flu all the time. MS has both remitting and chronic progressive forms, however. Which one Mr. Edwards had was not yet determined.

Doran: Was his confusion the result of the MS or was it something unrelated to the MS? Was there any reason to think his state of mind would have improved, or deteriorated, if he had followed the treatment plan?

Warren: His confusion could've been the result of his MS, but that only happens in a minority of cases. It was also possible that he was suffering from dementia from organic causes. It was possible that his confusion could have stabilized. We just don't know. It is a feature of the disease, however, that MS patients often disbelieve their diagnosis.

Doran: What do you mean "his confusion could have stabilized"?

Warren: He might not have become progressively more confused. If his condition turned out to have been chronic progressive, he might have become more confused to the point of complete dementia. If he had the remitting form, he might even have improved for a while, and possibly have relapsed later.

Doran: What were his husband's views? It seems they had a good relationship, though Brad had little influence over Mr. Edwards's decisions. Is that right?

Warren: Yes, Brad tended to follow Mr. Edwards's lead rather than taking a position himself. Mr. Edwards's family agreed with him.

Patrick: His family agreed with him that he could eat solid food?

Warren: Yes.

Doran: Did his family understand that there was a good chance that eating solid food without a nurse's constant supervision could cause him to choke so badly that he'd become a vegetable?

Warren: Mr. Edwards's family accepted his position that this danger was exaggerated.

Doran: But they were mistaken?

Warren: Yes, they were mistaken.

Patrick: Why would his family accept his position, rather than the position of the medical professionals?

Warren: There was some history there of his brooking no opposition and having all the say in family matters.

Doran: Very sad. I assume the family realized they made a mistake. Is that true?

Warren: They realized the mistake too late.

Patrick: Did the family genuinely believe that the danger was exaggerated, or were they just afraid to speak up and tell Mr. Edwards what they really thought?

Warren: Mr. Edwards was always right. After a point in the family history, nobody disagreed with him because he could out-think them and browbeat them all. If they had opinions different from his, they did not reveal them.

Patrick: So the family might have thought he was mistaken, but felt that there was no point in trying to convince him of that?

Warren: Right.

Doran: In defence of the family, a psychiatrist found Mr. Edwards competent. Isn't that finding surprising though?

Warren: The psychiatrist saw Mr. Edwards at a good time for him and questioned him in ways that did not involve Nettles the cat. Before the examination, nobody talked to the psychiatrist about Mr. Edwards's odd behaviour, although it would have been noted in his chart. Perhaps the chart was not clear. For whatever reason, the psychiatrist did not take much notice of the apparent hallucinations.

Doran: Did the psychiatrist know the doctor's opinion that Mr. Edwards would likely choke again if he ate solid foods, like lamb chops, and that it could make him hypoxic, that Mr. Edwards insisted on eating the chops nevertheless, and that he denied that there was a serious risk of harming himself?

Warren: The psychiatrist did not talk to anyone before the examination. This particular psychiatrist thought that it was best to see a patient before getting prejudicial comment. In the hurly-burly of hospital life, there was no coordination or communication with the rest of the health care team, partly by accident and partly by the psychiatrist's design. However, he would have seen Mr. Edwards's chart, so he would have had some idea of Dr. Paladin's view of the matter.

Doran: Did anyone on Mr. Edwards's team meet with Brad and Mr. Edwards before he was released to explain the situation to them?

Warren: Before Mr. Edwards even tried to leave, Dr. Paladin had patiently explained the dangers of hypoxia to him, but Mr. Edwards was dismissive. Brad had been told about the dangers too, but did what Mr. Edwards told him to do, including smuggling in lamb chops.

Doran: Did the psychiatrist have Mr. Edwards sign an **AMA**?

Warren: No, but there is no doubt that Mr. Edwards was adequately warned and refused to listen. Charles even went to his home and thoroughly briefed him after he had been discharged from the hospital.

Patrick: Do you think that the psychiatrist would have reversed his decision that Mr. Edwards was competent if he had gotten to know him better?

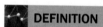

> **DEFINITION**
>
> **AMA** in this context stands for "against medical advice." Patients like Mr. Edwards who leave when their doctors tell them to stay in the hospital are asked to sign a form certifying that they know their physician wants them to stay. It gives legal certitude that the patient was warned against leaving.

Warren: Probably not. Psychiatrists are not usually willing to ask the courts to force involuntary treatment on patients. Dr. Paladin just thought they should have used the second evaluation to delay Mr. Edwards's departure. She wanted another chance for the staff to get through to Mr. Edwards about the dangers.

Doran: Okay. Patrick, do you have any more questions about the facts of the case?

Patrick: Not now, although more questions will probably arise once we start the debate.

MORAL ISSUES RAISED BY THE CASE

Doran: This case raises a number of ethical issues, but let's discuss the following proposition: It was a moral error for Mr. Edwards's health care team to allow him to discharge himself without further evaluation. They could not legally stop him, presumably, but they might have found practical ways to delay his departure.

Patrick: Good—this seems to be the main ethical issue raised by this case. So, what do you think?

Stating Our Positions

Doran: I agree with the proposition. It was a moral error for Mr. Edwards's health care team to allow him to discharge himself without first making a greater effort to protect him from harm.

Warren: You are saying that patient autonomy can be restricted even for a patient who has been certified as competent?

Doran: Yes.

Patrick: I also agree with the proposition. Although Mr. Edwards had been certified as competent, it seems the testing of his competence was incomplete. So it was not an accurate measure of his competence, right?

Doran: Right, that is what I was thinking, too.

Warren: Although I find this to be a very hard case, ultimately I disagree with the proposition. Imagine yourself having been certified as competent and having the staff tell you that's not good enough. They want a second opinion on whether you are competent. You would rightly feel that they want to keep trying until they can get you declared incompetent.

Patrick: Well, if I were in a situation relevantly similar to Mr. Edwards's, I probably wouldn't like the staff telling me that further evaluations were necessary. But that's not the appropriate question to ask. The question to ask is, Would you and I—or some other person whose competence is not in question—object now to future evaluations and restrictions on our liberty, if we were displaying symptoms similar to Mr. Edwards's? I suspect we wouldn't now object to future **paternalistic** interferences with our liberty if we were later to find ourselves in a situation like Mr. Edwards's.

> **DEFINITION**
>
> **Paternalism** is interference in the liberty of another for that person's good. There is an ongoing controversy about the extent to which paternalism may be morally justified. For a good brief overview, see the entry "Paternalism" in the *Stanford Encyclopedia of Philosophy*: http://plato.stanford.edu/entries/paternalism/.

Warren: Mr. Edwards's hallucinations were not clearly relevant to the determination of his competence to make medical decisions. Competence is context-relative. Mr. Edwards may not have been competent to judge the presence of Nettles, his cat, but he was competent to understand the risks he was running according to Dr. Paladin. He was competent to decide to dismiss those warnings. It was morally permissible for the staff to release him when they did.

Doran: I agree with Patrick that his health care team erred in releasing Mr. Edwards without further evaluation, but I would not agree that he should be kept indefinitely. If I were to be in his situation, I would not now agree to being kept in the hospital indefinitely, although I would agree to delaying my discharge for a short period of time to give caregivers a better opportunity to explain the situation to me, and to give me more of a chance to come to terms with my situation.

Patrick: Well, Doran and I have serious doubts about whether the hospital acted permissibly. So we affirm the proposition that *it was a moral error for his health care team to allow Mr. Edwards to discharge himself without further evaluation.* Warren, why don't you present your argument to see if you can convince us otherwise?

AN ARGUMENT FOR THE RIGHT TO IGNORE EXPERTS

Warren: The real issue here has to do with valid refusal of treatment by competent people. The right to have one's refusal of treatment respected is, in turn, dependent on the right to autonomy. In the **original position**, we would insist on a strong right to autonomy because without that, others would be able to limit us in ways they might think are in our interests. When others try to run our lives for us, they often make a bad job of it, despite good intentions. Our interests are best protected when we have the right to assert and protect those interests on our own. That is why one's competent, free refusal of treatment must be respected.

> **DEFINITION**
>
> **Autonomy** is derived from the Greek *autos* ("self") and *nomos* ("rule," "governance," or "law"). It has come to have many meanings, among them the capacity for, or the right to, self-government. We prefer to use *autonomy* to mean "self-determination." When the context is clear, though, we will also use *autonomy* to mean "the **right to self-determination**." For a good discussion of autonomy, see chapter 3 in Tom L. Beauchamp and James F. Childress, *Principles of Biomedical Ethics*, 5th ed. (New York: Oxford University Press, 2001), 57–112.

In this case, if Mr. Edwards knowingly chose not to respect the expertise of his doctor and nurses, and not to take precautions, he may still have given valid refusal of treatment. The idea that he was incompetent if he did not respect medical expertise or believe what experts told him is inimical to a basic right to autonomy. As a competent adult, he could have chosen what information he wished to accept or to consider. He could have also chosen what risks he wished to take, including the risk of ignorance. To deny this is to slip into a kind of paternalism that would not be tolerated by those in the original position.

> **BACKGROUND**
>
> Warren is relying on a version of **social contract theory**. See chapter 3 for an explanation of this approach.

Doran: That's an interesting argument. For purposes of evaluation, I would like to restate part of your argument in **standard form**:

(1) Actions are morally justified if they are consistent with the rules that would be chosen by people in the original position to form the ideal social contract.

(2) People in the original position would choose rules to protect their own interests in the real world.

(3)   In order to protect their own interests, people in the original position would choose rules that secure a strong right to autonomy as part of the social contract.

(4)   This strong right to autonomy entails that competent patients have a right to information about their condition, a right to accept or reject that information, and a right to refuse treatment with or without use of the information that is available.

> **TECHNIQUE**
>
> Part of Warren's argument is put in **standard form** (a numbered list). This helps with clarifying the argument and makes it easier to consider targeted objections to specific premises.

(5)   Mr. Edwards was a competent patient who was given access to information about his condition, but deliberately chose to ignore that information and to leave the hospital against the medical recommendations of his physician and nurses.

(6)   As a competent individual who refused information, Mr. Edwards was within his rights to leave the hospital against the medical recommendations of his physician and nurses.

(7)   If Mr. Edwards was within his rights to refuse treatment, then his health care team was morally required to respect this choice.

(8)   Therefore, his health care team did not err in releasing Mr. Edwards.

Is that what you intended to argue?

Warren: That is a good start. There's more to it that I hinted at, but let's see what you think of this bit.

Clarifying Premise (3)

Patrick: Let's start with the third premise. You claim that people in the original position will pick rules granting them a strong right to autonomy. What do you mean by a right to autonomy?

Warren: Autonomy is a complex notion. But the basic idea is that an **autonomous** person is self-determining: autonomous persons make their own choices, free of external controls or internal compulsions. To say that people in the original position will want to make sure that they have a strong *right* to autonomy (or a strong right to self-determination) is to say that they

> **BACKGROUND**
>
> A classic defence of individual liberty can be found in John Stuart Mill's *On Liberty,* chapter 4. Mill, too, thinks that the strongest argument against interfering with a competent person's liberty for his own good is that such interference is likely to be done poorly.

will pick rules that protect their right to make their own decisions and to lead their own lives—that is, they will want to ensure that others are not justified in controlling their self-regarding choices; they may also want to make sure that they have the social conditions necessary to make their own decisions.

Doran: I see why you think people in the original position would choose rules giving them a strong right to autonomy. But just how strong is this right?

Patrick: Good question. In the original position we would of course want to secure a right to autonomy, but presumably we wouldn't want the right to be so strong that we'd end up undermining others' autonomy, and presumably we would want to limit our autonomy so as to prevent serious harms to ourselves through foolish, uninformed, or irrational choices.

Warren: Since people in the original position are purely self-interested, they would not concern themselves directly with the autonomy of others. Nonetheless, they do not know who they are in the real world; therefore, people in the original position would want to limit everyone's right to autonomy in order to protect their own autonomy. On this point, I agree with John Rawls that people in the original position would choose what he calls the **liberty principle**.

> **DEFINITION**
>
> John Rawls's **liberty principle** states: "Each person is to have an equal right to the most extensive basic liberty compatible with a similar liberty for others" (*A Theory of Justice* [Cambridge, MA: Harvard University Press, 1971], 60.

A more difficult question concerns identifying the conditions, if any, under which people in the original position would agree to limit their right to autonomy for the sake of self-protection. For, on the one hand, people in the original position would certainly not want to be treated like children whenever experts think their choices are foolish. Yet, on the other hand, it also seems that people in the original position would want to protect themselves from their reckless, ill-conceived choices.

Patrick: Under what conditions, then, would people in the original position accept paternalistic interferences with their liberty?

Warren: I think that when interferences in one's liberty are relatively minor and when the benefits of interference are great, then paternalism would be accepted by people in the original position. Seat belt legislation is a case in point. Here the benefits of seat belt wearing are clear and substantial, while the interference in a person's liberty is relatively minor, so requiring seat belt use could be justified for paternalistic reasons.

Contrast this with interferences that are significant—say, total bans on tobacco use, or on gambling, or on backcountry skiing. Likewise, preventing people from acting AMA—against medical advice—would be too great an interference with liberty. Unlike the case of seat belt legislation, where there is at most minor frustration of preferences and minor interference with liberty, not allowing people to discharge themselves from the hospital when it is against medical advice would constitute a major interference with liberty, and would likely greatly frustrate the satisfaction of preferences.

Patrick: I still wonder, though, why simply warning people about the risks of not wearing seat belts is not enough on your view. Why wouldn't people in the original position just accept a rule that they be warned of harms to self, and then let competent people make their own decisions?

Warren: We would recognize, in the original position, our vulnerability to rash decision making. Seat belt legislation is an instance of insurance against such decisions. Not wearing a seat belt can be a moment of foolishness for no significant personal gain that leads to huge personal pain. Booking out AMA is different, and much more complex.

Patrick: All right, but given that acting AMA can also be foolish and lead to great personal pain, wouldn't it be justified to also take steps to protect patients from their own rash choices?

THEORY

Here Warren assumes that seat belt legislation could be justified on paternalistic grounds. Of course, other reasons could be given in defence of seat belt laws. For example, one could argue that such a law is justified on the basis of trying to reduce economic costs to society. Whether a piece of legislation is paternalistic or non-paternalistic depends on why it was passed. Legislation is often considered paternalistic only if it is justified at least partly on the ground that it prevents people from harming themselves.

 UP FOR DISCUSSION

How would you distinguish a minor interference in a person's liberty from a significant interference in a person's liberty? What do Warren's views on justified paternalism imply about total bans on cocaine or heroin use? Do you agree with these implications?

Warren: I agree that some limited steps would be agreed to by people in the original position to protect themselves from reckless decisions when it came to acting AMA. They would agree to testing for competence, and perhaps to brief delays to allow a person to change their mind. But they would accept only limited interference with their autonomy. The decision to act AMA is too important to a person to have it indefinitely interfered with by others. Ultimately, it must be up to the competent patient to determine what information to accept, believe, and act on.

Doran: I am beginning to get a clearer idea of your view of the right to self-determination as it relates to those who are competent, but what about incompetent individuals? I imagine that paternalism is more easily justified for those who are unable to competently decide for themselves.

Warren: I agree that with respect to those who are not competent to make their own decisions, such as young children, paternalism is easier to justify. The state, for instance, may be justified in requiring those who are not competent not only to wear seat belts, but also to refrain from tobacco and alcohol use, to receive an education, to undergo certain medical procedures, and so on. But, here too, there has to be clear evidence that the incursion on liberty is necessary to protect the important interests of those whose liberty is restricted.

> **BACKGROUND**
>
> Philosophers sometimes distinguish between different sorts of paternalism. For example, **hard paternalism** is the interference in a *competent* person's liberty for their own good. **Soft paternalism** is the interference in an *incompetent* person's liberty for their own good. It is generally recognized that the latter sort of paternalism is much easier to justify than the former. It should also be noted that different philosophers differ slightly on how they define these terms.

Doran: Okay, you have suggested two ways in which paternalism may be justified. With respect to competent individuals, liberty may be interfered with for paternalistic reasons only when there is very clear evidence that the interference will be greatly in the person's interest, and the interference is slight. Both conditions are necessary for the competent. With respect to incompetent individuals, such as young children, interference with a person's choices for that person's own good can be more extensive and will be easier to justify. Is that right?

Warren: Right.

Patrick: Although a lot more could be said about when paternalism is justified, perhaps we should now turn back to Mr. Edwards's case, and consider what your view implies about his case.

 UP FOR DISCUSSION

When, if ever, do you think hard paternalism is justified?

Assuming Mr. Edwards Was Competent, Did His Health Care Team Err in Releasing Him from the Hospital When They Did?

Patrick: Given that you think that Mr. Edwards's health care team did not err in releasing him from the hospital when they did, I assume you think that he was competent to make the decision to act AMA and that his decision to refuse care was valid. I have serious doubts about Mr. Edwards's competence and whether his refusal of care was valid. But let's set that aside for the time being. It seems to me that his health care team should have done more to protect Mr. Edwards from his reckless decision not to follow a soft diet, even if we assume he was competent to make that decision. I think it was pretty clearly a foregone conclusion that Mr. Edwards would not do well. Everyone knew that he would continue to eat meat, and everyone but him (and perhaps his husband) knew that this would kill or seriously harm him. Letting him discharge himself from the hospital when they did seems rather irresponsible to me.

Warren: Some staff thought Mr. Edwards would be killed or seriously harmed, but nobody knew. Patients surprise the experts often enough. The staff took the key steps to protect Mr. Edwards from his reckless decisions. They obtained a competence evaluation; they repeatedly warned him about what they took to be the dangers of his eating solid foods. In other words, they discharged their duty of

> **TECHNIQUE**
>
> It is common for philosophers to grant a claim *for the sake of argument*—that is, to accept a claim not because they think it is true, but because they want to focus on another aspect of the argument. In this case, Patrick is not agreeing that Mr. Edwards is competent; he is only assuming it for the sake of argument. For he wants to consider whether it was wrong for Mr. Edwards's health care team to discharge him from the hospital if he was competent. Later, Patrick and Doran will challenge Warren's premise that Mr. Edwards was competent to make his health care decisions.

protecting persons from harming themselves. Given this, it was up to Mr. Edwards to decide what he preferred and to act on what he took to be in his best interest.

Patrick: But surely there was undeniable evidence that restricting Mr. Edwards's liberty—in particular, forcing him to remain in the hospital—was in his best interest in this case. Being forced to stay in the hospital may have frustrated some of his preferences, but it may well have enhanced many of his other preferences and interests. For instance, if Mr. Edwards was kept in the hospital, this would have frustrated his strong preference to go home, but it would also have furthered his interest in living. And by giving him a longer life, it would also have furthered other preferences he has—such as the preference for taking risks. One can't do that when one is dead. So it's not clear to me that we would oppose limitations on our liberty if we were to find ourselves in a situation relevantly similar to Mr. Edwards's situation.

Warren: Medical expertise gives us good predictions about a patient's future, not undeniable evidence. I do not deny, however, that the evidence was strong that Mr. Edwards would suffer harm. To keep Mr. Edwards in the hospital any longer against his will would have constituted a great incursion on his liberty. And, as I argued, I believe that in the original position, people would not agree to great incursions on the liberty of competent persons for their own good. We would want to have our competence tested and to be duly warned by the experts of the risks we were taking, but we would ultimately want to preserve our right to self-determination.

Doran: I agree, Warren, that after due warning, competent people should have the right to self-determination; however, among other things, I question whether Mr.

Edwards was adequately warned. In the original position, I think people would agree to more consultations and psychological evaluations before allowing a person to take such great risks for so trivial a reason. If risks were less than life and death, then the warnings would have been sufficient, but when the stakes are so high, greater interferences with liberty are justified.

Warren: I think people in the original position are not going to want to surrender their autonomy unless absolutely necessary. They know that generally a person knows their own interests best. The warnings, delays, and competence evaluations were sufficient in Mr. Edwards's case. It was time to let him make his own decisions. Being allowed to continue his high-risk lifestyle and not being treated like an infant were far from trivial matters to him.

> ### THEORY
>
> An **act utilitarian** might consider the whole discussion wrong-headed. Any restriction on liberty would be automatically justified, in that view, if it maximized happiness. Very likely, in this instance, happiness would be greater for everyone affected if Mr. Edwards had been prevented from becoming hypoxic and, as a result, demented. However, it should be noted that in *On Liberty*, John Stuart Mill presents a complex utilitarian argument against any paternalistic interference in a competent person's voluntary choices. He argues that for several reasons, in the final analysis, competent people will be happier if left free to make their own voluntary decisions in matters that do not harm others.

Doran: So, to sum up: In your view, people in the original position would want to give themselves a strong right to autonomy in order to protect their interests. This strong right to autonomy entails a strong presumption in favour of competent individuals making their own decisions, provided they do not violate others' autonomy. This is why Mr. Edwards, if competent, would have the right to reject his doctor's and nurses' medical advice. The right is not absolute, however, since people in the original position would want to protect themselves from, for instance, their ill-considered rash decisions. Paternalistic restrictions are justified when the benefits are significant and the loss of liberty insignificant. And in situations where the loss of liberty is significant, warnings are still appropriate, but not prohibitions. Mr. Edwards had sufficient warning, though, and so the decision to follow or to reject the doctor's advice was now properly his to make.

Warren: Yes. In this case, Mr. Edwards's right to autonomy gave him the right to book out AMA, but staff members were right to delay and to try to dissuade him. They were also right to order a test of his competence. That done, they were right to let him go.

Patrick: Well, I think people in the original position would agree to greater restrictions on their liberties when the choice to be made is clearly so dangerous and so at odds with their overall preferences. These greater restrictions seem to be in people's interest in the original position. But let's move on. Thus far we have been granting for the sake of argument that Mr. Edwards was competent to make his health care decisions. I, however, think Mr. Edwards was probably not competent to make his health care decisions, and this again leads me to think that his health care team erred in the moral duty to protect him from harming himself.

 UP FOR DISCUSSION

Do you think that Mr. Edwards's health care team did enough to protect him from harming himself? Why or why not?

Doran: I agree with you, Patrick, that people in the original position would agree to greater restrictions on their liberties when the choice to be made is clearly so dangerous and so at odds with their overall preferences. And I also think Mr. Edwards was not competent to make his health care decisions. So why don't we hear Warren's defence of his premise (5), the premise that claims both that Mr. Edwards was competent to make his health care decisions and that he gave a valid refusal of care?

Patrick: Right, I have concerns about both of those. Let's start first with the issue of competence.

OBJECTIONS TO PREMISE (5)

Was Mr. Edwards Competent?

> **BACKGROUND**
>
> Premise (5) states: Mr. Edwards was a competent patient who was given access to information about his condition, but deliberately chose to ignore that information and to leave the hospital against the medical recommendations of his physician and nurses.
>
> Medical professionals assess the capacity of a patient for rational self-determination with respect to their future medical care. The courts call a person competent in a different sense: to be competent means to have the legal authority to make those decisions. We are interested in the notion of competence as capacity rather than as authority.

Warren: Okay, but let me first clarify what I mean when I say that Mr. Edwards was competent. To say that someone is competent is to say that they have certain capacities or abilities. Individuals may be competent relative to some tasks, but not others. For instance, someone may be competent to drive a car, but not competent to fly a plane. When I say that Mr. Edwards was competent, I'm saying that he was competent to make decisions about his health care. He may, however, have been incompetent in other areas, but these are not directly relevant to our present concerns.

Patrick: That sounds right. Competence is a relation: people are competent relative to certain activities. But I have serious doubts about whether Mr. Edwards was competent to make important decisions about his health care. My doubts stem in part from the fact that he wanted to live, but at the same time insisted on eating solid food rather than a soft diet. If the medical professionals were right, these preferences were blatantly inconsistent. If Mr. Edwards ate solid food, it was quite likely that he'd choke and either die or suffer serious brain damage. So I have concerns about whether Mr. Edwards had the capacity to understand his situation and to decide what to do about it. If he was not competent in this context, then the right to autonomy would not entail that Mr. Edwards had a right to refuse treatment.

Warren: I agree that if Mr. Edwards was not competent to refuse treatment, then his health care team should not have accepted his refusal of treatment, but let's look carefully at what makes you doubt his competence in this respect. It is that he had blatantly inconsistent goals, and this shows that he did not adequately understand the nature of his condition and the consequences of his actions. I disagree, however, that his goals were blatantly inconsistent *to him*. They may have appeared so to the doctor and to others. He just didn't accept expert medical advice. Mr. Edwards chose not to believe the experts, but surely that does not entail that he was incompetent.

Doran: I agree that *to him* these goals were not blatantly inconsistent, but the doctor was obviously right that his goals were, *in fact*, blatantly inconsistent.

Patrick: Right. His goals were not inconsistent *to him*. But that's just the problem—he *should have* recognized that his goals were actually inconsistent. The mere fact that Mr. Edwards chose not to believe his doctors does not, of course, show that he was incompetent. The problem is that he did not see what everyone else saw: that he could not eat solid food *and* avoid serious harm. It is not as if, for instance, the experts disagreed about the consequences of his eating solid food. His belief that he could eat solid food, despite his condition, seemed entirely baseless—it flew in the face of all available evidence.

Warren: That is only so with hindsight. At the time, the nature of his condition was not obvious. Physicians sometimes disagree about a diagnosis of MS or dysphagia. A layperson cannot be expected to just see that the diagnosis is correct.

Doran: I think you miss the point. It's not about a diagnosis of MS. It's about the danger of choking on solid food. Surely any reasonable person would accept what the medical professionals say in this case, especially given that Mr. Edwards had recently choked and recently failed a motility test. It was his refusal to accept what should've been obvious to any reasonable person that shows that he was in denial and not competent to refuse treatment. He *denied* that he was likely to choke if he ate solid foods, he *denied* that medical expertise was needed if he did choke, and he even *denied* that he had MS or that he was ill at all.

Patrick: Well put, Doran. The concern about his competence stems from his denial of facts that any reasonable person would see as obvious. He refused to admit that he was ill or that choking was a probable and very serious threat to his health, and his denial of these things, given the available medical evidence, was baseless and therefore irrational.

Warren: Yes, Mr. Edwards had choked once in the past. Most of us have done that sort of thing. But that is not enough to convince a reasonable person that the medical professionals were right about a diagnosis of dysphagia. Make no mistake about it, this is a complex medical diagnosis, not something any reasonable layperson must understand. So it comes down to this: must any reasonable person accept what medical professionals say when the evidence is not clear to that person? I say, no.

 UP FOR DISCUSSION

Do you think Mr. Edwards was competent to make his own health care decisions? Why or why not?

The Gangrenous Foot Example

Doran: Let me give you an actual case on which we can probably agree about incompetence to refuse treatment, so we can compare that to Mr. Edwards's case. A homeless woman was taken to the hospital with a horrible infection in her foot, caused by frostbite. The foot had turned gangrenous. It needed to be amputated or she would die. The woman refused to admit it was gangrenous, however, and said she wanted to live and wanted to keep her foot. The doctors showed her the foot, but she never wanted to look, and when she did, she said it was just dirt, or that it was getting better, when plainly it was getting worse.

She was insensitive to clear and overwhelming evidence, and this led her to state two goals that were in blatant conflict (even though she did not realize this): "I want to live" and "I want to keep my foot."[1] Now, I agree that a competent person could say, "I would prefer to die rather than have my foot amputated, so I reject the medical advice." But this is different. Do you think this homeless woman was competent or incompetent?

Patrick: I think she was quite clearly incompetent.

Warren: I admit that, in this case, we have clear incompetence to refuse treatment. Once you see your foot washed and then try to pretend that the discoloration is from dirt, you really are in denial. Mr. Edwards's denial was different. It was a denial of a complex medical diagnosis of dysphagia on evidence that he did not see and understand. Mr. Edwards, moreover, had a successful career built partly on strong skepticism about expertise of others and on a damn-the-torpedoes attitude to danger. That was his preference as well, to live on the edge. He thought the doctors were exaggerating their own importance and the dangers. His life experience gave him some evidence for this being so. He competently made a choice that was mistaken.

Denying the probability of his choking in the future is a matter of denying an expert prognosis, not a denial of facts obvious to any reasonable person. As for his saying he wasn't ill, that was a denial of the obvious, but perhaps exaggeration rather than incompetence. Patients often say, "I'm fine," when this is pure hyperbole.

I think we agree on the principle that denying facts that any reasonable person should see is a sign of incompetence; however, I do not take his denials as indicating that he was incompetent in this way. He was refusing expert medical advice, but if we are compelled to accept the views of experts, our autonomy would be very severely restricted. We could never refuse treatment. In this case, it was about a diagnosis of dysphagia and the prognosis, the medical expert's claim that Mr. Edwards was in heightened danger of choking in future. This was not something that a reasonable person would have to accept as true.

 UP FOR DISCUSSION

Do you think Mr. Edwards's denial of the risk of choking is a case that falls under the principle of denying facts that any reasonable person should see?

Incompetence to Refuse Medical Care: Skepticism without Reason

Patrick: It's not just what Mr. Edwards believed, but *why* he believed it, that makes me doubt his competence. I agree with you that rejecting the advice of experts is not necessarily a sign of incompetence. But this is a case where his doctor and nurses seemed to agree on the dangers of eating solid food, given his condition. And, as far as I can see, Mr. Edwards had no good reason at all to doubt what the medical experts were telling him. If Mr. Edwards was competent to make decisions about the treatment of his condition, he must have been capable of giving reasons in support of his decisions.

Warren: I agree that doubt without reason is irrational and a sign of incompetence. That kind of baseless skepticism could make a person incompetent to refuse treatment. Strong skepticism and a strong preference for taking risks, however, had served Mr. Edwards very well throughout his life, as we know from Charles Nolet's descriptions. He had a successful life and business because he took great risks, believed in himself, and ignored experts. That success was his evidence. He used to ride a motorcycle without a helmet to feel the wind in his hair. He was an outlier, not an incompetent. The same can be said of star snowboarders. What is irrational given your preferences was rational given his.

Patrick: To be clear, I'm not at all suggesting that a willingness to take risks is a sign of incompetence, so I'm not arguing that athletes who take extreme risks in pursuit of their sport are incompetent. My point with respect to Mr. Edwards is that this wasn't a situation in which Mr. Edwards recognized the risks of eating solid food but chose to eat solid food anyway because he had a preference for risky behaviour. If that were the case, I might agree that Mr. Edwards was competent. In this case, however, he *denied* the risks, despite everyone's telling him that eating solid food was likely to seriously harm or kill him, and his denial was without good reason. Mr. Edwards is like the inexperienced adventurer who denies that climbing Mount Everest is risky, simply because his ignoring of experts has served him well.

Warren: Are you incompetent if you don't agree with experts for no reason except that skepticism about expertise has served you well through your life? We let people choose prayer over chemotherapy, for instance. We don't call them incompetent, although we may think they are stubborn and mistaken.

Patrick: Well, I may have doubts about the competence of people who would choose prayer over chemotherapy. But, setting that issue aside, it seems to me that there's an important difference between people who choose prayer over chemotherapy and Mr. Edwards's denial of obvious facts and refusal of treatment. The choice of prayer over chemotherapy makes sense, perhaps, given other beliefs such people have—for example, the belief in God and God's power to heal. I think these beliefs are mistaken, but they are beliefs reasonable people hold. And given these beliefs, the choice of prayer can, I suppose, make sense. Similarly, a person's preference for alternative treatments over conventional therapies isn't a sign of incompetence if that person has a reasonable network of beliefs supporting their choice. Mr. Edwards's case seems different, however. There's no background set of reasonable beliefs from which his denial of what all the experts are telling him makes sense.

 UP FOR DISCUSSION

Imagine an inexperienced mountain climber whose skepticism in business and in other matters has served him well. He now wants to climb Mount Everest, but is told by very experienced mountaineers that this is extremely risky and could result in his death. He is skeptical of the risks, however, since his ignoring of experts has served him well in life. Is this individual competent to decide whether he should climb Everest? What implications does your answer have for the case of Mr. Edwards?

Warren: The two cases aren't different. Mr. Edwards's choice to reject the expert assessment of two nurses and one physician made sense in his world view, just as the religious person's choice to reject expertise makes sense in their world view. As I have explained already, Mr. Edwards built a successful business, in part, by being domineering, independent, eccentric, and skeptical of expert claims. His rejection of expert medical advice was part and parcel of the skepticism that had guided him well much of his life. Indeed, Mr. Edwards's refusal was more rational than that of the religious believer. Mr. Edwards had experience of the success of his views in this life—not in some promised, not evidenced, afterlife.

Patrick: Okay. Perhaps, then, his skepticism was not entirely baseless, given his background beliefs and experiences. But I'm not sure his "world view" is one that a reasonable person could hold, so I still have doubts about his competence.

Doran: Interesting. But even if his world view was unreasonable, Patrick, perhaps we can still judge him to be competent, provided that he was reasoning well from that perspective?

Warren: That's right. We don't want to say that he was incompetent just because he has a set of beliefs that others regard as unreasonable. He was capable of understanding his situation. And he was capable of making health care decisions that were reasonable from his point of view. Surely, then, he was competent.

 UP FOR DISCUSSION

Do you think that Mr. Edwards's skepticism regarding the expert medical opinion that he was at great risk of death from choking is more analogous to holding a controversial world view or to holding an unreasonable view such as that one is made out of glass? Can one be incompetent because one holds unreasonable world views? Consider, for example, the case of Mr. Faithwards, who is like Mr. Edwards except that the reason he gives for refusing medical care is not life experience but his religious food rules. He denies the risk because he thinks God will save a God-fearing man. Is he competent to refuse care? If we say such a person is incompetent because of his strange views, can we deny that others are incompetent because of their unusual religious views—for instance, the view that medicines are unnecessary since God's will alone decides who will live and who will die?

Competence and Psychiatric Evaluation

Warren: Here is one additional reason why one ought to think Mr. Edwards was competent. He received a psychiatric evaluation and was found to be competent. Surely, if one believes in a strong right to autonomy, one is going to want to let people exercise that autonomy if they have been found to be competent by a psychiatrist.

Doran: Yes, it seems that a finding of competence by a psychiatrist should count as a reason in favour of thinking that a patient really is competent. But that presupposes that the evaluation was adequate. And there is reason to doubt the adequacy of the psychiatrist's evaluation of Mr. Edwards.

Patrick: I agree, Doran.

Warren: Why would you question the adequacy of Mr. Edwards's evaluation?

Doran: The psychiatrist, apparently, did not take into account all the relevant facts about Mr. Edwards's case. This is why, I suspect, Dr. Paladin believed that staff failed to adequately protect Mr. Edwards when he was allowed to leave the hospital without further delay. Presumably the psychiatrist had access to Mr. Edwards's chart, and this would have included his medical history and diagnosis, but presumably it did not include clear enough information about his hallucinations about Nettles the cat, nor enough details about his denial of his condition. Either that, or he failed to take account of these things. Given these problems in the evaluation, I think that the psychiatrist's findings were not, by themselves, a strong reason to believe Mr. Edwards was competent.

Moreover, even if the psychiatric evaluation was done adequately, it would be a mistake to count the psychiatrist's finding of competence as conclusive. For, as we know, psychiatrists can err in such judgments; moreover, different psychiatrists can reach conflicting conclusions about a patient's competence. So, I would say that the psychiatrist's declaration of competence in Mr. Edwards's case was not enough to conclusively prove that he was indeed competent.

Patrick: Again, I agree with you, Doran. The psychiatric evaluation gives us *one* reason for thinking that Mr. Edwards was competent. But the evaluation was incomplete, as just noted, and the psychiatrist's assessment of Mr. Edwards was at odds with Dr. Paladin's doubts about Mr. Edwards. Dr. Paladin, it seems, thought that Mr. Edwards was *not* competent, and as his physician, she presumably had a broader and deeper understanding of Mr. Edwards's physical and mental condition.

Warren: I agree that a psychiatric evaluation, even when adequately performed, is not decisive proof of competence. But few judgments in medicine are decisive. They just have to be sufficiently decisive, like this psychiatric evaluation. I believe, however, that an adequate evaluation finding that a patient is competent to make health care decisions needs to be treated with a great deal of respect. In the original position, we would want to be allowed to exercise our strong right to autonomy if we were found competent, and we would not want to be under continual examination in the real world just because somebody disagreed with the earlier examinations.

Psychiatric evaluation is the best way we currently have of determining whether the patient can competently choose. So, I believe that, given a psychiatric evaluation that shows the patient is capable of deciding freely to accept and understand information or not accept it, the patient counts as competent to reject medical treatment.

If one adequate psychiatric evaluation determines that the patient is competent in this sense, then that is all the proof the health care team should seek. Patients should not be under **double jeopardy** when it comes to evaluation of their competence.

Patrick: But given the psychiatrist's lack of relevant information, he arguably wasn't in a position to decide whether Mr. Edwards was capable of these things.

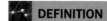

DEFINITION

Double jeopardy is the name of a legal rule that prohibits being tried twice for the same crime on the same set of facts. Here, Warren is applying the term to health care, and saying that a patient should not be required to prove their competence twice.

Doran: That's right. If the psychiatric evaluation is a key reason for thinking that Mr. Edwards was competent, then one had better be confident that the psychiatric evaluation was well done. But for the reasons I mentioned previously, I do not have this confidence.

Moreover, I think people in the original position will want to ensure that they really are competent when they are deciding to reject or accept medical treatment. They would thus want there to be an adequate, thorough evaluation. Given the questions about the adequacy of Mr. Edwards's evaluation, I therefore do not think people in the original position would object to a second, more thorough evaluation.

Patrick: Right. I think that in the original position, people would accept a rule that required further testing and restrictions on liberty, if necessary, in situations like the ones under discussion. The psychiatrist said Mr. Edwards was competent. His physician—who had much more interaction with him—thought otherwise. Surely people in the original position would want further testing to ensure competence in such situations.

Warren: How many evaluations must one have before one is deemed competent to refuse treatment? Dr. Paladin would never have been satisfied. Nurse Charles Nolet, on the other hand, already was satisfied about Mr. Edwards's competence. He cared deeply about his friend and knew him

THEORY

It is very important from the point of view of the ethics of care that there was this strong, caring relationship between the nurse, Charles Nolet, and the patient, Mr. Edwards. Charles displayed the primary virtue of care in his relationship with Mr. Edwards.

The very closeness of the two is a problem from other perspectives. Some might worry that Charles would not be impartial enough to treat all his patients with the same degree of care. Partiality might also blind him to things that an impartial observer would recognize in Mr. Edwards.

very well, much better than Dr. Paladin. Charles's opinion of Mr. Edwards's competence and preferences weighs more heavily with me for that reason. Charles was convinced that Mr. Edwards was competent to refuse both expertise and treatment, and Charles knew that Mr. Edwards was running a risk by not listening to medical advice and ran that risk with relish.

Doran: But how confident can one be, given that this is a "hard case"? And part of the concern is that the psychiatrist may not have known about Mr. Edwards's hallucinations. So, there seems to be a big difference between the case where his entire team agrees that he is putting himself in grave danger by eating solid foods, and this one psychiatrist who may have had an incomplete picture of Mr. Edwards's condition. But if a second careful psychiatric evaluation also agreed that Mr. Edwards was competent, then I would agree with you.

Warren: I admit that Mr. Edwards was on the cusp. That is what drives us to clarify our views about competence and autonomy. Perhaps the evaluation could have gone either way in a case like this. What we find by this debate, however, is that competence cannot be measured by the patient's willingness to accept a doctor's diagnosis or prognosis. If we always treat unwillingness as being in denial, we end the possibility of competent refusal of treatment.

Doran: I agree with that.

Patrick: I agree, too. We shouldn't *always* treat unwillingness as being in denial, and hence a sign of incompetence. But sometimes unwillingness does show incompetence, and I believe this is one of those times, for the reasons given.

Warren: Well, perhaps that is a good stopping point. We seem to agree in theory, but not in the application to this particular case. I agree with you two that there are serious concerns about Mr. Edwards's competence, but we draw the line in different places.

▨ UP FOR DISCUSSION

Warren argues for two points above: (1) an additional reason to think Mr. Edwards was competent to make his own health care decisions was that he received a psychiatric evaluation, and was found to be competent; and (2) if one believes in a strong right to autonomy, one is going to want to let people exercise that right if they have been found to be competent by a psychiatrist.

Discuss these two points as they relate to Mr. Edwards's case. Do you think that the fact that Mr. Edwards was deemed competent by the hospital psychiatrist is a strong reason to think that he was, in fact, competent to make the decision to leave the hospital?

Doran: Agreed. You make a lot of good points about competence.

Patrick: Let's move on now to consider a further issue. Besides the question of whether Mr. Edwards was competent, there is the question of whether his refusal of care was **valid**. For even if you managed to convince me that he was competent, I worry that his refusal of treatment was not valid, since he was not adequately informed.

Did Mr. Edwards Give a Valid Refusal?

Warren: I believe that his refusal was valid.

Patrick: Well, it is generally agreed that a patient's consent or refusal is valid only if it is informed. And a patient's consent or refusal counts as informed only if the patient is given relevant information and understands that information. The patient may accept or reject the information provided. But in cases where the rejection is based on obviously false beliefs, as it appears to have been in Mr. Edwards's case, it's hard to see how we can regard his refusal as *informed*.

Warren: It's still valid—ignorant consent and refusal may well be valid.[2] For instance, suppose a patient says to a physician, "I don't understand the treatment you have explained, but I trust you. Go ahead." Deliberate ignorance does not render the patient's acceptance of treatment invalid. The flip side is that if a patient says, "I don't trust you, so I don't wish any further information or treatment," deliberate ignorance should not render the patient's refusal invalid.

Doran: Well, I must say that your proposal seems right to me, but that it is an adventurous view. The literature on this subject emphasizes the need for freely informed consent to accept or reject treatment.[3] The idea seems to be that one's acceptance or refusal of medical treatment is not valid if one does not understand what various treatments are available, what the major risks are, and so on.

Warren: Yes, I realize that I am in a distinct minority here, but I think the majority is wrong. It seems to me to be false that a person must understand the relevant facts about their situation in order to make a valid choice, for a competent person might reasonably prefer not to know the facts. Let me be clear, though, that I believe the patient should be given access to the relevant medical information in an understandable form. The patient is not, however, required to accept or understand the information to give valid acceptance or refusal of treatment.

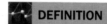

DEFINITION

The term *valid* has different meanings when we speak of valid arguments and valid consent. To say that a patient's decision to consent to or to refuse medical care is valid is to say that it is a legitimate reflection of the patient's free choice. What is necessary for consent or refusal to be valid is, of course, a matter of much debate.

THEORY

Because Patrick is using a common criterion for the validity of either acceptance or refusal of treatment—that it be informed—Warren's position is unorthodox and the onus is on him to provide strong reasons for rejecting the criterion.

Patrick: So you deny that consents and refusals must be informed to be valid?

Warren: If being informed means retaining explanations, understanding, and accepting the relevant facts, then, yes, I'm denying that valid consents and refusals must be informed. In my view, none of these things is necessary for a valid consent or refusal.

Patrick: None of these is required for valid consent or valid refusal? That seems mistaken. While I don't think it's necessary that a patient agree with their doctors and accept their advice and recommendations, it does seem plausible that valid consents and refusals must be informed at least in the sense that the patient has been provided with the relevant information about their condition and understands this information.

Warren: The patient must have access to the relevant information in an understandable form. If, however, Dr. Paladin gave Mr. Edwards a good pamphlet on dysphagia, Mr. Edwards would not have to keep it or even read it. In my view, if the patient is capable of deciding freely to accept or reject information and is capable of understanding that information as well as capable of seeing obvious facts that any reasonable person would accept, the patient's rejection or acceptance of medical treatment counts as valid. In Mr. Edwards's case, I believe that he had adequate access to information, but he did not accept it, try to understand it, or believe it. His decision was deliberately ignorant of the basis of the diagnosis and prognosis before he checked out of the hospital. He freely and deliberately chose not to follow medical expertise.

Doran: That's a plausible outline of a view of valid consent (and valid refusal). If the purpose of obtaining patient consent is to make sure that the patient's right to self-determination (that is, autonomy) is respected, and if the patient freely says, "I don't want to know the details," then respect for autonomy might reasonably require not making the patient know the details. Given this, I guess I would like to clarify what is needed to be "capable of deciding freely to accept or reject information," and to be "capable of understanding that information."

> **TECHNIQUE**
>
> It is generally a good idea to seek clarification of a view before considering its truth or falsity.

Patrick: I'm not sure it sounds plausible to me. But I'll reserve final judgment until Warren clarifies his view.

Warren: Okay, so there are two main points that require clarification. The first is what I mean when I speak of being capable of deciding freely to accept or reject information. The second is what is meant by being capable of understanding that information as well as being capable of seeing obvious facts that any reasonable person would accept.

Let's take the first point and look at what we normally expect in a competent adult's free decisions to see if that helps to clarify things. Part of what it is for people to decide freely is that we think their decisions flow from themselves, not from someone or something else like a hypnotist or a brain disease. We think that those decisions reflect their preferences and that those preferences are not themselves induced in some way incompatible with that person's ownership of them. There are, of course, some deep questions about free will that are not answerable here, but I am looking for something more on the surface of our thinking about deciding freely.

Doran: Okay, although it is somewhat vague, I am prepared to grant your claim about what is involved in deciding freely to accept or reject information. But what about your idea that patients must be capable of understanding information to give valid consent or refusal? Is the idea that patients are capable of understanding their alternatives, understanding their preferences, and judging in a reasonable way that a certain alternative will best promote their preferences?

Warren: At some level I would accept that, but, as I have explained, it might be at the level of choosing which kind of expertise, if any, to accept rather than understanding the alternatives as the experts describe them.

Doran: So, in your view, a competent person's consent or refusal is valid if she can freely choose some alternative based on her preferences, and where she makes this choice in light of her understanding of her situation and the alternatives. This may include accepting the physicians' and nurses' view of her situation, or it may include accepting her own view of the situation, provided that it is not a view that any reasonable person could see as false. Is that it?

Warren: Yes.

Patrick: But there's more to the view you proposed, Warren. The choice to refuse treatment can be valid even if the patient refuses to hear what the medical experts have to say about her condition. That is, she can choose to be ignorant about medical opinion, and still her refusal of treatment can be valid.

Warren: Yes, that's my view: uninformed consent or refusal may be valid. Suppose you say to your doctor, "I am in pain. I don't want to hear all about my condition right now. I trust you. You've never steered me wrong. Go ahead with the operation." That would surely be valid consent. Similarly, refusal can be valid without the patient's accepting information as long as the information is available. As long as one is competent and freely chooses to ignore information, one may accept or refuse treatment validly.

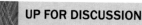 **UP FOR DISCUSSION**

Warren says that it "would surely be valid consent" if a patient says to her doctor, "I am in pain. I don't want to hear all about my condition right now. I trust you. You've never steered me wrong. Go ahead with the operation." Do you agree? Why or why not?

Doran: I think I agree with that—but, of course, we disagree on whether Mr. Edwards satisfied this principle, because we disagree on whether he was competent.

Patrick: I'm not sure I agree. Warren suggests that a valid consent or refusal requires the *capacity* to make free choices, and the capacity to understand the relevant information. I'm sure that in some sense Mr. Edwards had the capacity to understand and appreciate what the experts told him about his condition and the dangers of eating solid food. But, in fact, he did *not* understand this: his arrogance, stubbornness, and foolishness prevented him from seeing the facts as everyone else saw them. For a refusal to count as valid, one needs more than the capacity to understand relevant information; it seems one needs an actual understanding of the information. How can my consent be valid if I don't even know what I'm consenting to?

Warren: You could be saying, "I trust you. Go ahead with the operation." What one needs to give valid consent is the ability to freely decide whether or not one wants to know the relevant information. As my example of consent based on trust illustrates, it can be quite reasonable for a competent person not to want to know the details of their treatment options, especially if such knowledge will only do that person harm. Mr. Edwards freely decided not to believe the experts' advice, yet his refusal was valid.

Doran: Well, Warren, your view definitely challenges the prevailing view that valid consents and refusals must be informed, and you present a compelling case for your position. There are still lots of unanswered questions, but time is short, so why don't we move on now?

Warren: Sure.

> **BACKGROUND**
>
> "Some commentators have attempted to define *informed consent* by specifying the elements of the concept, in particular by dividing the elements into an *information* component and a *consent* component. The information component refers to disclosure of information and comprehension of what is disclosed. The consent component refers to both a voluntary decision and an authorization to proceed. Legal, regulatory, philosophical, medical, and psychological literatures tend to favor the following elements as the components of informed consent: (1) competence, (2) disclosure, (3) understanding, (4) voluntariness, and (5) consent."
>
> *Source:* Tom L. Beauchamp and James F. Childress, *Principles of Medical Ethics,* 5th ed. (New York: Oxford University Press, 2001), 79.

 UP FOR DISCUSSION

Must consent be fully informed to be valid? If not, to what degree, if any, must it be informed?

Patrick: Why don't we turn to an examination of premise (7) in your argument, Warren, which states: If Mr. Edwards was within his rights to refuse treatment, then his health care team was morally required to respect this choice. I have some doubts about this premise.

Warren: Let's hear your objection.

OBJECTIONS TO PREMISE (7)

Virtue May Overpower the Right to Refuse

Patrick: Even if you can satisfy me that Mr. Edwards was competent and adequately informed, I may part company with your premise (7). For even if Mr. Edwards had the right to refuse treatment, it does not follow that his health care team was morally required to respect that decision. The right to refuse treatment is not absolute. In cases where exercising this right is likely to defeat a patient's chosen health care goals, it seems his health care team may be justified in restricting a patient's liberty. Mr. Edwards presumably wanted to continue living. But because he was stubborn, foolish, reckless, and arrogant, he rejected the advice of his doctors and nurses and, as a result, was likely to die if he was dismissed. If Mr. Edwards did not want to die, and his actions were very likely to kill him because they were based on mistaken beliefs, then perhaps the responsible and beneficent thing to do was to force him to stay in the hospital. So Mr. Edwards may have had a right to refuse treatment, but respecting this right may not have been the virtuous thing to do, all things considered. Beneficence can sometimes outweigh autonomy.

Warren: That is a very interesting objection. You say even if the patient is competent and has a clear right, by way of autonomy, to refuse treatment, we might still be morally required to

> **BACKGROUND**
>
> The questions of competence, valid refusal of care, and whether the right to self-determination should win out over protecting the patient from harm and premature death are poignantly raised in the story of Donald (Dax) Cowart. Dax's case was made into two documentaries. These documentaries tell the story of a man who suffered third-degree burns to 68 percent of his body. Dax's recovery required that he submit to excruciatingly painful baths and treatments. Dax refused to consent to these treatments, yet they were performed against his will. He was held against his will for 14 months. Eventually, Dax was able to leave the hospital and go on with his life. Although he now says that he is happy, he still insists that his wishes should have been respected and that he should have been allowed to die.

force treatment on that patient. The reason is that it would be virtuous to do so in cases like Mr. Edwards's. According to my theory, of course, if the patient has a right that is not outweighed by other rights or duties, then we must accept his refusal. A right to refuse that can be ignored seems a poor right. Let me, however, try to meet you on your territory, virtue theory, as you have often met me in my theoretical realm.

Accepting, for the sake of argument, what I take to be your view, that virtues may outweigh rights, I would have to question the responsibility and charity you see here. It is irresponsible to treat a patient as incompetent when that patient is known to be competent. This undermines not only the dignity of that patient but can lead to paternalism becoming entrenched to everyone's detriment. It is, by the same token, not charitable. We know that Mr. Edwards would have been outraged to be treated in this way and had already found ways around the soft diet restriction. It does not appear that attempting to force treatment would do any good. The only alternative the staff had was pursued thoroughly when Charles did his best to educate Mr. Edwards at home after his release. That was charitable, but applying force that was both impractical and an outrage to the patient's dignity would not, all things considered, have been virtuous.

Patrick: Those are good points, and I recognize that there is much room for argument here as to what was the virtuous thing to do. But I'm not convinced that you've got things right. You suggest, for instance, that it is irresponsible to treat a patient as incompetent when that patient is known to be competent. Given this, it's not clear to me why you see seat belt laws, or virtually any other paternalistic interference with our liberty, as justified. Aren't these also irresponsible, since they involve treating competent people as if they were incompetent?

It seems to me that it is irresponsible *not* to restrict our liberty in cases where our freely chosen acts are based on clearly false beliefs and the acts are likely to undermine very important goals we have—like the goal to continue living!

> ### THEORY
>
> Recall that paternalism is interference in the liberty of another person for that person's good. Patrick is here arguing for what is often called **weak paternalism**. This is the view that interference with liberty is justified in order to prevent people from behaving in ways that are likely to defeat their goals. By contrast, **strong paternalism** is the view that we may legitimately prevent a person from attempting to realize irrational or mistaken goals. See Gerald Dworkin's entry "Paternalism" in the *Stanford Encyclopedia of Philosophy*, http://plato.stanford.edu/entries/paternalism/.

Warren: Beliefs that are clearly false to Dr. Paladin may not be clearly false to any reasonable person, so we cannot respect the dignity of Mr. Edwards if we require him to accept Dr. Paladin's views because Dr. Paladin is an expert. Further, seat belt legislation and the like are different from forcing health care on someone. The latter is a much more important interference and so is not the kind of thing that should be forced on a competent person, but the former interference is so trivial, and the benefits so huge, that it is more easily justified on grounds of virtue. Kindness and caring for others, for instance, require that we ignore trivial liberties to prevent massive suffering that obviously results.

Patrick: Well, I suppose that what I'm suggesting is that significant interference may be justified in cases where a person's actions are likely to undermine that person's freely chosen significant goals. If, for instance, people prefer to avoid injury, it may be legitimate to force people to wear seat belts. Similarly, if patients have a strong preference to continue living, then it may be permissible to prevent them from leaving the hospital if we are quite certain they'll engage in behaviours that are likely to kill them. Notice that I am not arguing that it *is* permissible to prevent them from leaving the hospital, only that it may be. These are tough cases. My point is that it's just not obvious to me that respect for personal autonomy ought to prevail over beneficence and other values in these cases.

> **THEORY**
>
> Notice the opportunity to use care ethics in this situation. The caring thing to do might well differ from the requirements laid down by rights theories.

Doubt Justifies Delay

Doran: Here for me is the concern. As you know, I have serious doubts about whether Mr. Edwards was competent to make his decision to refuse treatment. This is especially so in Scene 4, after his choking incident in the hospital. He seemed very confused about where he was, and what he was saying—though I agree his was a hard, borderline case. Given that it was a borderline case of competence, it seems to me that we should consider whether his health care team did all it ought to in order to enable Mr. Edwards to make the right choice for himself.

For instance, I notice that there were a couple of patient-care conferences to discuss Mr. Edwards's situation. This is good, but I think it would have been better if these conferences had been more inclusive, and had brought together Mr. Edwards and his husband, as well as a mental health professional, to discuss with everyone what was important to Mr. Edwards, as well as the medical history, the doctor's diagnosis, the risks of releasing him, the importance of getting a home nurse if he were to decide to leave the hospital, and so on. A more inclusive group effort would have been best. I am not necessarily claiming that Mr. Edwards ought to have been forced to stay in the hospital on a soft diet, but I am suggesting that it would have been better for his health care team to have taken a different approach toward Mr. Edwards. A more caring approach toward Mr. Edwards ought to have been followed. I believe such an approach would have had a better chance of respecting Mr. Edwards's choices while protecting him from the gravest risks.

Warren: Brad, his husband, seemed to be totally under Mr. Edwards's influence, so he would not have tried to dissuade him. Mr. Edwards might have been included in such a conference, but enough was done in the actual event whether or not there was such a conference. His health care team got a psychiatric evaluation. The balance between protection of the vulnerable and respect for autonomy was achieved. As Charles noted, Mr. Edwards was not to be persuaded.

Doran: Yes, I am not saying the hospital staff members were grossly negligent, or that they did nothing. But it is pretty clear from the get-go that Eva and Dr. Paladin had grave concerns about Mr. Edwards's competence, and about the risks he was willing to take for the sake of a lamb chop. At the end, after Mr. Edwards chokes and becomes hypoxic, Dr. Paladin thinks that they ought to have done more. I am trying to think about what that "more" ought to have been. I am suggesting that more efforts should have been made to talk with him and with his family about their concerns. Doing so may not have worked, but it should have been tried. They should also perhaps have gotten him to sign an AMA. Perhaps these extra meetings or conversations would have persuaded Mr. Edwards's husband, Brad, if not Mr. Edwards, to hire a home nurse.

Warren: Brad was not about to oppose Mr. Edwards. One could always do more for almost any patient, but the team has to balance that against neglect of other patients who are willing to be helped. As for signatures, that is a legal issue rather than a moral one. The staff members working with Mr. Edwards all knew his mind plainly enough. To be treated as a child would be horrific for someone of his temperament. He did not become hypoxic for the sake of a lamb chop but for the sake of his independence and personal dignity. It is doubtful that any different outcome could have been achieved with additional efforts.

Doran: I think the hour or two of extra meetings to try to ensure that Mr. Edwards knew the risks, to hear his wishes, and to persuade him to try to mitigate those risks would have been well worth their time. At the very least, it would have helped the medical team know that they did all they could. The signature is in a sense a legal issue, but it does have a moral point: namely, it helps the patient see the gravity of his choice. (I agree, though, that the moral issue is not one of actually signing an AMA document, but of understanding that one is going AMA. The extra meetings would just help underscore that fact.) You say they all "knew his mind plainly enough," but that seems wrong. Charles, and apparently the psychiatrist, thought Mr. Edwards was competent to make his health care decisions, but others on the team thought he was not competent and in denial. Lastly, to consult with him and his husband further was not "to treat him as a child"; it was simply the caring, responsible thing to do.

Warren: In the coarse exigencies of day-to-day health care in a busy hospital, doing what is required is hard enough. They knew his mind insofar as they knew what he wanted and knew that there was no changing his mind. Delay was what Dr. Paladin hoped for—and a possible reappraisal of his mental status. That would, if successful, have treated him as a child, for if he could be declared incompetent he could perhaps have been forced to follow the treatment regime.

Remember, too, that Charles did go to Mr. Edwards's home and give him the whole nine yards of warnings. I'm content that enough was done to establish Mr. Edwards's competence.

Doran: Yes, Charles was very caring, though some may wonder whether his past relationship with Mr. Edwards clouded his judgment and constituted a conflict of interest. That is not my view, however.

Perhaps we could step back from the facts of Mr. Edwards's case. Can we agree on a general principle, if not always on the application of that principle, about what hospital staff ought to do in cases where a patient of borderline competence makes a decision AMA that is likely to put his life in danger? Can we agree that we want the patient to have autonomy, but also to be protected from rash decisions that could be very harmful to himself or others?

 UP FOR DISCUSSION

In the drama, Charles Nolet has himself transferred to take over the care of his friend Jonathan Edwards. Is this morally laudatory since he is expressing gratitude and fulfilling a special obligation to a friend, or blameworthy as partiality not befitting a health care professional?

Warren: I think we are agreed on that. It is just that in this case we do not see the same balance point between protecting the vulnerable and respecting autonomy. I am emphasizing autonomy a little more because I believe that, in the original position, we would see it as in our interest generally to be able to direct our own lives. This interest is so strong that we would prefer to err on the side of autonomy rather than that of protection from ourselves.

Doran: Yes, what we are debating is this: How much protection should be given to patients to protect them from their rash choices? I want to recommend that in potentially serious medical situations, the hospital staff should, among other steps, discuss (as a team) with the patient (and perhaps immediate family and/or caregivers) what the patient's wishes are, and explain to the patient what their recommendations are, so that an agreement can be struck, or failing that, so that steps can be suggested to patient and family to protect the patient somewhat in case they go AMA. Here I think the insights of care ethics are to the point.

UP FOR DISCUSSION

How would you describe the ideal balance between patient safety and patient autonomy?

We recognize the autonomy of competent patients, but we want to demonstrate concern that the patient exercises their autonomy safely and in an informed way.

Patrick: Right. That is the kind of position I have been arguing for from my virtue ethics perspective. The right to autonomy is not absolute; it must be balanced against virtues such as compassion, charity, and beneficence. Even if Mr. Edwards had a right to refuse medical care, it was very foolish of him to exercise this right, given the situation. The medical professionals working with Mr. Edwards recognized the foolishness of his decision to refuse care, and so more should have been done to prevent him from harming himself.

Warren: The general suggestion seems fine to me. In cases like this, however, if one has to choose between hopeless attempts at persuasion of one adamantine patient and doing what will get results for other, more co-operative, patients, the choice is clear. One should attend to the other patients. Mr. Edwards was so obdurate that no meeting to discuss his case was likely to be fruitful. He was a hard man, and that made this a particularly hard case. Consequently, I come down on the side of the right to autonomy with some hesitation, not with total confidence.

Patrick: Well, this looks like a good point to end our debate of this case. Warren, it looks like Doran and I remain unconvinced that it was morally permissible for Mr. Edwards's health care team to release him when they did without at least some further attempt at delay.

Warren: Yes, it seems my arguments have failed to persuade you.

Doran: Right, but by critically examining your argument, I think we were able to shed much light on the difficulties involved in clarifying the concepts of autonomy, competence, and valid consent in a medical context.

SUMMARY

Here is a summary of the main questions, concepts, and arguments covered in this chapter:

- In this chapter, we debate the proposition *It was a moral error for the staff to allow Mr. Edwards to discharge himself without further evaluation.* Warren denies the proposition; Doran and Patrick accept it.
- Warren defends his view by appealing to his favoured approach to ethics, social contract theory. He argues that in the original position people would want to protect their interests by insisting on a strong right to autonomy in the real world. This right to autonomy, while not absolute, would prevent others from significant paternalistic interferences in a competent person's liberty. Warren then argues that Mr. Edwards was a competent person who made a valid refusal of care. To continue to hold him in the hospital against his will would be

a significant paternalistic interference, and therefore the hospital staff did not err when they allowed him to discharge himself when they did.

- Defence of Warren's argument requires an examination of several difficult topics: What is competence, and how is it related to autonomy? When is paternalism justified? And what is valid consent?

- Warren thinks that only minor interferences in a competent person's liberty can be justified, whereas Doran and Patrick think that more substantial paternalistic interferences with competent persons can be justified.

- Warren argues that Mr. Edwards was competent, but Patrick and Doran disagree.

- Warren advances an argument that valid consent need not be informed consent, and Patrick disagrees.

- Warren thinks that Mr. Edwards's refusal of care was a valid refusal, although neither Doran nor Patrick thinks his refusal was valid.

- Patrick argues that even if Mr. Edwards had a right to refuse care, it does not follow that the hospital staff should have allowed him to exercise that right, given that it could seriously harm him. The virtuous thing to do may have been to restrict Mr. Edwards's liberty to prevent him from serious harm or death.

- Doran argues that more efforts were required to ensure that Mr. Edwards and his family understood his circumstances and the consequences of him refusing care. Warren thinks that enough efforts were made, and further efforts would have been fruitless.

REVIEW QUESTIONS

1. What is autonomy?
2. Why does Warren think that people in the original position would want to protect their right to autonomy in the real world?
3. What is paternalism?
4. Explain Warren's reason for rejecting paternalism in Mr. Edwards's case. Explain why Doran and Patrick think that some paternalism is justified in Mr. Edwards's case.
5. How is *competence* defined?
6. When it comes to health care decisions, what do Warren, Patrick, and Doran think is necessary to be a competent patient?
7. Why does Warren think Mr. Edwards was competent to reject medical advice and to discharge himself from the hospital?
8. Why do Patrick and Doran think that Mr. Edwards was not competent to reject medical advice and to discharge himself from the hospital?
9. Why, according to Warren, does valid refusal or acceptance of medical care not require that one understand the medical advice being given?

10. What does Patrick think is necessary for valid consent or refusal of medical care?
11. Explain Patrick's argument for the view that the health care team was not morally required to accept Mr. Edwards's decision to discharge himself from the hospital, even if his decision was competent and adequately informed. What is Warren's response to this argument?
12. What concerns does Doran raise about Mr. Edwards's health care team's behaviour when it came to allowing him to leave the hospital? Explain Warren's reply to Doran on this point.

———

NOTES

1. Thomas Grisso and Paul S. Appelbaum, *Assessing Competence to Consent to Treatment: A Guide for Physicians and Other Health Professionals* (New York: Oxford University Press, 1998), 42–43.
2. Warren's views on consent are influenced by Benjamin Freedman, "A Moral Theory of Informed Consent," *Hastings Center Report* 5, no. 4 (1975): 32–39, reprinted in *Readings in Biomedical Ethics: A Canadian Focus,* 3rd ed., ed. Eike-Henner W. Kluge (Toronto: Pearson-Prentice Hall, 2005), 161.
3. See, for example, Tom L. Beauchamp and James F. Childress, *Principles of Biomedical Ethics,* 5th ed. (New York: Oxford University Press, 2001), ch. 3.

5 EUTHANASIA

INTRODUCTION

Medical assistance in dying **(MAID)** is when a health care professional assists a patient in dying, either by providing the patient with the means to commit suicide (assisted suicide) or by performing **euthanasia** on the patient. The term *euthanasia* is most often used to refer to bringing about another individual's death for that individual's own good through some act or omission. Philosophers and health care professionals commonly distinguish *active* **euthanasia** from *passive* **euthanasia**. The distinction is based on an alleged difference between *killing* and *letting die*. Our main concern here is with *voluntary* **active euthanasia** (VAE), in which a patient freely consents to and receives active euthanasia, and *non-voluntary* **active euthanasia** (NAE), in which a patient who cannot express a wish to live or die is actively euthanized. In Canadian law, **competent** adults have long had a legal right to have medical treatment stopped, or to refuse treatment altogether even when this might lead to the death of that competent adult. As of 2016, competent adults near death have a conditional legal right to receive MAID, either through physician-assisted suicide or physician-provided voluntary active euthanasia.[1] NAE is still forbidden under Canadian federal law. Although Canadian law is clear in supporting some VAE, considerable debate remains about the *morality* of VAE and NAE, and about whether the laws permitting some VAE and prohibiting all NAE ought to be changed.

To explore these issues, we summarize a real case of MAID received by Tim Regan. It is unclear whether Mr. Regan's case is an instance of VAE or physician-assisted suicide; however, a recent analysis indicates that almost all cases of MAID involve VAE as opposed to physician-assisted suicide.[2] Given this, and the controversy around active euthanasia, we will assume that Mr. Regan received VAE. Our debate focuses on the question of whether VAE, in this case and in general, is morally permissible. We then turn our attention to consider the moral status of NAE.

Doran, Patrick, and Warren agree that VAE is morally permissible under certain conditions. They agree, moreover, that NAE is also morally permissible under certain conditions, although they concede that the arguments here are less decisive. That the authors reach the same conclusions, despite their different theoretical approaches, provides broad support for the moral permissibility of some cases of VAE and NAE.

LEARNING OBJECTIVES

After completing this chapter, you should be able to:

- Define *euthanasia*
- Distinguish the different types of euthanasia
- Explain why considerations of autonomy and best interests are not, without qualification, sufficient to show that voluntary active euthanasia is permissible
- Outline Doran's, Patrick's, and Warren's arguments for the moral permissibility of voluntary active euthanasia
- Describe the Sanctity of Life and the God's Ownership objections to active euthanasia and why they fail
- State the Best Interest argument given in support of the moral permissibility of non-voluntary active euthanasia
- Explain Philippa Foot's argument against the moral permissibility of non-voluntary active euthanasia and why her argument is rejected
- Develop your own arguments for or against the permissibility of voluntary active euthanasia and non-voluntary active euthanasia

---

CASE DESCRIPTION

Please note: This case description is based on Dr. Brian Goldman's interview of Tim Regan and his family including the moments leading up to Mr. Regan's being given MAID by Dr. Sandy Buchman.[3] The facts in this case are a matter of public record, so privacy is not invaded. Mr. Regan wanted his case to inform the further liberalization of laws concerning euthanasia, in particular VAE based on advance directives.

Case Description: Tim Regan's Voluntary Active Euthanasia

Tim Regan received MAID in 2017, after he was diagnosed with inoperable liver cancer. Mr. Regan took advantage of a law enacted in Canada in 2016 that legalized MAID, including VAE, under certain restrictions. These restrictions include being terminally ill and being competent to consent to VAE at the time it is administered. In Mr. Regan's case, these restrictions on when VAE can be administered led him to receive MAID before he would have preferred. Mr. Regan was at risk of becoming incompetent from the toxins being released into his system from his failing liver. We are assuming he asked for and received VAE rather than physician-assisted suicide. He affirmed that he wanted VAE before his disease progressed to a point where he could no longer consent, because he did not want to risk becoming incompetent. He would have preferred that an **advance directive** be honoured so that he could receive active euthanasia once he was no longer competent to consent. But since Canadian law does not allow for active euthanasia in cases where a patient is no longer competent, he opted for the earlier death.

Mr. Regan was a long-time supporter of VAE. As a teenager, he witnessed his aunt suffer a lingering death. She was denied the right to refuse life-prolonging treatment, and, as a result, her death was drawn out and agonizing. At that point, Mr. Regan became a supporter of VAE. His views were reinforced decades later when he watched his father-in-law endure a protracted death. He objected to pointless suffering and to what he viewed as a waste of health care resources in cases like his aunt's and father-in-law's; therefore, when he was diagnosed with inoperable liver cancer in the summer of 2017, it was no surprise that he sought MAID.

Mr. Regan enlisted the help of his daughter, Honor Regan, to navigate the MAID bureaucracy. Finding a physician willing to take a request of this kind seriously can be trying. After a difficult search, the Regans were able to find Dr. Sandy Buchman, a palliative care specialist, who is active in MAID. Even if one can find physicians who will help, MAID is heavily regulated. For instance, MAID is allowed only if the patient's death is reasonably foreseeable. Thus, those who are suffering from non-lethal but agonizing conditions are not eligible for MAID in Canada. As we noted above, current law in Canada also requires one to affirm one's choice *at the time of* MAID. Advance directives asking for MAID are not honoured in Canadian law. Since Tim Regan had already needed some treatment for confusion, he could not risk any delay. Dr. Brian Goldman, who interviewed the Regans, quotes Honor Regan as saying, "To me, that was such a cruel twist of fate that you have my dad, who since the age of 16 knows that he wants MAID. It finally becomes legal the year before he gets this diagnosis, and he's given a cancer that's going to degrade his mind." Tim Regan could not enjoy his family's company until his mind faded. He had to make use of MAID while he was still competent. He and Honor believed that he should be able to give an effective advance directive requesting MAID in the event of his losing competence. His competence was also tested eight times from when he requested MAID up to the moment before MAID was given. Mr. Regan thought this excessive.

On December 12, 2017, with loving support from his wife and extended family, Tim Regan died quickly and peacefully with Dr. Buchman's help.

What Is Euthanasia?

Doran: Before we turn to the specifics of Mr. Regan's case, let's start with a general definition of *euthanasia*.

Patrick: Consider the etymology of the term *euthanasia*. It derives from the Greek prefix *eu*, which means "good," and the word *thanatos*, which means "death." This suggests that *euthanasia* means "good death."

Warren: Right, but that definition is much too vague and ambiguous. Many things may be viewed as good deaths that would not qualify as euthanasia—dying for a just cause, for instance, may be a good death, but would not be euthanasia. So, we need a much more precise definition of the term.

> **TECHNIQUE**
>
> In this section, we illustrate a philosophical technique of conceptual analysis. Inadequacies of some common definitions are noted. Progressively better definitions of *euthanasia* are produced in response to objections.

Patrick: I heard an interesting discussion of euthanasia on the CBC, in which euthanasia was defined as bringing about the death of a terminally ill person through the omission or commission of an act. This definition is moving in the right direction, but needs refinement.

Doran: I agree that this definition moves us in the right direction, but it still is somewhat problematic. One problem is that euthanasia need not be performed on *persons*; we can and do euthanize non-persons—for instance, pets. Another problem is that euthanasia need not involve bringing about the death of *terminally ill* individuals. We can euthanize individuals who suffer from very serious disabilities or injuries, yet who are not terminally ill.

> **BACKGROUND**
>
> The Julia Lamb case brought to the Supreme Court by the BC Civil Liberties Association is a case in point. Ms. Lamb was not terminally ill, though her condition meant that she faced the likelihood of extreme suffering for decades if she continued to live.
>
> *Source:* British Columbia Civil Liberties Association, "Lamb v. Canada Case Documents," August 22, 2016, https://bccla.org/our_work/lamb-v-canada-case-documents/.

Warren: A third problem with that definition is that it does not acknowledge that euthanasia involves bringing about an individual's death *for the sake of that individual*. Ending the life of a person who is terminally ill in order to get her insurance money is certainly not euthanasia.

Patrick: Right, of course. In the light of these points, let's try this: Euthanasia is an intentional act, or omission, that brings about the death of an individual for that individual's own good.

Warren: That looks better. The definition rightly recognizes that the individual being euthanized need not be terminally ill, and it also correctly states that euthanasia is something performed with specific intentions. That is, one intentionally allows or brings about an individual's death with the intention of benefitting that individual.

Patrick: Given this definition, the intention behind the act will greatly affect whether some act is a case of euthanasia. For instance, if a physician gives a patient a large quantity of medication—say, morphine—with the intention to ease the patient's pain, while foreseeing that the drug will likely kill the patient, then this would not count as a case of euthanasia. However, if the patient was given the same dose of morphine with the intent to kill him for his own good, then that would be a case of euthanasia. Thus, the same behaviour could amount to an act of euthanasia or not, depending on the intention of the person who behaves in this way.

Warren: It is true that doctors, and others, often want to draw this distinction, so I suppose it is good that our definition allows for this distinction to be made. But a different concern is with the idea of "an individual's own good." Perhaps we need to limit the idea of an individual's good to health-related concerns, such as extreme pain or incapacity. For if we do not limit the idea, it may turn out that we would have to view certain killings as instances of euthanasia when they are not really cases of euthanasia. For instance, it could be for an individual's own good if he is killed rather than having to spend his life in a notoriously brutal maximum security prison, but it seems odd to count such an act as euthanasia, even if it was done at that person's request and intending his own good.

Patrick: Well, I am not so sure that it would be odd to count that as an act of euthanasia, if we assume that there was no other option for this person, and that life in that prison would be absolutely dreadful. But, given that our present concern is with health care situations, perhaps we would be wise to avoid controversy and to stipulate that whenever we speak of the individual's best interest, we mean the individual's *health-related* interests.

Warren: All right, just to stick with what we perceive to be common usage, let's stipulate that the benefits are health-related.

Patrick: In order to stick to common usage, we might also want to distinguish euthanasia from suicide, and this definition does not do that.

Doran: Right, Patrick. Our definition entails that some suicides can be cases of euthanasia, but I think that is fine.

> **UP FOR DISCUSSION**
>
> In Toni Morrison's novel *Beloved*, a mother kills her young child in order to prevent her from being enslaved by notoriously brutal slave owners. On the assumption that the child's life would have been not worth living, should we view the mother's actions as a case of euthanasia?

When one intentionally kills oneself for one's own good, one performs an act of euthanasia on oneself. For example, imagine a person who is diagnosed with an extremely painful cancer—say, mouth cancer. Suppose, after several surgeries, and much suffering, the cancer has returned and the end is near. Not wanting to face the horrific pain of untreatable mouth cancer, and not wanting to take so much medication that she would be rendered barely conscious for the rest of her natural life, suppose this person opts to take her own life by taking an overdose of barbiturates. I see no problem with viewing her act as a case of euthanasia. Indeed, to say she simply "committed suicide" would be to under-describe this act.

Nevertheless, I admit that my use of the term is idiosyncratic, and since our focus here is on euthanasia when performed on others, let's stipulate that when we use the term *euthanasia*, we mean it to involve intentionally bringing about the death of *another* individual.

UP FOR DISCUSSION

Do you think that some suicides should count as instances of euthanasia?

Warren: Agreed. Our definition is now this: *Euthanasia is an intentional act, or omission, that brings about the death of another individual for that individual's own health-related good.*

BACKGROUND

The Canadian Medical Association defines *euthanasia* as follows:

> Euthanasia means knowingly and intentionally performing an act, with or without consent, that is explicitly intended to end another person's life and that includes the following elements: the subject has an incurable illness; the agent knows about the person's condition; commits the act with the primary intention of ending the life of that person; and the act is undertaken with empathy and compassion and without personal gain.

Source: Canadian Medical Association, *Policy Document PD15-02—Euthanasia and Assisted Death* (Update 2014).

Different Kinds of Euthanasia

Patrick: Even though we now have a working definition of *euthanasia*, there is still more work to do in order to clarify the concept. This is because there are different types of euthanasia. Let's begin by noting the difference between active and passive euthanasia.

UP FOR DISCUSSION

The concept of euthanasia is closely related to another concept—**physician-assisted suicide**. Physician-assisted suicide occurs when a physician provides a hopeless, usually terminally ill patient with the means (such as a prescription for a lethal dose of a drug) to commit suicide. A noteworthy example of physician-assisted suicide is the case of Sue Rodriguez, a victim of ALS. After Canada's highest court denied her the right to VAE, a sympathetic physician assisted her to die. She was paralyzed and unable to take her own life, but she was clearly rational, competent, well informed, and willing to die.

Why would our definition of euthanasia not include physician-assisted suicide? Do you think there is a morally significant difference between physician-assisted suicide and euthanasia?

Active versus Passive Euthanasia

Doran: Roughly, active euthanasia occurs when one *directly causes* another individual's death—for instance, by administering a lethal injection—for that individual's own health-related good. Passive euthanasia occurs when one *allows* another individual to die—by withholding life-prolonging treatment, for example—for the sake of that individual's health-related good. It must be said that the boundaries between active and passive euthanasia are not always clear, however.

Warren: Yes, but in spite of the penumbral area, we can often agree on the distinction in health care contexts. For instance, it was a case of active euthanasia if Dr. Buchman gave Tim Regan a lethal series of drugs by IV. But it would have been a case of passive euthanasia if, instead, Tim Regan had a heart attack and Dr. Buchman had respected his advance directive, do not resuscitate.

Perhaps we can just say that intentionally refraining from treatment so that it will lead to death for the patient's good counts as passive euthanasia, while intentionally causing the patient's death for the patient's good counts as active euthanasia.

Doran: But what about cases where a feeding tube or respirator is removed from a terminally ill patient? In a sense this is active, since it requires action, and yet in a sense it is passive, since the act stops treatment and so allows the patient to die of a natural cause.

Patrick: Interestingly, such cases are usually viewed as passive euthanasia. Perhaps that is because what marks the distinction between passive and active is the cause of death. Roughly, the idea is that if one intends to let the disease kill the patient for the patient's own good, then it is passive. But if one intends to cause "non-naturally" the death for the patient's own good, then it is active. Thus, not treating the cancer or the infection, or removing the respirator and "letting nature take its course" are cases of passive euthanasia, while giving a lethal dose of drugs, for instance, is active.

> **BACKGROUND**
>
> The case of Nancy B. is a well-known Canadian example of voluntary passive euthanasia. Nancy B. was paralyzed by a rare neurological disease and refused to be kept on a respirator. The case came to court where a judge agreed that she had the right to refuse treatment. She was tranquillized and then removed from the respirator, and she subsequently died.
>
> *Source:* "'Who Owns My Life?' Asks ALS Patient Sue Rodriguez," *CBC Television*, November 24, 1992, http://www.cbc.ca/archives/entry/who-owns-my-life.

 UP FOR DISCUSSION

Explain why rationing health care—for instance, denying needed heart transplants to elderly people so that younger people can get them instead—is not passive euthanasia.

Warren: I think that drawing the exact boundaries between passive and active euthanasia is very tricky, but the basic idea is quite clear, and in many cases we can confidently judge whether it is passive or active euthanasia.

Voluntary, Non-Voluntary, and Involuntary Euthanasia

Patrick: Next, we need to note that active and passive euthanasia can be done either voluntarily, involuntarily, or non-voluntarily.

Doran: Right. **Voluntary euthanasia** occurs when a competent individual consents to his death; **involuntary euthanasia** occurs when a competent individual does not consent to his death; and finally, **non-voluntary euthanasia** occurs when it involves mentally incompetent individuals who lack the decision-making capacity to express a preference to live or die.

Patrick: Those definitions look good, but a few clarifications are in order. We should note, for instance, that voluntary euthanasia can occur with the patient consenting at the time of the euthanasia, or prior to that time, through an advance directive. So, it is important to realize that a person need not be competent at the time of their death for it to count as a form of voluntary euthanasia. Recall that Tim Regan wanted the law to respect his advance directive to receive VAE.

Doran: Right. And notice also that we've defined non-voluntary euthanasia in such a way that it applies to individuals who lack the ability to make a decision. This would include young children, for example, and the severely cognitively impaired.

BACKGROUND

A well-known Canadian example of non-voluntary active euthanasia is the case of Tracy Latimer. Tracy was a 12-year-old **quadriplegic** who functioned at the level of a three- or four-month-old infant. She suffered from excruciating pain, underwent repeated surgeries, and required further surgeries to remove her thigh bone. In 1993, her father, Robert, unwilling to see his daughter suffer any longer, placed her inside his pickup truck, ran a hose from the exhaust pipe to the inside of the cab, and watched as his daughter died. He then turned himself in to the police, admitting that he killed his daughter. Latimer was convicted of second-degree murder. The jury recommended parole, and the trial judge agreed, even though the minimum sentence for second-degree murder is 10 years in prison. This decision, however, was repeatedly appealed, going all the way to Canada's Supreme Court. In the end, it was ruled that the minimum sentencing laws needed to be followed, and Robert was sentence to life in prison, with no eligibility for parole for 10 years. In 2007, Robert was denied parole for failing to express remorse. In 2008, however, Robert was granted day parole, and he received full parole in 2010. See "Latimer Granted Full Parole," *CBC News*, November 29, 2010, https://www.cbc.ca/news/canada/saskatchewan/latimer-granted-full-parole-1.884458 for a brief overview. Non-voluntary euthanasia remains illegal in Canada.

Warren: Finally, there are cases of involuntary euthanasia. These would be rare cases, but they could happen. It is not unrealistic to think that a physician, or, more likely, a family member, might, on grounds of compassion, decide not to tell her competent patient or loved one that she is going to be allowed to die or to receive a lethal injection.

Patrick: True, Warren, but it takes some imagination to come up with cases of involuntary euthanasia that seem permissible.

Warren: Yes, of course.

Doran: I agree. And once again there can be grey areas that divide these different categories, but the distinction between these types of euthanasia usually seems quite clear.

Doran: I have one more question. What is the connection between medical assistance in dying (MAID) and euthanasia? Much discussion around this topic seems to prefer referring to the issue as "MAID" rather than "euthanasia."

 UP FOR DISCUSSION

Suppose there was someone who was mentally competent, yet totally unable to communicate any of his preferences as a result of permanent and complete paralysis. If this person was intentionally allowed to die or intentionally killed for his own good, would it be a case of nonvoluntary or involuntary euthanasia?

Patrick: I take it that MAID includes both assisted suicide and active euthanasia. In cases of assisted suicide, one is given the means to end one's own life. For instance, it would be assisted suicide if Dr. Buchman gave Mr. Regan some pills to swallow that would cause his heart to stop beating. In cases of active euthanasia, one directly causes another individual's death (for the benefit of the one who is killed). For instance, it would be active euthanasia if Dr. Buchman injected a lethal drug into Mr. Regan's body. Because we want to focus directly on the topic of euthanasia, we will stick to that term, rather than the more general MAID.

Warren: Good. With these definitions in hand, we can now turn to the moral questions about euthanasia raised by the particular case under consideration.

BACKGROUND

Here's a table that lists the six possible kinds of euthanasia:

Voluntary active (VAE)	Non-voluntary active (NAE)	Involuntary active (IAE)
Voluntary passive (VPE)	Non-voluntary passive (NPE)	Involuntary passive (IPE)

DECIDING WHICH ISSUES TO DEBATE

Doran: There are a variety of ethical issues surrounding euthanasia. These ethical questions concern the moral permissibility of the various kinds of euthanasia, as well as ethical questions over whether such actions should be legalized.

Warren: Right, moral and legal rights are two different issues that are best kept separate. One can think that certain kinds of euthanasia are morally permissible without also thinking that they should be legally permissible, and vice versa.

Patrick: Let's focus here on questions about the *moral* permissibility of euthanasia. We have assumed, for the sake of argument, that Tim Regan's case was an instance of VAE. He freely chose to receive active euthanasia, and Dr. Buchman intentionally caused Mr. Regan's death for his own health-related good. Was it morally permissible for Dr. Buchman to perform VAE on Tim Regan? More generally, under what conditions, if any, is VAE morally permissible?

> **THEORY AND DISCUSSION**
>
> Moral principles and their legal counterparts are two different things. Laws may be moral, immoral, or amoral, and moral principles may not be legally enforceable. Discuss an example of an act that is morally wrong but should not be illegal. Give an example of an act that is not morally wrong but should be illegal.

Warren: We should also consider the moral status of non-voluntary active euthanasia, since VAE and NAE are the most discussed in public debate.

Doran: Sounds good. Let's start with an examination of the morality of Tim Regan's case and of VAE in general. Later, we can debate the morality of NAE.

THE MORALITY OF VOLUNTARY ACTIVE EUTHANASIA

Warren: I think VAE is justified in some cases, including Tim Regan's. In the **original position** it would be in our interest to accept a rule that would allow us to choose the manner and time of our own deaths. There may be all sorts of restrictions we would want to put on the practice of euthanasia, however. Things like psychological evaluations and the availability of good comfort care including excellent pain control would be adopted to protect our interests as seen from the original position. But the basic right to VAE would be acknowledged in the original position as being obviously in one's interest for just the sort of reasons Mr. Regan expressed.

Patrick: I agree that VAE is permissible in many cases, including the case of Tim Regan. Compassion, kindness, charity, empathy, respect for personal autonomy, and other virtues speak in favour of VAE in this case and relevantly similar cases. And I also agree that various restrictions will likely be needed to protect people from such things as temporary depression, irrationality, and so on.

Doran: I also think VAE is morally acceptable in Mr. Regan's case, as well as in many other cases. I have many reasons for my view. One of my arguments is, roughly, that respect for autonomy and considerations of welfare constitute reasons in favour of euthanasia that, in many cases including Mr. Regan's, overwhelm any arguments against it.

Warren: Well, why don't we begin, Doran, by taking a closer look at your arguments in support of VAE?

Doran: Sure. I'd like to begin by identifying some fairly familiar reasons that speak in favour of VAE, and then I will point out that these reasons are not by themselves sufficient to justify VAE. I will argue, however, that, suitably modified, these reasons form the basis of a sound argument for the morality of VAE.[4]

Patrick: Sounds good.

The Autonomy and Best Interest Argument for Voluntary Active Euthanasia

Doran: Two basic sorts of arguments are frequently voiced in support of VAE. One sort of argument raises the idea of autonomy—the basic refrain is that competent people should have the right to determine their own futures, euthanasia allows for death with dignity, and so on. Another strain of argument in favour of active euthanasia emphasizes that sometimes it is in the best interest of a person to no longer continue living. Often this is because of the tremendous hopeless suffering, both physical and psychological, experienced by some patients, but it may also be because the patient is in a condition where life is no longer a benefit to her (say, because she is able to exist without horrible pain only if she is in a drug-hazed stupor). It is this appeal to the patient's best interest that constitutes another powerful reason in support of active euthanasia.

Patrick: Both strands of argument seem to introduce powerful considerations in favour of VAE, although without qualification they may not be sufficient to make the case for VAE.

Doran: I agree. Let's begin with an initial statement of what we might call the Autonomy and Best Interest argument. This version of the argument will be too simple, but understanding its weaknesses will enable us to revise the initial argument into something that I take to be sound.

(1)   If a person freely chooses some action, and that action is in that person's best interest, then the act is morally permissible.

(2)   In some cases, including Tim Regan's, a person freely chooses VAE and it is in that person's best interest.

(3)   Therefore, in these cases, including Tim Regan's, VAE is morally permissible.

Patrick: The argument is valid, but it is likely unsound. Some may try to reject this argument by attacking premise (2). The critic may deny, for instance, that a person could ever have a life that is not worth living and, hence, that death is ever in a person's best interest. But that objection is weak and is, I believe, refuted by Sue Rodriguez's case, and by other cases that are particularly grim, such as Tim Regan's would be if he waited too long for MAID and his body and mind became degraded.

Warren: Others will suggest, more plausibly, that VAE will be misapplied and performed on people who don't really freely choose it, or on people whose lives could still be a benefit to them. Of course, these are serious concerns, but they speak to the issue of whether VAE should be practiced, and to the dangers of legalization, and not to the present issue of whether VAE is, in principle, morally wrong.

Patrick: Agreed. The critic is better off attacking premise (1) of the argument. An act can be morally wrong even if it is freely chosen and in the best interest of those primarily concerned. One way it could be wrong is if such an act violated the rights of others. For example, it may be in the best interest of a person who just found out that he needed a liver transplant to have his friend put him at the head of the **queue**, but such an act—though freely chosen and in the best interest of the person primarily involved—would be wrong since it would violate the rights of those who had a prior claim to the transplant.

Warren: Notice further that freely chosen acts that are in a person's best interest can be wrong even if they do not violate anyone else's rights. Think of a case such as this. Suppose there is a person, call him Zeke, who is fabulously rich, and who is soon going to die. As a last act of pleasure for himself, he decides he will collect his millions and light it all on fire. The decision to burn the money may be an autonomous decision, and perhaps it is in Zeke's best interest to do so, since his choice will give him pleasure. But it also certainly seems wrong for Zeke to engage in such a wasteful, selfish action, given that Zeke could instead have used his wealth to benefit many people in great need. And if this is right, then we have another reason to reject premise (1).

The Revised Autonomy and Best Interest Argument

Doran: Your counterexamples show that premise (1) of the above argument is false. It is too simple to say that euthanasia would be justified if it was freely chosen and in a person's best interest. But suitably modified, I think this argument can be saved. So consider what may be called the Revised Autonomy and Best Interest argument for VAE.

(1) If a person freely chooses some action, and that action is in that person's best interest, and it neither violates anyone's rights nor sets back anyone's very important interests, then it is morally permissible.

(2) In some circumstances, a person freely chooses VAE, and it is in that person's best interest, and it neither violates anyone's rights nor sets back anyone's very important interests.

(3) Therefore, in those circumstances, VAE is morally permissible.

I believe that Tim Regan's case of euthanasia is a case where VAE is justified because it satisfies the conditions set forth in premise (1). He freely chose euthanasia, euthanasia was in his best interest, it did not violate anyone else's rights, and it did not set back very important interests of others. Therefore, it was permissible for him to receive VAE.

Of course, in other cases, euthanasia may not be permissible. For example, if euthanasia was not freely chosen, or if receiving it violated others' rights or seriously harmed others, then it may be wrong. But, other things being equal, the fact that VAE is sometimes an expression of one's deepest preferences and is necessary to serve one's best interests, and can be done without setting back even more important moral considerations, means that VAE is sometimes morally permissible.

Warren: It is good that your modified premise (1) can avoid our previous

TECHNIQUE

Frequently in philosophical debate, the response to a counterexample is to revise the statement that it attacked, explicitly stating exceptions so as to avoid the counterexample. The process may then be repeated until all the necessary exceptions are explicit in the statement. A concern with this sort of process, however, is that the revisions to the principle become merely ad hoc. One wants the principles one defends not only to avoid counterexamples but also to have an underlying rationale that is itself morally significant.

 UP FOR DISCUSSION

Note that some could still challenge premise (2). They might maintain that euthanasia violates God's right to say when we die. Is this a plausible position? What would that imply about other sorts of killing?

counterexamples. The revised premise (1) does not support putting one's name at the top of the transplant list, since such an act violates the rights of others. And the revised premise avoids the thrust of the case of Zeke, since his action would set back the very important interests of others.

Patrick: But there's still room for objections to premise (1), even with the revision.

Warren: I suppose that opponents of VAE will try to reject your premise (1) by arguing that freely chosen acts that serve a person's best interest and violate no one else's rights nor set back any very important interests of others, can still be wrong if they transgress other important values. For instance, they might think that such acts would be wrong if they violate the sanctity of human life or if they are contrary to God's will. We should, therefore, consider those arguments against VAE.

 UP FOR DISCUSSION

Do you think that the Revised Autonomy and Best Interest argument is sound?

The Sanctity of Life Objection to the Morality of Voluntary Active Euthanasia

Doran: Right. Those who oppose VAE often argue that it is wrong because it would allow for the intentional killing of innocent human beings, and that killing innocent humans is always immoral. Given that this is a common argument against active euthanasia, and given that it could be used to counter my premise (1), we should consider it.

Warren: Yes, that is a standard objection. It is derived from the **Sanctity of Life principle**.

Doran: I think the objection is mistaken.

Patrick: I do too, but before we look at problems with this objection, I think we need to spell it out in more detail. This view is often characterized as the view that it is wrong to kill, because life is sacred. But proponents of this view are surely not claiming that *all* life is sacred. The suggestion seems to be, rather, that *human* life—specifically, *innocent* human life—is sacred. But why do proponents of this view believe that there is something special about the lives of humans, and only humans? And how is it supposed to follow from this that it's always wrong to kill an innocent human?

TECHNIQUE

Notice that Patrick is pointing to frequently overlooked features of the Sanctity of Life objection to active euthanasia: (1) it applies only to human life; (2) it typically is said to apply only to innocent human life; and (3) it assumes that if a life is sacred it is always wrong to end it.

Doran: Various reasons are given for why human life is "sacred." Often, arguments that appeal to God are invoked in support of this claim. God created humans in His image, and so they are special, and deserving of special respect.

Other times, non-religious reasons are given for the view that human life is sacred. Kant, for instance, could be seen as (to some degree) relevant here, since he famously claims that humanity is an end in itself, and as such, has a special dignity. By *humanity*, however, he means "rational agents," not "human beings." So it is the lives of rational beings that are "sacred" for Kant.

But, Patrick, you raise an interesting question. What does it mean to say a human life is sacred? I take it the claim is not that human beings may

BACKGROUND

One statement of the Sanctity of Life view is expressed by Lutherans for Life–Canada, "whose mission is 'to witness to the sanctity of human life through education based on the Word of God.' Lutherans for Life–Canada believes every human life—from conception to natural death regardless of physical or mental challenges or condition of dependence—is precious in God's sight."

Source: "Who Are We," Lutherans for Life–Canada, http://lutheransforlife-canada.ca/who-are-we/.

never be killed, since, as you suggest, most who espouse this view accept the legitimacy of killing humans in some cases, such as self-defence, a just war, or maybe even capital punishment. So, most likely, to say that a human life is sacred is to say that an innocent human life may not be taken or may not be taken intentionally. Thus, perhaps the principle should really be called *the sanctity of innocent human life*.

Patrick: Yes, I think that better captures the principle behind the Sanctity of Life view, as I understand it.

Doran: Still, you're right that one may wonder why the sanctity of innocent human life entails that innocent humans may never be killed. After all, proponents of the view are willing to make exceptions in cases like self-defence. Why should they not make an exception when life is no longer a benefit to the person, and when that person no longer wants to live?

Warren: More to the point, there are compelling counterexamples to the principle that innocent humans may never be intentionally killed. Suppose that a totally incompetent patient has been infected with an incurable disease that is easily spread, and that the patient has escaped custody and is running toward a crowd. Now, suppose a police officer shoots and kills that patient to avert what could be a global disaster, a plague. In this case it would be permissible to kill an innocent human being so as to avoid a worldwide plague, and so the sanctity of innocent human life principle must be false.

Doran: I take it that this patient is innocent in virtue of being "totally incompetent," and so the doctrine that says it is always wrong to kill an innocent human being would imply that it was wrong to kill the plague victim. But it would clearly not be wrong to kill this innocent human being, given that it was necessary to avert a global disaster. Therefore, the claim that innocent human beings may never be intentionally killed must be false.

Patrick: Although I agree that it would not be wrong to kill the innocent person in this example, we should note that not everyone would agree with our conclusion concerning the permissibility of killing the plague victim in this case. A Kantian would argue, for instance, that it is always wrong to use persons as a mere means to an end. Assuming the innocent human is a person—which is questionable, I suppose, given his incompetence—then some may argue that it would be wrong to kill him, even if it is necessary to save the lives of others. So the example might be unpersuasive for some.

Warren: It is only problematic if we think, like Kant, that we must be so non-consequentialist that we would risk all of humanity to save one person who will die from his illness in any

UP FOR DISCUSSION

Do you think the case of the innocent plague victim is a successful counterexample to the claim that innocent human beings must never be intentionally killed? Why or why not? Develop your own counterexample to the principle that innocent human beings must never be killed intentionally.

THEORY

There are many definitions of *person*, most of which make persons a different class from the class of all humans. If one thinks, for instance, that rationality is essential for being a person, then some human beings would fail to be persons. For Kant, the hallmark of a person appears to be the ability to make one's own decisions, including the ability to follow moral rules. This is why Patrick questions whether a totally incompetent human would still be a person in Kant's view.

case. I think it presents a counterexample to Kantian thought and, more generally, to the principle that it is always wrong to kill innocent human beings intentionally.

Patrick: I agree, Warren. As you know, I'm no Kantian.

Doran: I believe your case presents a counterexample to most versions of the principle of the sanctity of innocent human life, Warren. Kantians maintain that it is wrong to treat rational beings merely as a means; they could then point out that a totally incompetent person is no longer a rational being, and so the injunction not to treat him merely as a means no longer applies. But a different case could serve as a counterexample even to the Kantian version of the sanctity of human life (that is, the sanctity of *rational* life).

Patrick: Let's hear your counterexample, Doran.

Suicide and Hare's Lorry Driver—More Counterexamples to the Sanctity of Life Principle

Doran: First, let me give a case that seems morally permissible but that involves suicide, rather than euthanasia. Do you recall the September 11, 2001, terrorist attacks in New York, and the heartbreaking cases of people jumping from the top floors of the World Trade Center in order to avoid burning to death? I take it that these were cases where suicide was both in one's rational self-interest and morally permissible. For clearly it was in the rational self-interest for these people to die quickly rather than to roast to death, and clearly it was morally permissible in such a case to end one's own life as painlessly as possible rather than being burned alive. But if you grant this, then it seems to me that you must reject the principle that it is always morally forbidden to intentionally kill an innocent human being.[5]

Warren: I agree, Doran, that this is a case of morally permissible suicide. But I suppose some would argue that there is a big moral difference between suicide and active euthanasia. For the former involves killing oneself, but the latter involves killing someone else.

Doran: Right, opponents might argue this. But I deny that there is always a significant moral difference between a rational and morally permissible suicide and active euthanasia. For there could be cases where a person is in a situation where suicide would be both rational and morally permissible, but where they are unable to do it. Surely, in such a case, it would be permissible for this person to ask for and to receive help from someone else.

Indeed, the Christian philosopher R. M. Hare gives this case: a petrol lorry driver (gasoline tanker truck driver) gets into an accident and is trapped in his vehicle as flames begin to engulf him. He screams for someone to kill him, so that he does not have to roast to death. A bystander, understanding the situation, takes action and ends the petrol lorry driver's life. Does the bystander act permissibly? It seems so. And if that is the case, then we have a clear counterexample to the Sanctity of Life principle. For the petrol lorry driver is an innocent person who is permissibly killed by another person.[6]

Patrick: Good. This example seems to be a clear case where it is not wrong to end the life of an innocent person, as it would be cruel not to comply with his request. Further, it is a useful example to show the implausibility of the claim that it is never in one's best interest to die.

Still, although we agree with Hare's counterexample, I suspect some would argue that killing the lorry driver is wrong, because it is sinful or cowardly for the driver to want to die.

Warren: That response to Hare's example confuses, as Nowell-Smith says, a right to live with a duty to live.[7] If one has a right to live, then one may sometimes waive the right and release others from their duty not to kill. That is what the driver does. The idea that it is sinful to want to die, however, probably rests on the mistaken view that one has not just a right to live but a duty to live. Those who think wanting death is cowardly are, moreover, being quite unrealistic about pain. What do you think, Patrick?

THEORY

Hare defends the permissibility of active euthanasia in the case of the petrol lorry driver by employing an idea that is similar both to the golden rule—"Do unto others as you would have them do unto you"—and to Kant's universal law version of the categorical imperative, "Act only according to that maxim which you can at the same time will that it should become a universal law." Kant's basic idea is that we should act only on principles that we can consistently will everyone to follow. Since we cannot consistently will to universalize a principle that prevents us from being killed were we in a situation like that of the lorry driver, we should reject a principle that prohibited killing in such situations.

There is considerable irony in using a Christian- and Kantian-inspired argument to support VAE, since many Christians think that their faith requires them to oppose active euthanasia, and since, as we have seen, Kant is usually interpreted as a defender of the principle of the sanctity of human life (at least as it applies to innocent rational beings).

For a more detailed discussion of Kant's ethics, see chapter 2.

Patrick: I agree, it is certainly not cowardly for the driver to want to be killed when the alternative is burning to death. If anything, it would perhaps be cowardly not to comply with the driver's request to be killed. I believe this case shows that it is sometimes morally permissible to intentionally kill innocent persons. If that's correct, then the main premise in the Sanctity of Life objection to VAE is false, and that objection is therefore unsound.

Doran: Beyond giving a clear counterexample to the Sanctity of Life principle, I would like to explain why it is a mistake to claim that the intentional killing of innocents is always wrong.

Warren: Go ahead.

 UP FOR DISCUSSION

Do you think that the case of the petrol lorry driver refutes the view that it is always wrong to kill an innocent human being because innocent human life is sacred? If so, is this because you think that the lorry driver's life is no longer sacred, or is it perhaps because you think that because life is sacred it ought not be left to such a miserable fate? Do you think that Tim Regan's case is importantly different from the lorry driver's? Explain.

An Argument That the Moral Reasons against Killing Do Not Apply to Voluntary Active Euthanasia

Doran: Normally, there are many reasons that explain why killing an innocent person is wrong. The thing is, though, none of these reasons speak against VAE, and some seem to actually support the moral permissibility of VAE.[8]

For instance, consider a typical murder—say, a drive-by shooting. Why is that act wrong? Reasons why it is wrong include the following: (1) it harms the victim—he is deprived the goods that his life had to offer and would have come to offer; (2) it goes against his preferences—he did not want to die, yet his preferences were disregarded; (3) it violates the victim's autonomy—he had various plans in his life, yet this killing took away his ability to control his life choices; (4) it spreads fear in the community—knowing that there is a murderer on the loose who kills people against their will is bound to terrify others. Perhaps there are other reasons that make the act of murder wrong, but these seem to be the principal ones.

But notice that none of these reasons apply to VAE. It does not deprive the "victim" of a good future (since it is only to be performed on individuals whose life is no longer a good for them); it does not act against the "victim's" preferences—it honours them; it does not violate the "victim's" autonomy—it respects it; and it need not spread fear in the community, since VAE is limited to people who both need it and want it. So the standard reasons that make killing people normally wrong do not apply to VAE, and that is why it makes sense to say that VAE is an important exception to the moral rule against killing innocent humans. Perhaps there is some other reason why killing is wrong that I have overlooked, and which applies to VAE, but the onus is on opponents of VAE to identify that reason.

An Argument That Euthanasia Is Wrong Because It Destroys What Belongs to God

Patrick: I agree with you, Doran, that the considerations that typically make it wrong to kill innocent human beings tend to speak in favour of VAE, rather than against it. Once this point is made explicit, it seems implausible to suppose that VAE is always morally wrong.

I doubt, however, that your argument will persuade many proponents of the Sanctity of Life view. This is because the reasons you cite for why killing is generally wrong are not the principal reasons why many advocates of this view think killing is wrong. What principally makes killing humans wrong, in this view, usually turns on the fact that humans are God's creation. So whether you kill someone in a drive-by shooting or you kill a terminally ill person, you are killing one of God's creations either way. This is often why both are regarded as wrong, according to their view.

Doran: You may be right, Patrick. But those who appeal to this theistic argument are in trouble, since, as we have seen, there are clear counterexamples to the Sanctity of Life view they wish to defend—the petrol lorry driver case, or cases of self-defence, or suicide for a worthy cause. Further, this argument has other problems.

Patrick: I agree—I think that this line of argument is indefensible. One additional and obvious problem is that it presupposes that God exists. This is something that I, and many others, would deny.

Doran: Yes, plus setting that question aside, notice that *everything* (or at least every "natural" thing) in a theological view is God's creation, and so it would turn out that it would be wrong to destroy anything (or any natural thing)—bacteria, plants, weeds, animals, and so on. Clearly, however, that is an absurd consequence. Instead, for this argument even to get off the ground, we should revise it so that it says that *human life* belongs to God, and so to destroy it (whether one's own or others') is wrong, because it destroys something that belongs to God.

Warren: Yes, one often hears that only God can take human life because human life belongs to God, but those who say this may nonetheless accept capital punishment, or killing in self-defence, or killing in defence of one's country, or killing the *innocent* plague-stricken incompetent in our earlier example. Instead of pointing to their view that our lives belong to God, they should face the justificatory arguments already given, if they are to be consistent, or deny that any killing of human beings, who are God's creation, innocent or not, is ever justified, even in self-defence.

> **TECHNIQUE**
>
> Warren is setting up an argument called **a dilemma**. A dilemma shows that one's opponent is faced with only two or more logical alternatives, none of which the opponent would accept. If these opponents insist that only God may destroy human life, then they have a problem, for they would not be able to explain why it is permissible to kill in cases of self-defence. But if they say humans may justifiably kill in some cases, then they have not yet provided an argument against active euthanasia.

Patrick: Right. To sum up, then, either it is always wrong to kill human beings or it is not always wrong. Proponents of the Sanctity of Life view would not—or at least cannot plausibly—hold the former view. They would, or should, accept that killing humans is sometimes permissible. But then they cannot object to VAE simply on the ground that human life is sacred or that human life belongs to God. Further argument is needed.

A Counterexample to the Revised Autonomy and Best Interest Argument

Warren: Before ending our examination of the morality of VAE, I want to raise a more direct challenge to your argument for VAE, Doran. Your first premise was that "If a person freely chooses some action, and that action is in that person's best interest, and it neither violates anyone's rights nor sets back anyone's very important interests, then it is morally permissible." But this principle faces counterexamples that have nothing to do with euthanasia.

Doran: It sounds like you've got one in mind. Fire away.

Warren: Consider this very unusual case: consensual private incest (say between two adult siblings). Imagine that these siblings freely choose to have sex in the privacy of their remote cabin. They enjoy their sexual encounter and no one ever finds out about it. Now granted, this is a really fanciful case. But the point of the example is it seems like your first premise implies that this case of incest would be morally permissible, but I suspect many people would find this case of incest to be morally wrong.

Doran: Obviously, most cases of incest are not like your imagined case. They are anything but consensual and they are extremely harmful. So here we have a *very* unusual case. I would also wonder whether both parties truly freely consented and were truly not harmed by the encounter, but *if* this case is really as you've described, then I'd have to admit that their actions were not morally wrong. For everyone's autonomy was respected and no one was harmed by their actions. Given this, I am willing to bite the bullet and assume that while their actions might be unpalatable, they weren't immoral.

Patrick: Interesting example, Warren. For this to work as a counterexample to Doran's principle, however, the act in question has to be in the person's best interest. Doran wonders whether the individuals might have been harmed by the relationship, and I suppose I share a similar concern. And even if they weren't harmed, it's far from obvious that this incestuous relationship genuinely was in either person's best interest.

Warren: Perhaps one could argue that it is impossible for it to be in their interest. That is what is required to fully defuse the counterexample, but that discussion would take us too far from our topic.

 UP FOR DISCUSSION

In the final analysis, do you think it was morally permissible for Dr. Buchman to perform VAE on Tim Regan?

THE MORALITY OF NON-VOLUNTARY ACTIVE EUTHANASIA

Doran: Okay, so it looks like we all agree that the Sanctity of Life objection fails, and that VAE is morally permissible in certain situations. There are, of course, other objections to VAE, but perhaps we should now consider the difficult issue of NAE, *non-voluntary* active euthanasia.

Patrick: Yes, it's one thing to say that if competent people regard their life as no longer worth living and express a clear preference for euthanasia, then it may be permissible to end their life. It's quite another thing, however, to say that it's permissible to euthanize individuals if they do not, because they *cannot*, consent to the act. This, of course, is different from Tim Regan's case. But we can easily imagine that he had left no advance directives and his failing liver released toxins causing brain damage that rendered him mentally incompetent to make his own medical decisions. In this imagined scenario, we might ask whether NAE would then be permissible to avoid a long dying process replete with suffering.

> **BACKGROUND**
>
> One of the most common arguments against VAE is the "slippery slope" objection. Roughly, this is the concern that if VAE is accepted, it will lead to other kinds of killing that are morally unacceptable, for example, killing patients who do not really choose euthanasia, or killing patients who could have had lives that were worth living. These slippery slope arguments raise serious concerns regarding legalization of VAE, but they do not show that any particular instance of VAE, such as Tim Regan's, is morally wrong.

Doran: Things are especially difficult when it comes to NAE, since my favoured argument for VAE appealed, in part, to people's right to control their own futures in matters that primarily concerned them. But this appeal to control one's own future, and the right to make one's own decisions, is not something that applies to human infants or to humans with severe mental incapacities. In general, we do not say that young children, for instance, have a right to make their own decisions about matters that could seriously affect their well-being. So this argument cannot be used to support NAE, where individuals cannot consent.

Warren: So, Doran, if your main argument for VAE won't apply to NAE, then what is your view on the morality of NAE?

The Best Interest Argument for Non-Voluntary Active Euthanasia

Doran: I think NAE is sometimes morally permissible. I think the crucial issue is what we should do for individuals who cannot make their own decisions. Here it might be instructive to consider one's beloved pet, when it comes to end-of-life decisions. It is quite clear that when it comes to one's dog, for instance, one has a moral duty to euthanize him, if continued existence harms the dog because he is in unremitting pain, or cannot do the basic activities that dogs do—like eat, play, move, and so on. In the case of one's dog, questions of what the dog wants, or getting consent from the dog, are obviously out of place. What is relevant is helping the dog avoid misery.

If we turn from one's pet to an incompetent human being, it seems that here, too, questions of respecting autonomy are out of place. When a child does not want to go to the dentist, or wants to eat a pound of junk food, the responsible adult should not be concerned with respecting the child's "autonomy," since children are not competent to make their own decisions about such matters, but rather should do what is in their children's best interest. Likewise, those individuals who are not competent to make their own decisions need others to do what is in their best interest. Similarly, when it comes to active euthanasia of incompetent human beings, I believe that the primary concern needs to be with doing what is in the best interest of the patient.

Warren: I have a caution to offer. I have noticed that examples of euthanasia of pets are red flags to some critics of a liberal position on euthanasia. They say that promoters of euthanasia value human beings no more than dogs. It bears emphasis, then, that the point is to look at the reasons for mercy killing, not to compare the value of the lives of humans and dogs.

Doran: Point taken. Nonetheless, I always find that reply odd, since it is tempting to say, "You would do it for your dog—why wouldn't you do it for a person?" Why should someone who is supposedly worth more have to suffer in ways that we would not dream of making a dog suffer?

Patrick: A related point is that we agreed that VAE is morally permissible in certain cases. Given this, it is arguably unfair to make certain individuals suffer needlessly, simply because they are unable to give consent.

Doran: That's an excellent point, Patrick. Let's now get back to the best interest argument for NAE. My argument is as follows:

(1)   If an action is in an incompetent patient's best interest, is performed for that patient's sake, and neither violates anyone's rights nor sets back anyone's very important interests, then it is morally permissible.

(2)   NAE is in an incompetent patient's best interest, is performed for the sake of that patient, and, in some circumstances, neither violates anyone's rights nor sets back anyone's very important interests.

(3)   Therefore, in some cases, NAE is morally permissible.

Patrick: Let's consider what premises (1) and (2) imply with respect to the modified case of Tim Regan in which he left no advance directives and became mentally incompetent.

Warren: Euthanasia is performed for his sake. It is consistent with both his best interests and his rights. If he is suffering, it is in his best interest and it is his right to avoid pointless suffering. He also has an interest in and a right to dignity. But a dignified existence is not possible in his current condition. Euthanasia would serve his right to avoid indignity.

Doran: Yes, and given the sort of family he has, Tim Regan's euthanasia does not violate anyone else's rights or very important interests.

Patrick: Well, it seems in this modified case that NAE would be justified for Tim Regan, assuming he is suffering pointlessly. Though I am not sure it is fundamentally a matter of respecting rights, as Warren suggests. I believe a virtuous person would be moved by considerations of mercy and charity to do what Tim Regan is unable to do for himself—put an end to his pointless suffering and allow a more dignified death.

Warren: Before we move on, though, the critic might attack the second premise of Doran's argument, specifically the part that asserts the moral claim that NAE can be consistent with everyone's rights. For NAE involves killing patients without their consent, and surely that would violate their right to life.

Doran: In response to that objection, I would deny the claim that killing violates the patient's rights in justifiable cases of NAE. We must remember that rights exist to protect one's important interests, and these include autonomy interests as well as interests in not being harmed. But in cases of the incompetent, autonomy interests do not apply since incompetent individuals lack the capacity for autonomy. And while they certainly have an interest in not being harmed, this is, in fact, respected by NAE. This may be borne out by a straightforward analogy with the vaccination of a young child. We do not (and should not) say it violates her rights because she never consented, and we do say that it is in her interest in not being harmed since the painful poke protects her from contracting a much more serious setback to her well-being. Similarly, we should not say that NAE violates the rights of the incompetent patient since the patient never consented. Instead, we should say that NAE is justifiable if it is in the best interest of the patient, done for the sake of that patient, and neither violates anyone's rights nor sets back anyone's very important interests.

Patrick: So you agree, Doran, that incompetent individuals have a basic right to life. But you deny that the right is violated in cases where death is in the patient's best interest?

Doran: That is a fair way to put my point. The right to life protects individuals who have an interest in living. But in justifiable cases of NAE, the patients—tragically—do not have an interest in living.

Patrick: I agree with you that NAE is sometimes permissible, though my argument might look a little different from yours. As I suggested above, I believe it is primarily virtues such as compassion, charity, and so on that justify NAE in certain situations. There are, however, other virtue ethicists who would disagree with me—and with your argument. Philippa Foot is one.

Doran: Yes, let's consider Foot's view. Opponents to my argument must either reject my claim that NAE does not violate anyone's rights, or reject my claim that NAE is sometimes in the patient's best interest. Why don't we begin with an examination of Foot's objection? She claims that NAE violates the patient's right to life.

Philippa Foot's Objection to Non-Voluntary Active Euthanasia

Warren: Okay. Philippa Foot, a prominent virtue theorist, argues that NAE is unjust since it violates the right to life of the incompetent individual who is euthanized. Her argument is that we should assume that an act that infringes a right violates that right unless that right is positively waived, or unless we can assume that it would be waived. In the case of NAE, the patient has not waived her right to life (obviously). So the question is whether or not we can assume that the right would be waived. She says we can make this assumption when it comes to NPE (non-voluntary passive euthanasia) but not when it comes to NAE: this is because there is a widespread feeling in society that one would not want to be kept alive indefinitely when there is no hope for recovery, but there is no widespread consensus that people would want to be killed if they were in a hopeless condition. Thus, in the end, she supports the permissibility of NPE but opposes NAE, on the grounds that the latter (but not the former) violates the individual's right to life.[9]

Patrick: I think Foot is mistaken. We must show compassion and sympathy for the suffering of incompetent individuals. When it is clear that continued life is of no value, the compassionate thing to do is to end the suffering by ending the life. Moreover, as I suggested earlier, it may well be unjust, or unfair, *not* to perform NAE in certain cases. Both competent and incompetent individuals have an interest in avoiding pointless suffering and dying with dignity. Given this, it seems rather unfair to grant active euthanasia to the former but not the latter.

Doran: I believe Foot is mistaken, too. In general, I think it is a mistake to decide what is right (or wrong) by appealing to prevailing consensus. It is odd to think that whether NAE is justified or not depends on prevailing social mores. Why should it be wrong in Canada, but right in Holland, for instance? Such relativism seems problematic.

Moreover, I think we can understand, as I tried to explain above, why a right to life is not relevant when speaking of non-voluntary euthanasia. Here, the function of rights is to protect the person's interests in general, to protect autonomy, and to ensure that a person has the ability to make his own decisions in matters that intimately concern his life. But in cases of euthanasia, it is not in the interest of the person to continue to exist, and when considering those who are not competent there is no autonomy to protect and no decision-making capability to honour. Instead, what needs to be done is to do what is most merciful for the person whose life is in a hopeless condition.

 UP FOR DISCUSSION

Do you think that NAE violates the individual's right to life? Why or why not? Discuss the case of Hare's lorry driver when the driver is too overwhelmed by pain to competently request euthanasia but a bystander is moved by compassion to kill the driver.

Warren: I also reject Foot's view. In the original position, we would not want to be at the mercy of the majority in the real world. At the same time, we would recognize that if we were permanently disabled to the point of being unable to make a decision, we would want others to make decisions for us in our best interest. These interests should be judged, with notable and rare exceptions, from the viewpoint of the patient.

Doran: I am glad to hear, Warren, that your argument from the original position also supports the moral permissibility of some NAE. Likewise, I am pleased that Patrick's appeal to considerations of virtue also supports NAE. This is a very difficult issue, so it is good to know that there is more than one support for my conclusion.

The Never-Best-Interest Objection to Non-Voluntary Active Euthanasia

Patrick: Even if the critic accepts your first premise, Doran, there's room to argue that your second premise is false, by insisting that killing a person can never be in the best interest of that person. The underlying idea is that NAE is never in a person's best interest, because death removes all possibility of future benefit for the patient. In a sense, this is a concern for any kind of euthanasia, but it is a particular concern for non-voluntary cases. For, in such cases, the sole justification is an appeal to the best interest of the patient.

Warren: Right. When discussing this in class, students often bring up cases of so-called miraculous recoveries, where seemingly hopeless people turn out to have good lives.

Doran: Yes, but this line of objection is unsound. We certainly think that actively killing a dying pet can sometimes be in the pet's best interest. Further, it is reasonable to say, "It was for the best," when a loved one dies after enduring the end stages of terrible diseases like throat cancer. And finally, virtually everyone thinks it is sometimes in the best interest of a person to be allowed to die (VPE or NPE). So, it is difficult to see how one could plausibly deny that it could be in one's best interest to have that death brought about by active, quicker, less painful means.

Patrick: It would also be rather cruel to expect people to hold out for a miraculous recovery when they are suffering horribly and the likelihood of such a recovery is virtually nil.

Warren: I agree. To demonstrate that NAE could be in the best interest of the person, we could adapt Hare's example of the truck driver in the burning cab. Suppose the driver hit his head in the accident and is no longer competent to request death but is still conscious and dying in unbearable agony. It seems clear that it would be in his best interest to receive euthanasia in this case, and cruel to allow him to burn to death instead. It would also seem strange to suppose that VAE would be right in the original case and that NAE would be wrong in this case just because the driver cannot ask for death. While it is somewhat less obvious, I think the same sorts of things can be said about Tim Regan concerning the modified case where he is incompetent.

Patrick: I agree. The modified example of Hare's lorry driver pretty clearly shows, I believe, that it would be both cruel and unfair not to kill the driver simply because he cannot express a desire to be killed, when it is quite clear that that is what he'd want. The examples considered defeat the objection that NAE can never really be in the best interest of the patient, and support the view that NAE is at least sometimes permissible.

UP FOR DISCUSSION

Opponents of NAE often argue that it is wrong because it discriminates against incompetent humans. However, Patrick argues that not supporting NAE actually discriminates against those who are not competent. What do you think?

Doran: Nevertheless, there remain serious objections to *implementing* active euthanasia, both voluntary and non-voluntary. At present, active euthanasia is criminal in Canada when the patient is not competent (NAE). Even if a patient has left a clear advance directive when competent (a form of VAE by our definitions) the law forbids euthanasia. Perhaps there are good reasons for this? If that is the case, then even if we are right that some instances of VAE and NAE are morally permissible, it could still be the case that it ought to be legally impermissible to perform active euthanasia.

Patrick: Right. It does not follow from the fact that VAE and NAE are morally permissible that they should also be *legally* permissible. But the question of whether active euthanasia should be legalized is exceedingly complicated, so perhaps we ought to leave that debate for another time.

Doran: Agreed.

Warren: Well, this is a good beginning to a debate about the moral permissibility of various kinds of euthanasia that could go on a long way yet.

Doran: No doubt there is much more that can be said both for and against VAE and NAE, and the other kinds of euthanasia we didn't address in this chapter.

Patrick: Right. But let's call it a day.

SUMMARY

Here is a summary of the main questions, concepts, and arguments covered in this chapter:

- The main questions explored in this chapter are: When, if ever, is voluntary active euthanasia (VAE) morally permissible? And when, if ever, is non-voluntary active euthanasia (NAE) morally permissible? These questions are partly motivated by the VAE case of Tim Regan.

- Euthanasia is defined as an intentional act, or omission, that brings about the death of another individual for that individual's own health-related good.
- Active euthanasia is distinguished from passive euthanasia.
- Voluntary, non-voluntary, and involuntary euthanasia are distinguished.
- Doran, Patrick, and Warren agree that both VAE and NAE are morally permissible in some circumstances. They also agree that Dr. Buchman acted permissibly when he performed voluntary active euthanasia on Tim Regan.
- Doran initially presents the Autonomy and Best Interest argument *for* VAE, but Warren and Patrick show this argument to be unsound. In its place, Doran defends the Revised Autonomy and Best Interest argument.
- Various versions of the Sanctity of Life and God's Ownership arguments *against* VAE are considered and rejected.
- The Best Interest argument *for* NAE is presented and defended against objections.

REVIEW QUESTIONS

1. Why is the definition of *euthanasia* as "a good death" rejected? How, instead, do Doran, Patrick, and Warren finally define the term?
2. What are the six types of euthanasia? Give an example of each.
3. Explain the distinction between active and passive euthanasia.
4. Why is the initial statement of the Autonomy and Best Interest argument for VAE unsound?
5. Explain the Revised Autonomy and Best Interest argument.
6. Explain the Sanctity of Life objection and explain why this objection is rejected. What example does Warren give to show that it is sometimes morally permissible, and perhaps morally required, to kill an innocent human being intentionally?
7. Develop the argument that goes from the moral permissibility of some suicides to the moral permissibility of some cases of active euthanasia.
8. R. M. Hare's case of the petrol lorry driver is a counterexample to what principles?
9. Why do the normal explanations of the wrongness of killing fail to show that VAE is wrong?
10. What is the Best Interest argument for NAE?
11. Why does Philippa Foot think that NAE violates the right to life of the individual who is to be euthanized?
12. What responses do Doran, Warren, and Patrick each give to Foot's argument against NAE?
13. Why might a chooser of rules in the original position want to include some access to active euthanasia in the social contract?

NOTES

1. For a summary of Canadian law regarding euthanasia and assisted suicide, see the Government of Canada's publication, "Medical Assistance in Dying," at https://www.canada.ca/en/health-canada/services/medical-assistance-dying.html.

2. See the Government of Canada's "Interim Update on Medical Assistance in Dying in Canada, June 17 to December 31, 2016," at https://www.canada.ca/en/health-canada/services/publications/health-system-services/medical-assistance-dying-interim-report-dec-2016.html.

3. Dr. Brian Goldman, "Going Out with My Boots On: Tim Regan Used His Last Days to Lobby for a Clearer Path to Assisted Death," *White Coat, Black Art*, CBC Radio 1, January 18, 2018.

4. Doran's argumentative strategy for VAE is modelled on a similar set of arguments offered by James Rachels, "Euthanasia," in *Matters of Life and Death: New Introductory Essays in Moral Philosophy*, 3rd ed., ed. Tom Regan (New York: McGraw Hill, 1993).

5. Jeff McMahan, "From Suicide to Euthanasia," in *The Ethics of Killing: Problems at the Margins of Life* (New York: Oxford University Press, 2002).

6. R. M. Hare, *Essays on Religion and Education* (Oxford: Oxford University Press, 1998).

7. Patrick Nowell-Smith, "The Right to Die," in *Contemporary Moral Issues*, 3rd ed., ed. Wesley Cragg (Toronto: McGraw-Hill Ryerson, 1992), 8.

8. On this point, see Peter Singer, "Taking Life: Humans," in *Practical Ethics*, 2nd ed. (Cambridge: Cambridge University Press, 1993), 175–217. Also available online: http://www.utilitarian.net/singer/by/1993----.htm.

9. Philippa Foot, "Euthanasia," in *Virtues and Vices* (Oxford: Oxford University Press, 2002).

6 ABORTION

INTRODUCTION

The legal and moral status of **abortion** in Canada has been hotly debated for over a century, and abortion continues to be an emotional and divisive issue in Canadian society. In 1892, Canada's Parliament passed its first Criminal Code, which prohibited abortion (as well as the sale of contraceptives). This prohibition was relaxed in the late 1960s, when Pierre Trudeau's Liberal government permitted abortion in cases where pregnancy threatened the mother's life or health. In 1988, the Supreme Court of Canada struck down legal restrictions on abortion as unconstitutional. Chief Justice Brian Dickson stated: "Forcing a woman, by threat of criminal sanction to carry a fetus to term unless she meets certain criteria unrelated to her own priorities and aspirations, is a profound interference with a woman's body and thus a violation of her security of the person."[1] Although there is at present no law in Canada restricting abortion, many Canadians feel that some legal restrictions are called for, because they believe that abortion is a serious moral wrong, at least in certain circumstances.

In this chapter, we cast a critical eye on arguments both for and against the moral permissibility of abortion. Our drama presents the case of Marissa and Don, a couple who run a successful business they have started on their own. It takes much effort to keep going, but they have a good income from the business. Marissa is 38 and Don is 37, and they're expecting their first child. A series of routine blood and ultrasound tests determines that Marissa is at high risk to have a fetus with **Down's syndrome**. As our drama begins, Don and Marissa have just received confirmation from **amniocentesis** that the fetus Marissa is bearing does indeed have Down's. Don is initially in favour of having the child, while Marissa is very strongly in favour of aborting the fetus in order to protect their marriage and the business they have worked hard to build. In the end, Don concedes and accepts Marissa's choice for an abortion.

Our debate focuses on the question of whether abortion is morally permissible in this case. Marissa's life is not endangered by the pregnancy, but she sees abortion as necessary in order to protect important relationships and projects. We agree that Marissa's abortion is morally permissible, although it turns out that we have very different reasons

DEFINITION

"**Down syndrome** (or **Down's syndrome**) describes a set of cognitive and physical symptoms that result from an extra copy or part of a copy of chromosome 21.... The extra chromosome disrupts the normal course of development and results in the physical features and intellectual and developmental disabilities associated with the syndrome.

"The degree of intellectual disability in people with Down syndrome varies but is usually mild to moderate. Generally, children with Down syndrome reach key developmental milestones later than other children. People with the syndrome also are more likely to be born with heart abnormalities, and they are at increased risk for developing hearing and vision problems, Alzheimer disease, and other conditions. However, with appropriate support and treatment, many people with Down syndrome lead happy, productive lives. In recent decades, life expectancy for people with Down syndrome has increased dramatically, from 25 years in 1983 to 60 years today."

Source: "Down Syndrome: Condition Information," *National Institutes of Health*, https://www.nichd.nih.gov/health/topics/down/conditioninfo.

Amniocentesis is a prenatal diagnostic procedure performed in order to detect fetal abnormalities. A needle is used to remove a sample of the amniotic fluid surrounding the fetus. The amniotic fluid contains skin cells from the fetus, which are analyzed to determine potential problems with the fetus.

in support of our common conclusion. Before we each present our own arguments, we examine several **conservative** arguments against abortion that imply that it would be morally wrong to have an abortion in Marissa and Don's situation. We explain why we think these arguments are unsound. Patrick then argues that the moral status of abortion cannot be settled just by considering the issue of whose rights trump whose; instead, we must reflect on whether having an abortion is consistent with acting virtuously, where this includes more than respecting rights. Importantly, Patrick argues that even if the fetus has a right to life, it would still be morally permissible to abort it in certain situations, including Marissa and Don's. A virtuous person, Patrick goes on to argue, would view abortion as a morally difficult matter, an act that requires good reasons in order to be justified, reasons that are present in Marissa and Don's case. Doran argues that a 16-week-old fetus lacks the right to life, and so Marissa has the right to control her body. Unlike Patrick, Doran thinks that early abortions (in normal circumstances) are morally permissible regardless of the pregnant woman's reasons. Warren reaches the conclusion that Marissa's abortion is permissible by applying his social contract theory. He thinks that a woman's right to autonomy renders abortions at early stages (in normal circumstances) morally permissible in most cases.

LEARNING OBJECTIVES

After completing this chapter, you should be able to:

- Explain and evaluate some important conservative arguments against abortion
- Understand Patrick's reasons for thinking that abortion is morally permissible in this case
- Describe the reasons why Warren and Doran disagree with Patrick's argument
- Explain Doran's argument for the moral permissibility of Marissa's abortion
- Discuss Patrick and Warren's reasons for rejecting Doran's argument
- Defend your own view on the morality of abortion, in general, and the morality of abortion in Marissa and Don's situation, in particular

DRAMA

Please note: This case is based on various true stories, although names, places, and some uncontroversial elements of the case have been changed to preserve anonymity and confidentiality. Discussions of this and similar cases with health care professionals have also informed this fictional case. The drama merely raises issues. The philosophical arguments are to be found in the debate following the drama.

CHARACTERS

Don: 37 years old, a businessman, married to Marissa

Marissa: 38 years old, a business-woman, married to Don

Don: I can't believe it. I hoped right up to the last moment it would be okay.

Marissa: Honey, we'll try again. Everything will work out next time. At least we know about this early.

Don: It doesn't feel that way to me, Marissa. For 16 weeks this child has been growing inside you. I feel like I need to protect her.

Marissa: It must be so hard for you, Don. You see yourself as the protector. This decision is awful. But Don, that's why we had the tests, so we wouldn't have a child with … problems. It's too hard to do. Look at Lawrence and Anne. They tried to tough it out and now I hear they're splitting up. It's too much. Everything changes. If we had a child like that, you couldn't work like you do now. We couldn't keep the house. Everything would be so different, but it doesn't have to be that way. We can try again. We can have a normal child. Don, Don—look at me. We can. That's why we had the tests, isn't it? Isn't it, Don?

Don: I guess. Still, it's different when it's real like this. When we were told to get the tests it was just something like a worry in the back of my mind. It wasn't going to happen to us. I don't know. Maybe I'm not as tough as I thought I was. Maybe I never really thought it through. It just isn't that easy. I care about her now, Marissa. She wasn't real to me then.

Marissa: Love, I know you're a strong and caring man. That's part of what I love about you. But you've got drive too. You're happy when you're creating our future in our company. You love our house and the kind of life we have now. We don't have to throw that all away. We don't have to. We have options. We can have it all, but not if we continue this pregnancy. Look, I talked to Lawrence yesterday, and he was really bitter. Anne is exhausted. It takes so much work to raise a child with Down's, and the work is never-ending. The government help they thought they could get never seems to materialize. They've already burned through all their savings. I think of Lawrence and Anne, and it gets me.

Don: But maybe it won't be that bad. Lawrence and Anne's son is particularly low functioning. The doctor says there's a huge variation in Down's. Maybe she'll be really high functioning.

Marissa: Sweetheart, I can see how you're torn by this. But think about what you're saying. High functioning! Is that what we want to hear about our kid? I can't bear the thought of it. We want a daughter who will go to university some day, who will be independent and able to lead a normal life.

Don: But there are families with kids like this who are so loved and it isn't all bad, honey. We don't know what it might be like. She doesn't have any really severe physical things showing up on ultrasound. Maybe she won't be so badly off mentally, either. We don't know what we can do until we try.

Marissa: Love is what moves you now, but I don't want a life of sacrifice just because of the feelings that move you for a while. You're the one who is always so bugged by uncertainty. You've stopped us from taking risks time and time again because things were too unpredictable. What's different now? Only that we are betting our whole way of life, and the odds are terrible. Don't do this to yourself. Don't do this to us, honey. Please don't.

Don: Take it slow. We don't have to decide this minute.

Marissa: You're right. We have to be careful and deliberate about this. Still, I want to talk about something else. Nobody would be patting us on the back saying how heroic we are for doing this. Look at Anne and Lawrence. They come in for some really tough criticism behind their backs. People say they got themselves into this. It's like they're letting the side down. They didn't have to have a child that would be a drain on them and everyone. You know we both felt they shouldn't have done it.

Don: I feel guilty for that now. There are lots of ways kids give back to their parents, and they aren't all money or appreciation or gaining fame as a feminist. I've read that people with Down's syndrome can be poets and painters, they are mostly happy people, and so emotionally intelligent. We are all differently abled. Give her a chance.

Marissa: Oh honey, don't feel guilty. You were right when you said Anne shouldn't have gone through with it. It's not fair to the kid or anyone to have a kid like that when you can *avoid* it. That's why society supports the whole medical thing with tests and ways of dealing with it when things go wrong.

Don: Just call it what it is—abortion. We want to kill someone here.

Marissa: Okay, it's abortion we're talking about, and that's not a bad thing. There's a fetus that could become someone, but it's not someone yet. Abortion gives us much better options than we would have otherwise. I just don't want you to blame yourself. Someday we're going to be celebrating our child graduating, not celebrating her learning to feed herself when she should be graduating. We've planned our lives. We've had a real curve thrown at us, but we're not out yet. There's nothing wrong with abortion to do something good for ourselves and everybody. There's nothing wrong at all. We have a choice, and that's a good thing.

Don: I'm not saying abortion has to be wrong, but it isn't wrong to have the child either. It may be a very good thing to do. Maybe it's a good thing just because she would be helpless and we are strong and can take care of her. Maybe that's not such a bad life.

Marissa: It is for me. I look at Anne and Lawrence, and I say, "Not me." Maybe it's my weakness, but it's tough enough being a parent without that extra challenge. I want a strong, independent daughter. I can't do this. Maybe it seems right for you now, but please, please think about what you would have to give up.

Don: What are you saying, Marissa? Your body, your choice? Or is it just that you want this child but you are afraid of the challenge? I swear I would take on the child care while you ran the business.

Marissa: Don, I don't want to do this. I really don't. And you know you're essential to our work. I don't think deliberately having a wounded child is right either, not just wrong for us but plain wrong. Do you remember that deaf couple that deliberately had a deaf child? We were sure they shouldn't do that, weren't we? I'm still sure.

Don: Everyone should have a chance, including those who are disabled, but I can't make you keep her, Marissa. We can't keep her. Even if you tried, you'd be resentful. You wouldn't be in it. It would be hopeless. I can't fight you on this, Marissa. All I can do is cry.

DEBATE

Clarifying the Case and Identifying Relevant Facts

Doran: Okay, so Don and Marissa are trying to decide whether or not to abort given that their fetus has Down's. Marissa is unwilling to take on the rigours of parenting a child with Down's. She considered another family's difficulties with raising a disabled child and is unwilling to live like that.

Warren: Marissa is also very concerned that their lifestyle would be drastically altered if they had a disabled child. Don is willing to raise a child with Down's, but realizes that it will probably break up the marriage. In the end, he gives in, accepting abortion reluctantly.

Patrick: It is not just the marriage and their lifestyle—they have built a business, and it requires their constant concern, but Don is uncertain, as he has bonded emotionally with the fetus.

Warren: Yes.

Patrick: Do we know how long Don and Marissa have been together, and how solid their relationship is?

Warren: They have been together two years.

Patrick: And we can assume that their relationship is strong?

Warren: They have bought a house and built a business together. They are pretty solid, but cracks are showing over the abortion decision.

Doran: I think we can assume their relationship is solid, but Marissa is clearly telling Don that it would destroy the relationship if they chose to have the disabled child. For her, that was understood from the start. Marissa says that this is why they did genetic testing in the first place.

Patrick: If they have the baby, is that the end of their business? They can't have both?

Warren: Yes, it takes two people to manage the business. Marissa could not do it if Don was dealing with a child full-time indefinitely.

Patrick: Could she not get someone else in to help run the business? Or is Don himself needed?

Warren: Like most family businesses, it requires more work than a business partner would normally commit to. Marissa can't see how to keep the business without Don.

Patrick: How far along in the pregnancy was Marissa when the abortion was performed?

Warren: At the end of the case it has not yet been performed. It is just after the amniocentesis at 16 weeks.

Patrick: What is the level of fetal development at 16 weeks?

Warren: At 12 to 16 weeks from the last menstrual period, quickening occurs. The mother feels the **fetus** moving within her. At 26 weeks the length is about 18 centimetres.

Doran: The fetus's development is in that middling range—it is not a **zygote** or an **embryo**, it has a brain and functioning nervous system, but it is not yet conscious. It is also incapable of surviving on its own, since vital organs, like lungs, are not yet formed.

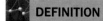

> **DEFINITION**
>
> A **zygote** is a single diploid cell that results from the merging of a sperm and ovum through a process of fertilization. The developing organism, from the moment of conception until about the end of the eighth week, is called an **embryo**. From that point until birth it is called a **fetus**.

Patrick: So I take it the fetus is unable to feel pain at 16 weeks.

Warren: It is very unlikely that the fetus is able to feel pain at that stage. Studies show that the fetus may respond to painful stimuli by around 16 weeks, but doctors generally believe that this is simply an unconscious response to the stimuli. Conscious awareness of pain requires neural connections that do not form until the third trimester.

Patrick: Interesting. So the fetus may be able to respond to painful stimuli at 16 weeks, even though it does not *feel* pain.

Warren: Yes, that's right. The fetus's withdrawal response is controlled by lower brain structures that have formed by 16 to 20 weeks. But the neural pathways required for the *perception* of pain are not developed until 23 to 30 weeks.[2]

> **UP FOR DISCUSSION**
>
> On what basis can one determine whether another individual is conscious? Using those criteria, how confident can we be that a 16-week-old fetus is or is not conscious?

Patrick: Okay. If Marissa does not abort, do we know, or have any reasonable idea of, how serious their child's mental disability will be?

Warren: One cannot tell in advance. The Down's syndrome is evident, but it can be very severe or produce a high-functioning Down's child or anything in between.

Patrick: So there's a range of possible disabilities. If their child was born with severe disabilities, couldn't they put the child up for adoption?

Warren: Don would not do this. As for Marissa, she may also have been concerned that her child would not be adopted, given that she believes it can be difficult to find homes for children with Down's and other disabilities.

Patrick: Okay, I see. So, formally, it may be an option, but it's unrealistic to think Don could do that, and Marissa would not risk trying it.

Warren: Yes.

Patrick: This case, like the others, raises a number of difficult moral questions. Why don't we now decide which of these we want to debate?

MORAL ISSUES RAISED BY THE CASE

Warren: The central question is whether it is morally permissible for Marissa and Don to obtain an abortion. And more generally, when, if ever, abortion is morally wrong.

Doran: It's odd to speak of Marissa *and Don* obtaining an abortion. We have to recognize that it's her body. She is the one who would have the abortion. So it seems to me the central question is whether it is morally permissible for Marissa to obtain an abortion.

Patrick: That seems right, Doran. But the decision to abort is one they are making together. Don is on the hook here, too!

Warren: Agreed. My point was to recognize shared responsibility. Don shares some responsibility. At the same time, your point has merit, Doran.

Patrick: Let's just follow Doran's usage throughout, but announce that we think Don shares responsibility for the pregnancy, and therefore for the abortion.

Warren: Good. So, what do you guys think? Is it morally permissible for Marissa to obtain an abortion in this situation?

Stating Our Positions

Doran: I believe it is morally permissible for Marissa to obtain an abortion. I believe this because I believe that the fetus, at this stage of development, does not have a moral right to life. The woman's right to control what happens in and to her body should prevail.

Warren: I agree that it is morally permissible to have an abortion in this case. My reason is that this is in accord with rules we would choose if we were in the original position. In the original position we would have a difficult choice. On the one hand, we would not want to be forced to use our bodies or other resources to bear, have, and raise a child who might present us with great difficulties and require heavy sacrifices. On the other hand, sympathy, among other considerations, would inhibit us from making rules that treat the fetus as having no value. I come down, ultimately, on the side of the right of the woman to choose.

> **UP FOR DISCUSSION**
>
> Opponents of abortion think that social contract theory stacks the deck against their view because people in the original position know they are rational beings. They cannot be fetuses. They cannot be the victims of abortion in the real world. Is this a reasonable objection to social contract theory? Can you think of a reply?

Patrick: This is a very difficult case, but I agree with you two that it would be permissible to abort, though I agree for different reasons. From my virtue ethics perspective, I don't think the moral status of having an abortion can be settled just by looking at the rights possessed by the fetus and the mother (and father). For even if Marissa has a right to control her body, abortion may still be wrong. And even if her fetus has a right to life, this abortion may still be permissible. To determine whether this abortion is wrong, we need to consider whether Don and Marissa's reasons for aborting manifest vices. We need to consider, for instance, whether having an abortion would exhibit cruelty, selfishness, injustice, and so on. All things considered, I conclude—though somewhat tentatively—that having an abortion in this case would not be vicious, and hence, not wrong.

Warren: Your approach sounds interesting, Patrick. Why don't we proceed as follows? Let's first consider some important arguments *against* the morality of abortion.

Since none of us accepts these arguments, we should first raise them and explain why we think they fail. We can then turn to Patrick's virtue-based argument and see whether we accept his argument as sound. If disagreement persists between us, perhaps we can also look at Doran's pro-choice argument on abortion and see if it is any more conclusive.

UP FOR DISCUSSION

What do you think? Is it morally permissible for Marissa to have an abortion? Why or why not?

Patrick: Sure.

Doran: That sounds like a good plan.

LEADING ARGUMENTS AGAINST THE MORALITY OF ABORTION

Doran: Many conservatives—those who generally oppose abortion—claim that abortion is wrong in all, or virtually all, cases. This is because they believe that it involves the unjust or wrongful killing of the fetus.

Patrick: Right. But conservatives have different, sometimes *quite* different, reasons for thinking this.

Warren: Let's consider some of their reasons.

Noonan's Argument

Doran: We cannot consider all of their arguments, but let's look at some of the most influential. For instance, John T. Noonan, in his widely read paper on abortion, argues as follows:[3]

(1) Any being with human **genetic code** is a human.
(2) Fetuses receive human genetic code at conception.
(3) Therefore, fetuses are human at conception.
(4) Being human (i.e., having the right genetic code) is sufficient for having moral rights, including a right to life.
(5) So, fetuses have moral rights from conception.
(6) It is, presumptively, seriously immoral to kill a being that has moral rights.
(7) Therefore, abortion is, presumptively, seriously immoral from conception.

Warren: Yes, that seems to be his argument, although your description of the argument contains premises that he does not explicitly state. For instance, he never explicitly states premise (4), that being genetically human is sufficient for having moral rights; however, it is quite clear that premise (4) is implicit in his argument. Noonan focuses much of his energy on supporting premise (1). Specifically, he gives a couple of reasons why he thinks that having a human genetic code is sufficient for something to be a human being. First, by maintaining that all who have human genetic code are human, he thinks we will guard against the tendency to discriminate against some on the basis of their abilities, or lack of abilities. Secondly, he thinks that genetic humanity—what we might now call human DNA—is morally significant since it is the material that is the "biological carrier of human wisdom."

> **TECHNIQUE**
>
> Students of logic will see that this is an argument in the broad sense, sometimes referred to as a derivation. An argument in the narrower sense has only one conclusion. Here a series of arguments is used to derive a final conclusion using earlier conclusions in the derivation as premises.

Patrick: And I take it he maintains that it is only *presumptively* seriously immoral to kill a human being because he wants to allow for the possibility that killing in self-defence, or perhaps applying the death penalty, may be morally permissible.

Doran: Yes, that's right. He maintains that intentionally killing an innocent human being can *very* rarely be justified. When it comes to abortion, he appears willing to recognize its permissibility only when necessary to save the pregnant woman's life.[4]

> **UP FOR DISCUSSION**
>
> Suppose a woman discovers that the child she is carrying has a serious disease such that the child's life is likely to contain much more pain than pleasure. Noonan's view seems to imply that having an abortion in this situation would be wrong. Do you agree? Why or why not?

Warren: So he would certainly contend that it is wrong for Marissa and Don to procure an abortion.

Patrick: Right. This is an interesting argument, but I believe it fails.

Evaluating Premise (1) of Noonan's Argument

Patrick: Premise (1), which states that any being with human genetic code is a human, looks especially suspicious. Non-humans can have human genetic code.

Doran: I agree. Cattle are sometimes injected with human genetic code to make their milk more digestible, but the mere fact that they have this genetic code does not make them human. Likewise, pigs are sometimes injected with human DNA so they can grow tissue that can be transplanted to humans, yet we would not call these pigs human.

Warren: These counterexamples might not be persuasive. For Noonan might say that individuals that have *only* human DNA are human. The cattle and pigs you mentioned do not have all and *only* the human genetic code, so they need not be viewed as human in this interpretation of his premise.

Patrick: Yes, I suppose that is the charitable way to interpret Noonan.

Doran: But I don't think this interpretation of his premise will help his argument very much, for it, too, is vulnerable to clear counterexamples.

Warren: That's true: some human cells have all, and only, human DNA, but we do not consider human cells to be human beings.

Doran: I agree that it is implausible to think that the mere possession of all and only human DNA is sufficient for being human. To see this, consider some analogies: Think of an acorn. It has the DNA of an oak tree, yet no one would consider an acorn to be an oak tree, merely in virtue of the fact that they share the same DNA. Likewise, imagine you come over for breakfast and I serve you an omelet.

> **TECHNIQUE**
>
> Warren is employing a methodological principle called **the principle of charity**. This principle instructs us to interpret an author's claims and arguments in the best possible light. The general aim is to arrive at a fair and sympathetic understanding of the author's position in order to critically evaluate it. In this case, Noonan appears to be relying on a premise that is clearly false. The principle of charity requires that we try to find a more plausible understanding of his premise. Employing the principle here will help Warren, Doran, and Patrick avoid making weak criticisms that Noonan could easily escape by a more careful statement of the premise in question.

You say that the eggs are delicious. I, however, correct you. I point out that the eggs you're eating were fertilized. Thus, what you are eating are (three) chickens! Surely this would strike you as absurd. Similarly, it seems absurd to suggest that a one-celled organism could be a human being, merely because it happened to contain all and only human DNA. At best, such an organism has the potential to become a human being, but it is not one yet!

Patrick: Right, and further, possessing all and only human DNA is not even *necessary* for being a human being. To see this, consider **xenotransplantation**—the transplantation of non-human organs into humans. If I received, say, a heart valve from a pig, then I would not have all and only human DNA. So the modified premise would then imply that I ceased to be human!

Warren: It appears, then, that premise (1) in Noonan's argument, whichever way it is interpreted, is quite clearly false.

> **UP FOR DISCUSSION**
>
> Do you see a way of defending Noonan's claim that a being with human DNA is a human being? Can you think of other objections to this premise?

Evaluating Premise (4) of Noonan's Argument

Warren: Interestingly, even if we grant Noonan's claim that one is in some sense human in virtue of possessing human genetic code, I think Noonan's argument is still in trouble, since premise (4) looks dubious.

Doran: I agree. Premise (4) says that being human is sufficient for having rights. This is dubious because if we really think that human DNA is sufficient to make one human as is claimed in premise (1), then we would also have to say that having human DNA is sufficient for having rights. But that seems much too strong. As Warren noted previously, many human cells have all and only human DNA, but we do not grant individual human cells human rights. Similarly, the process of IVF (in vitro fertilization) requires the creation and subsequent loss of many human fertilized ova, but it seems to be mistaken to regard this process as one that involves mass manslaughter.

 UP FOR DISCUSSION

Do you think that the possession of human genetic code ought to give a being moral rights? Do you agree that those who think human genetic code is sufficient for moral rights ought to oppose IVF, insofar as IVF results in the creation and death of large numbers of fertilized human ova?

Marquis's Argument for the Wrongfulness of Abortion

Warren: Given the many problems with claiming that the possession of human DNA is sufficient for being human, or being a rights holder, some conservatives on the abortion issue give rather different reasons for their opposition to abortion. One of the most interesting is an argument by Don Marquis:[5]

(1) It is, presumptively, seriously immoral to kill you and me because it deprives us of a future of value.

(2) In standard cases of abortion, abortion deprives the fetus of a future of value—a future like ours.

(3) Therefore, standard cases of abortion are, presumptively, seriously immoral.

The novelty of Marquis's argument is that he is not claiming that fetuses are human or that they have rights, and so forth; instead, he asks a different question. Why is it wrong to kill you or me? After identifying a principal reason why it is wrong to kill you or me, he then says that this reason also applies to the killing of fetuses—so it is wrong too, and for the same reason.[6]

Patrick: So Marquis's view is that the principal reason it is presumptively seriously wrong to kill you or me is because it prevents you or me from having a future of value. And that since fetuses (in standard cases) are individuals with a future like ours (i.e., futures of value), he concludes it is also presumptively seriously wrong to kill fetuses.

Doran: Yes, that's the basic idea. Marquis thinks it is wrong to kill us because it robs us of our valuable future. That is, it robs us of experiences, activities, and so on that we value now and would have come to enjoy in the future. And so he would say that Marissa's abortion is morally wrong for the same reason that killing one of us is wrong—it robs one of a valuable future.

 UP FOR DISCUSSION

Would an act utilitarian agree with Marquis's account of why aborting a fetus in a normal pregnancy is morally wrong? Why or why not?

Evaluating Premise (2) of Marquis's Argument

Patrick: When discussing this argument in class, my students often target premise (2). They reject the premise that, in standard cases of abortion, the fetus is deprived of a future of value. They suggest that children that are unwanted are not likely to have good futures. But this objection is rather weak.

Doran: Yes, this objection seems wrong to me, or at least exaggerated. Often, indeed probably most of the time, even if a child is unwanted, it is doubtful that her future would be so bad that it would be not worth living! As a case in point, it is doubtful that if Marissa

were to continue with the pregnancy, their child's life would be so bad as to be not worth living. We would be unlikely to think, once the child was born, that it would be a blessing for the child if she were to die prematurely.

Evaluating Premise (1) of Marquis's Argument: The Contraception Objection

Warren: Okay, then, if one is to reject Marquis's argument, it seems that one needs to question his first premise. Has he identified a reason that is sufficient for making killing someone immoral, namely, that it causes the individual the loss of a future like ours?

Doran: There is reason to suspect not. First, if we accepted premise (1), it seems that it would imply that contraception is immoral, since it seems that contraception also prevents a future of value. Of course, contraception is not immoral, so premise (1) must be rejected.[7]

Warren: Marquis, however, denies that his premise entails that contraception is seriously immoral, for he claims that prior to implantation, there is not yet an individual that exists who has a possible future of value. He never says it is wrong to prevent potential individuals from existing who will then have futures of value; rather, he says it is wrong to prevent individuals who already exist from having futures of value.

Patrick: Well, to make this sort of reply, I think Marquis owes us an account of what constitutes an *individual* in the relevant sense. Sperm and ova are not individuals, in his view, but a zygote is? Why? This is not an easy question to answer.

Warren: The response might be that the zygote or embryo will develop into a human being who could be a person unless it is prevented from doing so, while the sperm or ovum, left alone, will not do so. That, however, is weak.

Patrick: Yes, it is weak. We use contraceptives to prevent sperm and ova from developing into human beings. And nobody would say, moreover, after reflecting on the care needed for a successful pregnancy, that the fetus is simply left alone for a human being to emerge.

Warren: Yes, the enormous contribution of the mother seems typically forgotten in such arguments.[8]

Patrick: As you noted earlier, Warren, the novelty of Marquis's argument is, in part, that it does not rely on the premise that the fetus is a human, or a being with rights. But his notion of an "individual" is equally problematic.

Challenging the Logical Validity of Marquis's Argument: The Equivocation Objection

Doran: Well, I agree with your points, but I want to add the following even stronger objection. As we have seen, Marquis argues:

(1)   It is seriously immoral to cause the loss of a future of value.
(2)   In standard cases, fetuses are caused the loss of a future of value when aborted.
(3)   Therefore, in standard cases abortion is seriously immoral.

But one might object that this argument commits the **fallacy** of **equivocation**.[9] Specifically, the phrase "cause the loss of" is ambiguous—it has more than one meaning.

To see this, consider some uses of the phrase "cause the loss of":

DEFINITION

To commit the **fallacy** of **equivocation** is to use a term in two different senses so as to make an **argument** that is not valid appear valid.

Case 1. Patrick and I run a race. Patrick loses because I outrun him. I *cause the loss of* something of value for Patrick, namely, his winning of the trophy.
Case 2. Patrick and I run a race. Patrick loses because I tied his shoelaces together before the starting gun went off. I *cause the loss of* something of value for Patrick, namely, his winning of the trophy.

Now, in the first and second cases, I caused the loss of something of value. But only in the second case is the cause of the loss morally problematic. Let's consider a couple more examples:

Case 1. I am *caused the loss of* much happiness because Patrick gets a job that I dearly wanted after we both applied for it.
Case 2. I am *caused the loss of* much happiness because Patrick gets a job that I dearly wanted after we both applied for it, but he got it because he sabotaged my resumé.

Case 1. Your landlord does not renew your lease, *causing you the loss of* your beloved apartment.
Case 2. Your landlord does not renew your lease, *causing you the loss of* your beloved apartment, even though she had promised you that she would renew your lease.

In each of these cases, a loss of something of value is caused. But only in case 2 is the causing of the loss morally objectionable.

Thus, we might distinguish *neutral losses* from *moral losses*. Both neutral losses and moral losses involve causing the loss of something of value. They differ only in that it is not wrong to cause neutral losses, while it is wrong to cause moral losses.

Warren: So, Doran, what, in your view, makes it wrong to cause a moral loss and not wrong to cause a neutral loss?

Doran: It appears that the moral loss involves a violation of someone's rights or involves some unfairness, while the neutral loss cases do not involve violations of rights or any unfairness. This is confirmed by each of the cases above. It is not morally objectionable if I beat Patrick in a race, or if he beats me in a competition for a job, if we both fairly competed, but it becomes morally objectionable when one of us acts in ways that make the competition unfair. Similarly, the landlord's decision not to renew your lease seems only to be wrong in the second case, where she violates her duty to you to keep her promise to renew the lease.

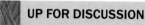

UP FOR DISCUSSION

Natural advantages might be unfair, too, since it is a matter of luck whether one has good genes. For example, is it fair if Doran beats Patrick in a race because he has superior natural athletic ability?

Warren: Okay, with this distinction between neutral losses and moral losses in mind, I'm sure you can generate problems for Marquis's argument.

Doran: That's right. Premise (1), which states that it's wrong to cause the loss of a valuable future, is true only if a moral loss is intended. But then for the argument to be valid, premise (2), which states that abortion causes the fetus the loss of a valuable future, would also have to be read as a moral loss. However, Marquis **begs the question** if he merely assumes that abortion causes a moral loss. He could only do that if he assumes that fetuses have a right to their futures, or that it was somehow unfair to the fetus to abort it, but Marquis never proves that such rights are violated or that it is somehow unfair. Indeed, it is precisely the issue of whether fetuses have rights that he hopes to avoid by giving his future-like-ours argument.

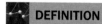

DEFINITION

To **beg the question** is to presuppose what you want to prove. See **circularity** in chapter 1.

Patrick: Of course, Marquis could instead argue that abortion causes a neutral loss. This would be true, in standard cases, but this, of course, wouldn't help his argument much.

Doran: That's right, because if he used neutral loss in premise (2), he'd then have to use neutral loss in premise (1)—and that would make premise (1) false, for as we have seen, it is not wrong to cause merely neutral losses.

Thus, I think Marquis's argument fails because of the fallacy of equivocation. He uses the phrase "cause the loss of" with two very different meanings.

In order for his argument to succeed, he first needs to show that fetuses have a right to their futures, and then that this right is violated if the pregnant woman obtains an abortion, but these are precisely the issues that he had hoped to sidestep.

The Argument That This Abortion Discriminates against the Disabled

Doran: Some might agree with us that these arguments are unsound, and that abortion is sometimes morally permissible, yet still object to abortion in this particular case.

Warren: Why is that? What's the objection you have in mind here, Doran?

Doran: Well, the couple in this case are seeking an abortion because the fetus has a disability. They would not abort if their child were going to be "normal." But because their fetus has Down's, they have chosen to abort. So, the objection is that their choice to abort discriminates against the disabled.

Warren: So I take it the argument would go something like this:

(1) It is wrong to discriminate on grounds of disability.
(2) Abortion in this case discriminates on grounds of disability.
(3) Therefore, abortion in this case is wrong.

Doran: That looks right, Warren.

Warren: What do you guys think about the argument?

Doran: Premise (1) claims that it is wrong to discriminate on grounds of disability; however, discrimination for reasons of sex, race, disability, and so on is not always wrong. For instance, if one were casting for the part of Martin Luther King in a play, it would not be wrong to favour black actors over non-black actors.

Patrick: Agreed. And it would not be wrong to discriminate against the blind, for example, if one were interviewing candidates for occupations that require excellent vision—a commercial airline pilot, for example.

Doran: Discrimination is not wrong in these cases, I believe, because it is not *unjust* discrimination. It is not depriving the individuals discriminated against of anything they have a right to.

Warren: Do you think discrimination is unjust, Doran, only when it violates rights? If an act of discrimination didn't violate anyone's rights, but caused serious harm to a person, that could also be unjust, couldn't it?

Doran: Yes, that sounds right.

Patrick: It seems to me that discrimination can be wrong, even when it is not unjust in the sense of violating anyone's rights or seriously harming them. For example, suppose Smith allows most of his neighbours to borrow his garden tools now and then. But suppose Smith does not allow his neighbour Jones to borrow his tools, simply because Jones is black. Now, none of the neighbours has a right to use Smith's garden tools, nor would they be seriously harmed by Smith's refusing to let them use his tools. So there's no injustice here. Still, Smith's discriminating against Jones in this case seems wrong. For Smith is refusing to provide a benefit to Jones that he generously provides to his other neighbours, simply because Jones is black.

Warren: So discrimination is certainly wrong when it is unjust, as Doran argues. But it can also be wrong for other reasons that don't involve violating people's rights or causing serious harm. What seems to make acts of discrimination wrong, when they are wrong, is that they discriminate on the basis of reasons—race, sex, disability, and so on—that are not morally relevant, or relevant but not sufficient to justify the action.

Patrick: Agreed. Whether or not one can see *is* relevant to whether one is qualified to be a commercial airline pilot. So discriminating against the blind is not wrong in that sort of case. But whether one is physically disabled is *not* relevant to whether one can hold public office, for instance. So, in that sort of case discrimination on grounds of disability would be wrong.

Warren: Since discrimination on grounds of disability is not always wrong, it looks like premise (1) is false. It should be revised to say: It is wrong to discriminate on grounds of disability, *where disability is not a morally relevant or sufficient consideration.*

Patrick: If disability is not a morally relevant consideration, then, of course, it cannot be a morally sufficient consideration—a consideration that justifies the discrimination. So premise (1) could simply say: It is wrong to discriminate on grounds of disability, *where disability is not a morally sufficient consideration.*

Doran: Right. But then premise (2) must also be revised in a similar way, otherwise the argument would be guilty of equivocation and therefore invalid. Premise (2) must be read as asserting that abortion in this case discriminates on grounds of disability, *where disability is not a morally sufficient consideration.*

Warren: When revised in this way, premise (2) is true only if the following two claims are true: (i) Abortion in this case discriminates against the disabled, and (ii) disability is not, in this case, a morally sufficient reason.

Patrick: I assume you think the fetus's disability is a morally sufficient consideration in this case, Doran, because of the negative impact the raising of a disabled child would have on Don and Marissa's business and marriage.

Doran: Yes, that's part of the reason.

Patrick: Marriage is an important good, likely the most important good, in the couple's lives. And they have invested considerable time and money building a business together. If having a disabled child threatens these goods, then this fact may be sufficient to justify the abortion.

Warren: So the two of you argue that premise (2) is false, because if this particular abortion discriminates against disabled people as a class, it does so for reasons that morally justify the discrimination.

Patrick: Right.

Warren: There's another way of thinking about this argument that we should consider. We've been focusing on the question of whether the couple's abortion wrongfully discriminates against disabled people as a class. But "pro-life" conservatives would object that abortion in this case discriminates *against this particular fetus* for reasons that are not morally sufficient. The fetus has a right to life, they would argue, whether or not it is disabled. So, since Don and Marissa are aborting the fetus *because* it is disabled, the couple is discriminating against the fetus by violating its right to life for reasons that are not morally sufficient to justify their actions.

Doran: This reading of premise (2) assumes that the fetus has rights. I would deny this. In my view, only beings with the capacity for consciousness have rights. Since Don and Marissa's 16-week-old fetus lacks this capacity, it does not have a right to life. So their abortion does not unjustly discriminate against their fetus.

Warren: Rather than focusing on consciousness only, I would argue for a larger set of capacities as essential to persons, so the woman's rights would all the more outweigh those of the fetus, who is human but not yet a person.[10] Persons in the original position would, moreover, be ignorant of their features in the real world, including gender. Among the rules they would approve would be a strong rule against using, without consent, another person's body. This would protect their interests by providing a strong right of bodily integrity that would prevent a woman from being required to continue a pregnancy. Knowing how vulnerable women may be in the real world, but not knowing if they themselves are women behind a veil of ignorance, the choosers of rules would be motivated to accept this strong right to bodily integrity—so the decision to end or carry on her pregnancy rests with Marissa.

Patrick: Even if we grant that all fetuses, disabled or not, have a right to life, it's not obvious to me that aborting on grounds of disability would be wrong. Disability might still be a consideration that carries sufficient weight to justify abortion. It is probably even a sufficiently good reason to justify abortion in this particular case.

UP FOR DISCUSSION

Some argue against sex-selective abortions on the grounds that they unfairly discriminate against women. Is there a morally relevant difference between abortion due to sex selection and abortion due to Down's syndrome? Might it be argued that abortions due to Down's syndrome discriminate against those with Down's syndrome?

Doran: If you grant that the fetus has a right to life, Patrick, I don't see how you could say that abortion in this case, or pretty much any other case, could be morally permissible. But it would be very powerful if you could show that it is not morally wrong for Marissa to have an abortion even if conservatives are given their claim that the fetus has a right to life. Let's hear your argument.

Patrick's Virtue-Based Argument for Why Abortion Would Be Permissible in This Case

Patrick: From my virtue ethics perspective, questions of right and wrong are settled by considering how the virtuous person would see things.[11] And this question directs us to consider whether an individual's actions in a given situation are consistent with the virtues. So, in the present case, we need to consider whether abortion is consistent with the virtues. When abortion is done to protect and promote other central and worthwhile goods in one's life, then abortion may be permissible. I don't accept any general rules about when abortion is or is not permissible, however. Each case has to be decided on its own merits. In Marissa and Don's case, the particular case under discussion, I believe, somewhat tentatively, that abortion is permissible. One way of putting my argument is like this:

(1)   It would be wrong for Marissa to have an abortion in this situation if and only if virtuous persons would see Marissa's having an abortion as wrong.

(2)   Virtuous persons would not see Marissa's having an abortion in this situation as wrong.

(3)   Hence, it is not wrong for Marissa to have an abortion in this situation.

Doran: Can you offer some explanation and support for your premises?

Patrick: Sure. The first premise follows from my view that an act is morally wrong (or prohibited) if and only if virtuous persons would perceive the action as morally wrong (or prohibited). Put briefly and roughly, perceiving an action as wrong is a matter of seeing the action as vicious (that is, as exhibiting vices), all things considered. So, the idea is that Marissa's having an abortion is wrong if and only if virtuous persons would see her action as vicious, all things considered.[12]

Warren: How about the second premise? Why do you think virtuous persons would not see Marissa and Don as acting viciously in this situation?

Patrick: The difficulty of answering this question is what makes my position in this case somewhat tentative. We need to consider what virtues and vices Marissa and Don would be manifesting in choosing to abort in this situation. All things considered, they do not seem to be acting viciously. Marissa's reasons for having an abortion do not reveal her to be selfish, shallow, greedy, callous, and so on. Rather, her aborting in this situation arguably shows a reasonable concern to preserve and protect very important and worthwhile goods in her and Don's life. If she has the child, it will likely destroy their marriage and the business they've built together. In short, the life Marissa and Don have worked hard to build would likely be ruined.

UP FOR DISCUSSION

Do you agree with Patrick's assessment of this case that Marissa and Don's decision to abort is not vicious, all things considered?

The Right to Life Weighed against Marissa and Don's Virtues

Doran: Given our different ethical perspectives, Warren and I would of course challenge your first premise. But let's set that issue aside and focus on the second premise. You claim Marissa and Don's choice does not manifest various character flaws, such as being selfish, shallow, greedy, and so on. But on the negative side, some people may quite reasonably say that her act is unjust, since it violates the fetus's right to life.

Warren: That's right. You have assumed, for the sake of argument, that the fetus has a right to life. But it is hard to see how Marissa and Don's reasons are sufficiently weighty to justify the killing of an individual with a right to life. Surely, in a case of conflict between saving one's lifestyle, business, and marriage, versus killing someone with a right to life, a virtuous person must choose to respect and protect the right to life. Marissa and Don's reasons are certainly not frivolous, but are they sufficient to permit killing an innocent human being? Surely that is not a way to act lovingly, as you put it earlier.

Doran: I am with you on this one, Warren.

Patrick: I don't think the right to life has the sort of force that you two think it has. This point is illustrated nicely by Judith Jarvis Thomson's renowned fanciful example of the famous violinist.[13] Suppose you are captured by a group of fanatics that arranges to have you surgically attached to a famous, unconscious violinist, an innocent person whose life can only be saved by this form of attachment to you. You must stay attached for nine months until the violinist is able to function on his own, or the violinist will die. Thomson argues that it

TECHNIQUE

Health care professionals may wonder why anyone takes this science fiction example seriously. The point is not that this is an example of something currently medically possible or likely to happen at any time in the future. The example, instead, helps us to see that if people other than pregnant women had some human being physically dependent upon them, they might view their rights rather differently than many tend, traditionally, to view the rights of pregnant women. The example is designed to put the shoe on the other foot and shake some people out of complacent acceptance of moral tradition.

would not be wrong to detach yourself. For you have a right to control what happens in and to your body. And the violinist's right to life does not entail a right to use your body against your wishes. So, there is no violation of the right to life and, hence, no injustice in detaching yourself from the violinist.

Warren: I'm not sure Thomson is of much help here insofar as you're trying to show that Marissa's abortion is not wrong. Assuming Thomson's violinist analogy has merit, it shows only that abortion is permissible in cases of rape.

Doran: I agree with Warren. Thomson uses the violinist analogy to argue that in cases of rape a woman has not given the fetus a right to use her body, so she may refuse to sustain its life without violating its right to life. Once you grant that the fetus has a right to life, I think it will be very difficult to avoid the conclusion that Marissa's abortion is wrong. For, if we're to take the right to life seriously, we have to say that it is very wrong to kill beings who have this right, except in extremely rare circumstances. Thomson's examples involve such special circumstances—for example, rape and, elsewhere, self-defence and failed contraception—but Marissa and Don's situation is different.

Patrick: You are right to note that Marissa and Don's case is different from Thomson's own examples. Her examples involve cases of unintended pregnancy, whereas Marissa and Don's case is one in which the pregnancy was intended. But I don't think the difference here is morally significant.

Doran: Why not? After all, since Marissa's pregnancy was intended, haven't they tacitly consented to the fetus's use of her body?

Patrick: Perhaps so; I'm not entirely sure. This depends on complicated issues related to the notion of tacit consent. But suppose the fact that they voluntarily intended to conceive constitutes tacit consent to use Marissa's body. It still doesn't follow that the fetus has an absolute and unconditional right to use Marissa's body such that aborting the fetus violates its right to life. For consider David Boonin's revised version of Thomson's violinist case.[14] Suppose that you voluntarily agree to have the violinist plugged into you for nine months. After a month or so, complications arise and, in order to keep the violinist alive, you will have to undergo a series of extremely painful bone marrow transplants. After the first round of transplants, you find the pain is more than you are willing to bear. Boonin argues that it would surely be permissible to unplug yourself at this point, and I agree. If this is correct, then it may be permissible for Marissa to have an abortion in this situation. For having a disabled child imposes significant burdens and costs that she is unwilling to bear.

Doran: Interesting case. I am not so sure it would be morally permissible to kill the violinist in this case. Think about it. To be analogous to abortion, it would not be an "unplugging of the violinist" (a withdrawal of treatment) but an intentional "killing." And it is not clear to me that intentionally killing the violinist would be okay if the violinist had a right to life and you volunteered to care for him for nine months, knowing that there was this risk of complications. This is especially the case in your virtue-based view, where the question is not what most of us would do in this sort of case, but what a *virtuous* person would do.

Moreover, it is not clear how analogous Boonin's case is to abortion in general, and Don and Marissa's case in particular. In a case of abortion, the individual that is killed is no stranger/violinist, but one's own "child." And, if we are assuming for the sake of argument that this child has a right to life, then I don't think it would be permissible to abort any more than infanticide would be permissible if one had given birth to a child who unexpectedly turned out to have Down's in a country where adoption was not allowed.

Warren: Don and Marissa's case would be a conditional contract—that is, a contract with conditions—made with the violinist. A virtuous person can opt out of a contract if her prior conditions are not met, can't she? Marissa clearly thinks the medical tests for Down's are used to see if her conditions are met. She agreed to carry a normal fetus to term and, as long as she keeps that promise, should be perceived to be virtuous by a virtuous person.

Patrick: Right, that's along the lines of what I was thinking, Warren. Any consent the couple has tacitly given would have to be understood as conditional. So, even if Marissa tacitly consented to the fetus's use of her body, it doesn't follow that aborting the fetus would be wrong. For it is not plausible to suppose that voluntary conception amounts to tacitly consenting to bear a child at all costs. In this particular case, the costs are significant—more than Marissa is willing to bear. Her abortion therefore does not deprive the fetus of anything it has a right to. So, Don and Marissa's abortion is not unjust.

Warren: Actually, I do not know if there is any objective answer to what a virtuous person would perceive. The pro-life supporter sees vices of selfishness, greed, cruelty, weakness, and shallowness in Don and Marissa's decision. I prefer to found my arguments on social contract theory, so I leave to Patrick this interesting problem of recognizing veridical perception of virtue where opposite perceptions are common.

Doran: I think you make a very interesting case for the moral permissibility of Marissa's abortion even if the fetus has a right to life, though I am not convinced. While Marissa is not willing to bear these costs, it is not so clear that a virtuous person would be unwilling to bear these costs, on the assumption that the fetus has a right to life. But like I say, you have made a very thought-provoking argument for your view.

I take it your view about the permissibility of abortion is a lot more straightforward if it turned out that the fetus lacked the right to life. Right?

Patrick: Well, I think abortion can be wrong even when it does not violate the fetus's rights.

Warren: Why do you say that, Patrick?

Patrick: I don't think the permissibility of Marissa's abortion, and the question of abortion more generally, can be settled simply by looking at the rights possessed by the relevant parties. In addition to looking at questions of rights and justice, we need to consider other virtues and vices that are relevant in cases of abortion.

As other virtue ethicists have noted, rights can be exercised virtuously or viciously.[15] In the case of abortion, even if a woman has a right to control her body, and the fetus has no right to use her body against her wishes, refusing the fetus the use of her body can be wrong if done for the wrong sorts of reasons.

Doran: Can you give an example to illustrate what you have in mind?

Patrick: Sure. Suppose that Marissa became pregnant from a drunken one-night stand, and wanted to have an abortion, not to save their marriage and business, but to protect her "party hard" lifestyle. In this sort of situation, it might well be vicious to have an abortion, since protecting a partying lifestyle is not in general a good enough reason to justify abortion. (However, that fact that "Partying Marissa and Don" may be unfit parents, together with the concern that their pregnancy could result in an unwanted child with fetal alcohol syndrome, provide reasons in support of abortion in this case.) But Marissa and Don's actual situation is very different from the one just imagined. She is having an abortion to save fundamental, worthwhile projects and relationships that are constitutive of living well.

UP FOR DISCUSSION

Do you think it would be morally wrong for a woman to have an abortion to preserve her "party hard" lifestyle? Why or why not?

Doran: For me, it pretty much all depends on whether the fetus has rights. If fetuses lack rights, and if no one else's rights are violated or there are not serious harms to others, then I don't think it is morally wrong for a couple to abort to preserve their party hard lifestyle. It may be "unseemly" or "unhealthy," but I don't think it is immoral. For I think that for an action to be wrong, there needs to be someone who is wronged, and if the fetus lacks rights, it cannot be wronged. And so, provided no one else is wronged or seriously harmed by the abortion, I think that such an abortion would not be wrong. Basically, if the fetus lacks rights, then abortion is morally on par with contraception. My views are more liberal than yours, Patrick.

Warren: I don't agree that the fetus has no rights at all. The strength of the rights of the fetus is determined by the probability of that fetus becoming a conscious person. And note that the increasing probability of becoming a conscious person as a fetus ages partially fits with the common tendency to think a greater justification is needed for abortion the later it occurs in the pregnancy. The upshot is that my view is more liberal than yours, Patrick, but more conservative than yours, Doran.

UP FOR DISCUSSION

What do you think? Is it permissible for Marissa and Don to obtain an abortion in their circumstances, if we assume the fetus has a full and equal right to life? If the fetus lacks a right to life, would abortion be wrong if done for trivial reasons?

Doran, why don't you give us your argument for why Marissa and Don's fetus lacks any right to life, and why you think her abortion is morally permissible?

DORAN'S ARGUMENT THAT MARISSA AND DON'S DECISION TO ABORT WAS MORALLY PERMISSIBLE

Doran: Though we all agree that Marissa and Don acted permissibly, you are right, Warren, that my position is more liberal than yours and Patrick's. My argument for thinking that Marissa may permissibly obtain an abortion is the following:

(1)   A fetus does not have a right to life at 16 weeks' gestation.
(2)   A woman has a moral right to control what happens in and to her body, provided she does not violate anyone else's rights.
(3)   In Marissa and Don's case, her decision would not violate anyone else's rights.
(4)   Therefore, Marissa has a moral right to obtain an abortion.

Warren: Well, clearly premise (1) would not be accepted by everyone. What reason can you give in support of this premise?

Doran: I believe the reason why a 16-week fetus does not have a right to life can most helpfully be explained if we ask a more general question: In general, what gives something a right to life? If we can answer this question, then we can apply it to fetuses and determine whether they have a right to life. In thinking about what gives something a right to life, we will eventually see the need to consider the question of whether rights to life can vary in their strength. When we do all this, we will end up seeing that at the time of Marissa's abortion, her 16-week fetus lacked any right to life and that even if her abortion happened later in pregnancy, the fetus would have had only a weak right to life that could be permissibly overridden in a circumstance like Marissa's.[16]

The Rationality Criterion for a Right to Life

Doran: Let's consider some obvious candidates for the basis of a right to life. One view says that one gets a right to life in virtue of being rational.[17] What is meant by "rational" varies, but the key idea is that you have the abilities to consciously set goals for yourself and to come up with a particular life plan, that you are self-aware, have reasonably sophisticated problem-solving abilities and communication skills, and so on. Of course, a normal adult human being is a paradigmatic example of a rational being, and so a normal adult human being would, in this view, be a paradigmatic example of someone who has a right to life.

Patrick: It seems right that being rational is *sufficient* for a right to life, but some may wonder if it is *necessary.* For if rationality were necessary for a right to life, many humans would not have a right to life.

Warren: Indeed, not only fetuses, but human infants and the severely cognitively impaired would, according to the proposed criterion, lack a right to life.

Doran: Agreed. A rationality criterion would also presumably exclude non-human animals, yet many believe that we have a duty not to kill them, unless there is sufficient justification. Although there is much more to be said by those who support rationality as necessary for a right to life, I think we ultimately have to conclude that the proposed criterion is too restrictive.

So, let's consider an alternative criterion. Some have suggested that a right to life should be given to all who are alive. If you are alive, you have a fundamental interest in living, and the right to life protects that fundamental interest.[18]

The Life Criterion

Patrick: The claim that all living things have a right to life is very counterintuitive. Bacteria are alive, but we do not think we are violating their rights when we take an antibiotic. Similarly, weeding a garden does not seem to be morally problematic, yet it would be, in this view, since weeds are alive and they're being killed.

Doran: I completely agree. Being alive is much too broad a criterion for a right to life. Moreover, I think we can *explain* why such a criterion is too broad. Rights protect interests—I agree with that—but to have an interest in the relevant sense requires that one be able to take an interest, or to have a point of view that one values or can value. Merely living things, however, like bacteria and weeds, do not have these kinds of interests, and so cannot be said to have rights.

Warren: Well, I am not sure that I agree with your analysis of interests and a right to life.

Patrick: Right, many would question this analysis. There's a clear sense in which plants, for example, have interests—it is in their interests to receive adequate sunlight, nutrition, protection from the elements, and so on. But your point, I take it, is that plants do not have interests *in the relevant sense,* since they are not conscious, and so do not have a point of view from which it matters to them how their lives are going.

Doran: Yes, that's right.

> **TECHNIQUE**
>
> Notice that the rationality criterion and the life criterion of moral rights are rejected by using counterexamples. Further, notice that an explanation is also provided for why these principles err. Whenever possible, one should go beyond the mere appeal to a counterexample to reject a moral principle, and one should try to provide an explanation for why the principle in question is false. For, ideally, one wants to discover not just that a particular principle is false, but also why it is mistaken.

Warren: This is an interesting issue, but let's leave it aside for now, and instead, let's hear what Doran thinks is the appropriate criterion of a right to life.

The Sentience Criterion

Doran: I believe that a necessary and sufficient condition for one to have a right to life is that one be sentient. By sentient, I mean that one is a conscious creature, capable of feeling pleasure and pain, and so can meaningfully be said to be benefitted or harmed. If a being can feel, then it has interests that ought to be respected. And the reason these interests should be respected is because it makes a difference directly to those sentient individuals.

Warren: It makes a difference directly to non-sentient beings when they are harmed as well. Both sentient and non-sentient beings may be unaware of the difference it makes.

Doran: Of course, in a sense, it makes a difference to a non-sentient being if it is harmed. If a weed is poisoned, its lifespan will be shortened, just as if a dog's throat is slit, its lifespan will be shortened. But surely there is a clear and important difference between these two sorts of cases. The clearest difference between them is that the one can suffer and enjoy, while the other can't. The *animal* cares not to be cut up in a way that a weed does not. That one is conscious has clear and important moral significance.

Patrick: I agree, Doran, that being sentient is morally significant for the reasons just mentioned. But I have doubts about sentience as a criterion for a right to life. Why do you think your view is more plausible than the other criteria for a right to life that we've considered and rejected?

Doran: My sentience-based view does not imply that taking antibiotics or weeding one's garden are morally objectionable, since we can assume that bacteria and weeds are not sentient. And it does imply that mentally challenged humans and newborn human infants have a right to life, since they are sentient.

Further, I believe that a sentience-based view ties in with a plausible conception of the proper role of morality—morality ought to be concerned with enhancing well-being or happiness, and with protecting the vulnerable from suffering or injuries to their well-being. A sentience criterion of rights tells us that all and only beings that can suffer and/or enjoy have a well-being, and that sentient beings are therefore to be protected from unwarranted harms. The newborn infant, for instance, can suffer and/or enjoy—it therefore has interests or a well-being that ought to be protected by morality.

Warren: As we discussed earlier, our best understanding of this is that fetuses are not capable of consciousness (and so are not sentient) before 23 weeks. And since Marissa's abortion happens well before this point, she is, in my view, not destroying a being with a right to life.

Doran: Right.

BACKGROUND

"In reviewing the neuroanatomical and physiological evidence in the fetus, it was apparent that connections from the periphery to the cortex are not intact before 24 weeks of gestation and, as most neuroscientists believe that the cortex is necessary for pain perception, it can be concluded that the fetus cannot experience pain in any sense prior to this gestation. After 24 weeks there is continuing development and elaboration of intracortical networks such that noxious stimuli in newborn preterm infants produce cortical responses. Such connections to the cortex are necessary for pain experience but not sufficient, as experience of external stimuli requires consciousness. Furthermore, there is increasing evidence that the fetus never experiences a state of true wakefulness *in utero* and is kept, by the presence of its chemical environment, in a continuous sleep-like unconsciousness or sedation."

Source: Royal College of Obstetricians and Gynaecologists, *Fetal Awareness: Review of Research and Recommendations for Practice (March 2010)* (London: Royal College of Obstetricians and Gynaecologists, 2010), https://www.rcog.org.uk/globalassets/documents/guidelines/rcogfetalawarenesswpr0610.pdf.

Warren: So, in your view, Doran, the capacity to experience is necessary for being sentient, and for having a right to life. Is your view that it is also sufficient for a right to life?

Patrick: And related to Warren's question, does the strength of one's right to life vary with how sentient one is? A mouse is sentient, so in your view does a mouse have as strong a right to life as you or me?

The Addition of Rationality to Sentience

Doran: Although I think sentience is necessary and sufficient for a right to life, I believe that it is reasonable to think that the magnitude of the right to life varies according to the level of sentience. In general, we think that adult human beings have a full right to life, since they are what we may call *fully sentient*, in virtue of their rationality. Not only do they have various interests in not suffering and in having their instinctive drives satisfied, but they also are capable of valuing their own lives and they are equipped with the ability to form preferences, including the preference not to be killed. Further, rational beings can imagine their future and consider various possibilities that non-rational beings cannot. This, in turn, expands the number of things they can dread, and desire.

Also, rational beings can be greatly affected by the success and failures of their loved ones, they can take pleasure in their children's accomplishments, worry about their parents' health, be concerned about the fate of their planet, and wonder about what will happen after their death. These, plus whatever is directly happening to them, are all things in which they can take pleasure or pain. All of this adds to a rational being's level of sentience, to the dimensions by which such a life can become better or worse, and helps explain why we believe it is especially awful (normally speaking) to kill a rational being. These facts make it reasonable to think that normal adult humans are much more aware than non-rational beings, and this helps explain why they have particularly strong rights to life.

Warren: None of the increases in sentience that you mention, Doran, require rationality. They require instead the ability to imagine one's future. Whether one does this in rational or irrational ways, one can have greatly increased sentience. The pains and pleasures of anticipation are among the most keen.

Patrick: Good point, Warren. It seems that irrationality, and various kinds of serious psychological disorders, can enhance sentience. Think about a psychotic individual suffering from delusions.

Doran: You guys are probably right. There are various ways one can become fully sentient—a robust (though irrational) imagination may be one way. Another way to become fully sentient is by having the psychological capacities of a typical adult human being—capacities that include rationality, imagination, empathy, and so on.

It must be admitted, though, that most other mammals are sentient, though not as fully sentient as typical humans. They lack many, if not all, the abilities I just mentioned. This means they have a significant, but not a full, right to life. Again, this matches what most of us believe on reflection: namely, that killing a non-human animal is not something to be taken lightly. It requires a justification, though this justification is more easily met than the justification required for killing a being with a full right to life. It also matches the idea that other things being equal, it is worse to kill a dog than a mouse, and, other things being equal, worse to kill a chimp than a dog, since a dog is more psychologically complex and so presumably more sentient than a mouse, and a chimp is more psychologically complex and so presumably more sentient than a dog.

Patrick: Okay, so I see now why you hold that sentient creatures have a right to life, and why this right can be stronger or weaker. Returning now to Warren's earlier question, what does your view imply about the rights of the fetus?

Doran: Embryos and early fetuses are clearly not sentient, though later fetuses probably are sentient insofar as they probably have the capacity to feel pleasure and pain. I believe this to be the case primarily because I think that sentience (in human beings) requires a certain neurological base—one that is absent in the first parts of pregnancy, gradually emerges later in pregnancy, and is more developed by birth. Because sentience emerges gradually sometime after 23 weeks, fetuses begin to acquire a right to life at that time; however, because they are never fully sentient, the magnitude of that right to life remains only partial.

Patrick: So, what does your view imply about the permissibility of abortion?

Doran: What this means for the morality of abortion is that early abortions do not involve the destruction of a being with a right to life. A pregnant woman is completely within her rights to have an abortion, during this period, for almost any reason.

An early abortion is morally on par with contraception. As the fetus develops and begins to acquire the capacity to feel pleasure and pain, then it acquires a right to life that deserves to be respected. Nevertheless, this right is not of full magnitude, and thus can be more easily overridden in cases of conflict. Thus, if a woman's life or health is in danger, or if continuing with the pregnancy would otherwise set back her important interests to a significant degree, then it would be within her rights to obtain an abortion. Finally, as the fetus matures and becomes more developed psychologically, it earns a more robust right to life, one that will be increasingly difficult to override.

Warren: What about Marissa and Don's case in particular?

Doran: Turning to Marissa and Don's case, she is carrying a fetus that is not capable of experiencing pleasure and pain. The right to life of Marissa and Don's fetus, then, is non-existent at 16 weeks. She therefore acts permissibly when deciding to opt for an abortion at 16 weeks.

Patrick: Interesting. But, as I argued earlier, I do not agree with your claim that in the early stages (prior to sentience) a pregnant woman may have an abortion for *any* reason. This seems too liberal a view to me. Even if the fetus is not sentient, it is a developing human being with the potential to become a sentient, rational being. Aborting such a being for trivial reasons would seem to be wrong.

Objections to Doran's Sentience-Based Criterion of a Right to Life

Is Sentience Sufficient for a Right to Life?

Patrick: I see how being sentient gives an individual an interest in seeking pleasure and avoiding pain. But how does sentience give one a right to life? Some sentient beings are not self-aware and have no concept of themselves as beings with a past and a future. It is plausible to suppose that such beings have a right not to suffer unnecessarily, but it's not clear why we should think these (minimally) sentient beings have a right to life.

Doran: Good question. I don't think that self-awareness and having a concept of oneself with a past and a future are necessary for a right to life, since I think newborn infants have a right to life, even though they probably lack these characteristics. As a thought experiment, consider a newborn infant that has some medical condition that will painlessly kill her in four months' time. Until the time of her death, the infant is expected to be happy and comfortable. It seems clear to me that such an infant has not only a right not to suffer, but also a right not to be killed. And a sentience criterion explains why. Though this baby will never be rational, and though it is doubtful that she is self-aware, she can still feel pleasure and pain, and so she has "a well-being." To kill her would go against her well-being, and so is *prima facie* wrong to do.

Patrick: You earlier rejected the life criterion for a right to life on the ground that beings who are alive, but not sentient, can't *care* about whether their interests are being satisfied. Now, minimally sentient creatures do care about whether they suffer, so again I see why you would think they have a right not to suffer. But since minimally sentient beings don't conceive of themselves as distinct living beings with a past and future, it seems they can't care whether they live or die. So merely being sentient does not seem sufficient to me to get a right to life.

Doran: You raise a challenging objection, Patrick. I suppose my answer is that there is a distinction between what is necessary for a being to have interests, and so rights, and what determines the particular interests (or rights) of a being that is a rights holder. I argued that in order to have interests (and so rights) at all, it is necessary for a being to be able to be benefitted or harmed in a way that matters to it (and this will require that the being be sentient or aware). However, the determination of the particular interests of an individual is a separate matter. It is in my dog's interests not to run in front of a passing truck, but she may not know it is in her interests. Likewise, it may be in an infant's interest not to be painlessly killed, though the infant won't know that.

Is Sentience Necessary for a Right to Life?

Warren: While Patrick has questioned whether sentience is sufficient for a right to life, others will question whether sentience is necessary. A person in a temporary coma is not sentient, but such a person surely has a right to life.

Doran: You raise a tricky issue. For obviously I think that a person in a temporary coma still has a right to life, even if this person lacks awareness. My response to this objection is to say that a person who falls into a temporary coma is still a sentient being, and thus still has interests that warrant protection, even if this person cannot access this capacity while in a coma. If I fall into a temporary coma (or otherwise become temporarily unconscious) later this evening, for instance, it seems clear that I will still have interests. It would still make sense to say, Doran has an interest and a right not to be killed because Doran values spending time with family, enjoys thinking about philosophy, and, if he is going to make a reasonable recovery, he prefers not to be killed. Thus, I think I can say that the coma objection does not work as a counterexample to my claim that sentience is necessary for having a right to life, for I believe that a sentient being who falls into a temporary state of unconsciousness retains their identity as a sentient being.

Warren: Note the difference if the coma is permanent. Does this not show that what is really functioning here is the potential of a being to have a certain kind of future?

 UP FOR DISCUSSION

If Doran argues that a person who falls into a temporary coma is still a sentient being, can he consistently say that a pre-conscious fetus is not a sentient being? Why or why not?

Doran: Well, my views on the rights of the permanently comatose are complicated, and we lack the space to go into that here. So, let me just address your question about potential. I do not think potential for further psychological development is what gives a sentient being a right to life. For I believe that many sentient beings clearly have significant rights to life, even if they are not fully sentient, and even if they do not have the potential to become fully sentient. Consider the case of the terminally ill infant discussed previously, or the case of a significantly mentally challenged human being. I would say they have significant rights to life, even if they lack the potential for significant psychological development. This shows that potential is not what is necessary for the right to life.

I also think potential is not sufficient for a right to life. Gametes and zygotes have the potential to become conscious, but they are not conscious yet. So, they lack a right to life. It is only once one is actually a being with the capacity for consciousness that one acquires the right to life. For it is only then (as I have tried to explain) that we have someone who can be benefitted or harmed in the way that I take to be morally significant.

The Objection That More Rational Individuals Will Have Stronger Rights to Life Than Less Rational Individuals

Warren: According to your view, a right to life becomes weaker as rationality declines. Wouldn't that have the unacceptable implication that humans who were more rational would have greater rights to life than those who were less rational?

Patrick: Right. So a brilliant scientist would have a greater right to life than the average soccer mom or dad?

Doran: No, this objection is based on a misunderstanding of my view. I am not saying that the more rational one is, the greater one's right to life. Rather, I think that a right to life is a threshold concept. This means that once one has the ability to form preferences about continued existence, and once one is self-aware, one meets the threshold for having a full and equal right to life. This is because, once one has these characteristics, one is a person, with a sense of who one is. This is equally the case even if one person is less rational, or self-aware, or imaginative than some other person. Thus, it is not an implication of my view that the average person has a weaker right to life than the brilliant scientist, even if the average person is less rational than the brilliant scientist.

What does follow from my view, however, is that a sentient individual who is not fully sentient has a weaker right to life than a fully sentient being. Killing a normal adult human being is normally worse than killing a normal dog or cat, in part, because

 UP FOR DISCUSSION

Does Doran's view imply that an adult chimpanzee has more of a right to life than a newborn infant? If so, how strong an objection would that be to his view?

the former has a stronger right to life than the latter. And killing a normal dog or cat is normally worse than killing a fish or a chicken, again, in part, because the former has a stronger right to life than the latter. This appears to accord quite well with most people's moral common sense.

Patrick: That seems right. But I think your view runs afoul of common sense when we consider the rights of infants and non-human animals.

Warren: I agree. Doran's view also runs into problems when we consider the rights of severely mentally disabled humans.

Doran: Okay, let me take these objections in turn, beginning with Warren's case.

The Objection That Rational Individuals Will Have Stronger Rights to Life Than Will Non-Rational Individuals

Warren: Isn't one of the conservatives' objections to the view that rights depend on degrees of sentience that it does not accord a full right to life to all humans? Specifically, severely mentally challenged humans would have a weaker right to life than you or I. This sounds like an objectionable form of *ableism.*

Doran: Yes, you have identified a principal objection to my view. My reply may not be fully satisfactory, but here goes. First, it is important to note that most mentally challenged humans are sufficiently sentient to have a full right to life. Most mentally challenged humans are capable of significant levels of understanding, have developed linguistic skills, are capable of participating in loving relationships, and so forth. Now, depending where the threshold for full rights to life is set, it can reasonably be maintained that most cognitively impaired humans surpass this threshold and so would have full rights.

Patrick: But there are of course humans who are so mentally impaired that they are only barely sentient.

Doran: Yes, it is true that some humans are so badly off that they are only minimally sentient, less than many typical non-human mammals. Here, consistency requires that I accept that they do not have a full right to life.

Patrick: But surely it can be just as wrong (and in some cases, maybe even more wrong) to kill a severely mentally disabled human than to kill another human without the mental disability.

Doran: While it is true that my view implies that a rational, sentient individual has a greater right to life than someone who is only barely conscious, it is consistent with my view to claim that non-rational humans warrant great, perhaps full, moral protection. It is just that a right to life won't be the reason for this moral protection. For example, one reason to extend special moral protection to the mentally disabled is that

UP FOR DISCUSSION

What do you think gives someone a right to life? What would your answer imply about the morality of abortion and the killing of non-human animals?

we tend to believe that we should give special moral concern to those human beings who are especially disadvantaged through no fault of their own. Also, another reason to protect the severely mentally disabled from harm is that other humans tend to care a great deal about them. Thus, even if I concede that the severely mentally challenged don't have a full moral right to life, I believe that they should receive strong moral protections because of a combination of their rights and other morally important factors.

Patrick: Okay, fair enough. And I suppose that you'd want to say something similar regarding infants. Infants are not rational, and so they are not fully sentient. So, in your view, they do not have a full right to life. But still, they deserve strong moral protection, for the reasons you just mentioned. Is that your view?

Doran: Yes, the remarks I just made in connection with the severely mentally disabled hold also in the case of infants. In such cases, the beings in question lack a full right to life, but they may be granted strong and perhaps full moral protection.

Warren: I agree with your policy, but for other theoretical reasons. Using my social contract theory, I would support your view requiring strong protection of the mentally challenged by pointing to the **sympathy metarule**. If we could steel ourselves to killing the severely mentally challenged, we would not have sufficient sympathy to make us follow our rules against killing of innocents. People with ordinary human sympathies abhor such killing. Rules permitting such killing would therefore be contrary to the sympathy metarule. By the same token, I would support your approach of gradually increasing the rights of the fetus as it develops, because human sympathy for the fetus gradually increases as it gains more and more similarities of various kinds to a newborn.[19]

> **THEORY**
>
> The **sympathy metarule** governing choices of rules in the original position says: Choose rules that people with ordinary human sympathies could follow.

The Objection That Rational Non-Humans Will Have Stronger Rights to Life Than Will Non-Rational Humans

Patrick: Though I suspect I know how you will reply, there's one last objection to your view that is worth considering. The objection is that your view implies that a mature adult chimpanzee, for instance, will have a greater right to life than an infant. This will strike many as highly counterintuitive.

Doran: Well, if we assume that a chimp is fully sentient, but a newborn infant is not, then, in my view, a chimp does have a greater right to life than a newborn human. And I admit that this is not likely to accord with people's intuitions, but this is not necessarily a problem with my view.

Patrick: Why not? Most people would hold that an infant has a much stronger right to life than a chimpanzee.

Doran: Even if the chimp has a greater right to life than the infant, there can be equally powerful (perhaps greater) reasons for not treating the human infant worse than the chimp. After all, since infants are sentient, they do have some significant rights in my view. Moreover, there are often very strong reasons against mistreating infants, based on the harmful effects this will have on other humans.

Patrick: That seems right. But if we ignore the effect that killing has on others, then, in your view, it is morally worse to kill an adult chimpanzee than it is to kill an infant. Killing the infant is made worse than killing the chimpanzee, in your view, only by the fact that more humans will be harmed by killing the infant. But I'm not sure this is the correct explanation for why killing an infant is morally worse than killing a chimpanzee.

Doran: I agree that on this point, my view parts company with most people's intuitions. But I am not sure that I should be too concerned about that. For, first, I think that any view of what gives someone rights is likely to run afoul of some of our intuitions, and second, I think that our moral intuitions when applied to other species are likely to be particularly biased, and hence unreliable.

I believe that the view of rights that I have defended is motivated by a plausible rationale, and that it is able to explain many of our deepest convictions about who and what has a right to life. Given this, I have more confidence in my analysis of the right to life than I do in our intuitions when it comes to the strength of the rights of newborn humans versus mature non-human primates. I repeat that in my view, it is, in itself, a morally serious matter to kill a newborn infant, for such an infant has a right to life. That my view implies that (in very isolated cases) it is an even more serious moral matter to kill a non-human of greater psychological abilities is an implication that I can live with.

> **THEORY**
>
> Note here that Doran is arguing that his views on the nature of moral rights and his moral judgments about particular cases are in **reflective equilibrium**. For more on this concept, see chapter 1.

Reductio ad *Vegetarianism?*

Patrick: Another concern many people have—though I'm not among them—is that your view, Doran, seems to imply that most of us are morally required to become vegetarians. I think the virtue ethics perspective suggests that most of us ought to be vegetarian, too. I don't see this as a problem with my view, and neither should you, I think.

Warren: I don't consider this a powerful objection either, but meat lovers will want to know how you respond.

Doran: Right. I think it is interesting that my rather permissive position on abortion turns out to be rather strict when it comes to the killing of non-human animals. In my view, non-human animals that are sentient have a right to life, and therefore ought not to be killed or harmed without just cause. Now, insofar as most of us do not have a compelling reason for eating meat—survival, health, and so on—and since most rearing and slaughtering of animals for food goes against the animals' most compelling interests, it follows that it is morally wrong for most of us to eat meat. There will be exceptions, of course, based on health or necessity, though I expect that for most people reading this book these exceptions will not apply, and a vegetarian diet would be morally required.

Warren: Although I agree with this implication of your view, many will consider it a reduction of the view to absurdity. I guess you just have to bite the bullet and accept what we believe to be the right answer in spite of the views of many meat eaters.

Patrick: I agree with you two that most of us ought to be vegetarian. But I don't base this on animals' having a right to life. I'm not sure they have any such right. But it is clear that animals have a serious interest in avoiding suffering. It's also true that most of us don't need to eat meat; we eat meat because it is convenient and we learn to enjoy its taste. The bottom line for me is that it is terribly cruel, callous, insensitive, and selfish to inflict tremendous suffering on animals simply for the fleeting pleasure one derives from eating them.

Doran: It must be admitted, though, that the question of what we owe to non-human animals would be a debate in its own right. So let's save a careful examination of this issue for another time.

> **UP FOR DISCUSSION**
>
> How might Doran's and Patrick's views diverge when it comes to such questions as abortion on demand for first-trimester pregnancies? In the final analysis, do you think Marissa and Don's decision to abort is morally permissible? Why or why not?

SUMMARY

Here is a summary of the main questions, concepts, and arguments covered in this chapter:

- Conservative arguments against the general moral permissibility of abortion are critically examined and rejected.
- Patrick provides a virtue-based argument for the permissibility of Marissa's abortion, while Doran and Warren state their objections.
- Doran considers various criteria for having a right to life and argues that Marissa's abortion was permissible. Warren largely agrees with Doran's views, although for very different reasons.
- Ultimately, Patrick, Doran, and Warren agree, for different moral reasons, on allowing abortion in the first trimester but requiring ever stronger justification as the pregnancy continues. Both Doran and Warren employ rights-based arguments.

- Patrick, in contrast, objects to general rules concerning abortion and insists instead on a principle of particularity: each case must be judged on its own merits for virtue. Nonetheless, a fetus's claim to life will generally increase as it develops and as the mother and father bond with it. So, Patrick agrees that late-term abortions will usually require stronger justification than early-term abortions.

REVIEW QUESTIONS

1. Why does Noonan believe that the fetus is a human being from the moment of conception?
2. Why do Doran, Warren, and Patrick reject premise (1) in Noonan's argument?
3. What is the distinction between being a human being in the biological sense and being a person?
4. Why does Marquis believe that abortion is (typically) wrong?
5. Doran objects that Marquis's argument is unsound, because it commits the fallacy of equivocation. What is this objection?
6. What is Patrick's argument for the view that Marissa's abortion is morally permissible?
7. Why do Doran and Warren object to Patrick's argument?
8. What is Doran's argument for the claim that Marissa's abortion is morally permissible?
9. What, according to Doran, is required for a being to possess a full right to life?

NOTES

1. Morgentaler, Smolling and Scott v. The Queen [1988] 1 SCR 30.
2. Susan J. Lee, Henry J. Peter Ralston, Eleanor A. Drey, John Colin Partridge, and Mark A. Rosen, "Fetal Pain: A Systematic Multidisciplinary Review of the Evidence," *Journal of the American Medical Association* 294, no. 8 (2005): 947–54.
3. John T. Noonan, Jr., "An Almost Absolute Value in History," in *The Morality of Abortion: Legal and Historical Perspectives,* ed. John T. Noonan, Jr. (Cambridge, MA: Harvard University Press, 1970).
4. Actually, his view is unclear on this point: He grants the permissibility of abortion when the fetus cannot survive and the mother's life is threatened; however, he is less clear about whether abortion of a viable fetus would be morally permissible even to save the mother's life.
5. Don Marquis, "Why Abortion Is Immoral," *Journal of Philosophy* 86, no. 4 (1989): 183–202.
6. In his analysis, Marquis excludes from consideration non-standard cases of pregnancy, such as pregnancy due to rape, pregnancy that endangers the woman's life, or cases of fetal abnormality. He simply takes no position on these non-standard cases.
7. Notice the objection raised here would apply equally to artificial and natural forms of birth control. Even the rhythm method, favoured by the Catholic Church, would be seriously immoral, for, if successful, it too prevents an individual from having a future like ours.
8. For more on this point, see, for example, Margaret Olivia Little, "Abortion, Intimacy, and the Duty to Gestate," *Ethical Theory and Moral Practice* 2, no. 3 (1999): 295–312.

9.   This point is made by Walter Sinnott-Armstrong, "You Can't Lose What You Ain't Never Had," *Philosophical Studies* 96, no. 1 (1999): 59–72.

10. More on Warren's view can be found in his book, *Persons: What Philosophers Say About You*, 2nd ed. (Waterloo, ON: Wilfrid Laurier University Press, 2003).

11. Readers interested in the application of virtue theory to the question of abortion should see Rosalind Hursthouse's "Virtue Theory and Abortion," *Philosophy and Public Affairs* 20, no. 3 (1991): 223–46. Patrick's argument owes much to Hursthouse's discussion of this issue.

12. See chapter 3 for the details of Patrick's virtue theory.

13. Judith Jarvis Thomson, "A Defense of Abortion," *Philosophy and Public Affairs* 1, no. 1 (1971): 47–66.

14. David Boonin-Vail, "A Defense of 'A Defense of Abortion': On the Responsibility Objection to Thomson's Argument," *Ethics* 107, no. 2 (1997): 286–313.

15. Hursthouse, "Virtue Theory and Abortion."

16. The arguments advanced by Doran on the morality of abortion are closely based on L. Wayne Sumner, "A Third Way," in *The Problem of Abortion*, 2nd ed., ed. Joel Feinberg (Belmont, CA: Wadsworth Publishing, 1984), 71–93.

17. Many ethical theories see a necessary connection between the possession of moral rights and being rational. For example, Kant argues that all and only rational beings have dignity and are proper objects of moral respect, while social contract theorists see morality as a kind of agreement that holds between rational agents. When it comes to the abortion issue, Mary Anne Warren appears to endorse the view that full moral rights require the possession of rationality. See her "On the Moral and Legal Status of Abortion," reprinted in *Biomedical Ethics*, 4th ed., ed. Thomas A. Mappes and David DeGrazia (New York: McGraw-Hill, 1996), 434–40.

18. Paul Taylor, "The Ethics of Respect for Nature," *Environmental Ethics* 3, no. 3 (1981): 197–218.

19. Jane English, "Abortion and the Concept of a Person," *Canadian Journal of Philosophy* 5, no. 2 (October 1970): 233–43.

7 C-SECTION BY CHOICE

INTRODUCTION

In this chapter, we examine moral issues raised by the practice of **Caesarean section by choice (CSBC)**. **Caesarean section**, or **C-section**, is the delivery of a fetus by surgical incision through the abdominal wall and uterus. While this method of delivery is commonly done for medical reasons, CSBC is C-section that is not medically indicated but rather chosen by the mother. CSBC has become popular of late among celebrities: in recent years, Christina Aguilera, Victoria Beckham, Britney Spears, and many other actors and musicians have chosen to have C-sections for non-medical reasons. The phenomenon is not just limited to stars, however, as statistics show more and more women opting for CSBC.

> **BACKGROUND**
>
> Legend has it that the C-section is so named because Julius Caesar was born that way.

Our drama focuses on Wendy, a woman who elects to have a C-section for a variety of non-medical reasons; these include convenience, preservation of her figure, and avoidance of pain. Wendy's doctor, Dr. Tan, refuses to provide her with a CSBC, because she believes the risks outweigh the benefits. Wendy then turns to a different physician, Dr. Tabor, who agrees to provide a CSBC. Although Dr. Tabor acknowledges that CSBC carries risks, she judges that it is very important to respect her patients' health care choices.

In the debate below, we focus on the question of whether Wendy's having a CSBC is morally permissible. The more general issue is whether it is morally permissible for any woman to have a CSBC. This debate pits the mother's right to **autonomy** against her duties to prevent harm to the baby, to herself, and to others. We also briefly consider the question of whether a policy that permits CSBC is justifiable in a publicly funded system of health care. These matters are complicated by disagreement among experts about the risks and benefits of CSBC.

 DEFINITION

Autonomy is used to refer generally to self-determination. Here, a right to autonomy means the right of the patient to choose her course of care without undue interference.

Doran argues that in the absence of clear and convincing evidence that CSBC poses significant harms to others, we ought to respect Wendy's autonomy. Since we are lacking such evidence, Doran therefore contends that Wendy's having a CSBC is morally permissible. Patrick and Warren agree that, in general, we ought to respect individual autonomy. But they argue that even if the evidence is not conclusive, it does indicate that CSBC may involve risks of very serious harms to the newborn child and to others, and that the duty to avoid unnecessary risks trumps Wendy's right to autonomy. The debate focuses on harms to the baby and the mother, and touches upon harms to others. Doran is not convinced that these risks are great enough to make Wendy's choice wrong. Patrick and Warren, in contrast, think that while some cases of CSBC are morally permissible, Wendy's CSBC is wrong. Patrick and Warren agree on much in this debate; however, they disagree on some of the likely harms of CSBC. In general, Warren thinks the harms of CSBC are likely to be greater and more varied than does Patrick.

LEARNING OBJECTIVES

After completing this chapter, you should be able to:

- Define *autonomy* and discuss the limits on the right to autonomy
- Explain why the ethical debate over CSBC is complicated by the fact that experts disagree about the risks and benefits of CSBC
- State Doran's autonomy-based argument for the permissibility of CSBC
- Understand Warren's good reason requirement, and what it implies for CSBC
- Outline Patrick's reasons for thinking that CSBC is wrong in Wendy's case, although not in all cases
- Explain why Doran rejects Warren's and Patrick's arguments that CSBC is wrong in Wendy's case
- Recognize how a general policy that permits CSBC may be wrong, even if Wendy's CSBC is not wrong

DRAMA

This case is based on various true stories, although names, places, and some uncontroversial elements of the case have been changed to preserve anonymity and confidentiality. Discussions of this and similar cases with health care professionals have also informed this fictional case. The drama merely raises issues. The philosophical arguments are to be found in the debate following the drama.

CHARACTERS

Wendy: an expectant mother and fitness trainer	**Dr. Tabor:** another family-practice physician Wendy visits
Dr. Tan: Wendy's family physician	**Helena:** Wendy's friend

Scene 1

Wendy consults her family physician to ask for a C-section for non-medical reasons.

Wendy: Dr. Tan, if it's good enough for Britney Spears and half of Hollywood, it's good enough for me. I want a C-section. Let's set one up. All joking aside though, Dr. Tan, I have considered this carefully, and C-section is what I really want.

Dr. Tan: But Wendy, there is no medical reason at all for you to have a C-section. We don't just do them on request.

Wendy: I'm not taking "No" for an answer, Dr. Tan. My body is my main business advertising. I can't afford to have less than the best, and I need predictability. I've got to schedule this, not wait for it to happen. I'm in business for myself.

Dr. Tan: What makes you think that a C-section is better?

Wendy: In my business, body aesthetics are crucial. My body is my main advertisement for my services to women. Clearly, if all the stars do it and look so good shortly after giving birth, it's the way to go. I know a number of trainers like me who have gone this route with excellent results.

Dr. Tan: There is no aesthetic advantage to this procedure, in spite of what you have heard, Wendy, and it is much harder on your body. The Hollywood crowd gets on lots of harmful bandwagons.

Wendy: Well, it just makes sense in other ways as well. Why should I go through the pain of labour and the uncertainty of scheduling when I can plan the time and day and avoid the pain? I'm a businesswoman. I like predictability.

Dr. Tan: Pain? A C-section is abdominal surgery. This is serious stuff. Recovering from a cut like that is not straightforward at all. The popularity of C-section has too much to do with fashion.

Wendy: Look, I promised my boyfriend I'd do this. Everybody knows it's better for sex if you don't stretch yourself out of shape.

Dr. Tan: That's a myth. Sexual function is not hampered by natural birth or improved by C-section.

Wendy: Yeah, tell Harry that.

Dr. Tan: Would you be willing to undergo dangerous surgery and avoid a wonderful natural process just because Harry is misinformed?

Wendy: Wonderful? What's wonderful about groaning in agony for hours?

Dr. Tan: If only you could know what it is really like. Most women who give birth naturally have a deep and significant experience—life-changing, in some cases.

Wendy: It was for my mom. She couldn't walk past a washroom for the rest of her life after having us kids. Then there was her **prolapse**.

Dr. Tan: It doesn't have to be that way. You can avoid **stress incontinence** and pelvic prolapse. In fact, there are exercises that are effective for lowering the risk of these problems. You, as a fitness trainer, should appreciate that. It might even form part of your business to help others do the training.

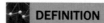

> **DEFINITION**
>
> A **prolapse** is a falling or sinking down of part of the body. Here it refers to a downward displacement of the uterus.

Wendy: I'm into achieving excellent health, not just prevention of illness. Vaginal delivery is full of dangers that can be avoided.

Dr. Tan: Wendy, you mustn't look at pregnancy as an illness. Many of my patients say that childbirth is one of the best things that ever happened to them. Talk to women who have experienced immense joy at giving birth naturally.

Wendy: Sorry, Dr. Tan. It's not like I really want to dismiss natural birth. Even if it is best for me, though, it may not be for my baby. Natural birth puts a baby through a lot more stress than a C-section. You know what's going to happen in a C-section, not like when things can go wrong and you use forceps and all that. I mean—it's so much safer for my baby. My friend Anastasia nearly lost her baby to **asphyxia** after a long and difficult labour. With C-section, you don't have to worry about that sort of thing.

> **DEFINITION**
>
> **Asphyxia** is a deadly condition caused by oxygen deprivation.

Dr. Tan: The evidence is, on balance, against that view, Wendy. C-section may be a lifesaver when there is serious fetal distress, but in a healthy pregnancy it is not safer than natural childbirth. In fact, children born by C-section are more likely to end up in the special-care nursery than children born naturally. Respiratory problems at birth and asthma in later life are greater risks with C-section. C-section babies are also less likely to be breastfed. Natural birth is better for your baby.

Wendy: Look, there are just too many pressures on me to do this. I want a C-section. "My body, my choice," right? If I can decide whether or not to procreate, I can decide how to give birth. My girlfriend from Brazil says everybody there gets a C-section if they can afford it. Please just set this up for me, Dr. Tan. Please.

Dr. Tan: I need a medical reason to do a C-section.

Wendy: Psychological stress counts as a reason for abortion, doesn't it? Why not say that is the reason? Let's just get this done.

Dr. Tan: I'm sorry, Wendy. You've been my patient for a long time, and I want to do my best for you. In this case, that amounts to giving you all the information you need to see what the best choice is for you and your baby. I can't give you what you want or are being pressured to request. I can give you lots of information that I think will persuade you that natural birth is the best course for you and your baby. Take these pamphlets home and please go over them carefully. I'll answer all your questions.

Wendy: Okay, thanks.

Scene 2

Wendy is at the office of a different physician, Dr. Tabor, to see if she will give her a C-section.

Wendy: Dr. Tabor, I *really* want a C-section.

Dr. Tabor: Well, I appreciate the reasons you have given. Physicians may very well disagree on this difficult issue, so there is nothing untoward at all about another physician refusing you even if I do not.

Wendy: So you're going to give me a C-section?

Dr. Tabor: Yes, if you still want one after you are fully informed. I accept a very strong right to patient autonomy.

Wendy: Dr. Tabor, I am informed to death. I read all this stuff my other doctor gave me and heard other opinions that favour C-section much more.

Dr. Tabor: Well, you must realize that physicians have been at odds about how to interpret the data you have been considering. Like Dr. Tan, I think the safest course is to try for vaginal delivery.

Wendy: But are you still going to let me have a C-section?

Dr. Tabor: While I favour natural birth in your case, I will accept your decision for C-section or natural birth once I am sure you are aware of the basic facts. I believe it's up to you once you know for sure what you are getting into. Let's go over the risks again, shall we?

Wendy: Good. Okay, let's.

Scene 3

Wendy discusses her decision with her friend, Helena.

Wendy: Helena, you're going to be proud of me. I really took control. My doctor didn't want to give me a C-section on demand, so I found somebody else who will do it.

Helena: Well, of course I'm glad you're sticking up for what you want. You know I'll always support you, so please don't take this the wrong way, Wendy, but why do you want a C-section?

Wendy: Oh, lots of reasons. The thing is that I know the risks and decided to take them. It's my body, my choice.

Helena: I certainly agree with the general idea, of course, but I worry that our choices are being constructed by others.

Wendy: What?

Helena: Well, I choose things sometimes and then wonder if the choice really came from me.

Wendy: Like what?

Helena: Like getting my tubes tied. I had all sorts of good reasons, but when it was done I couldn't help thinking they were other people's reasons, like Jim's and my doctor's, but not my reasons.

Wendy: Oh, Helena. I'm sorry. I didn't know how you felt.

Helena: But this isn't about me. It's about you. I think that we women are often at the receiving end of huge social pressures that make us choose things. The way we dress, the way we make ourselves up, the way we live seem to me sometimes to be chosen for us by others. Some of our freedom is an illusion.

Wendy: Honestly, Helena, I don't think this is like that. I want a C-section for myself. Okay, so tell me. Who do you think would be making me choose this, and how?

Helena: Sorry, Wendy, but you need to know that C-section on demand is a political issue. It's about physicians taking control of birth, taking it away from women.

Wendy: Hold it, Helena. How do you figure that? If we are doing the demanding, how are they in control?

Helena: Women weren't behind the C-section on demand thing, physicians were. There was no massive uprising of women demanding the procedure. Even now, most women go for vaginal birth if they've got the full story. Physicians want to talk you into a C-section when they want it. It reduces their medico-legal risk. If something goes wrong with the birth they can say, "I did everything I could," while with vaginal birth they can always be asked, "Why didn't you do a C-section?" The vast majority of births are good. The bad ones are lawsuits. C-section also serves physicians' convenience. Why hang around for eight hours or get woken in the middle of the night to attend labour when you can schedule it to fit your day? The fact is that it's major abdominal surgery for you instead of a joyful natural process.

Wendy: Do you know how hard I had to fight to get this? Nobody is telling me to do it, quite the opposite.

Helena: Wendy, I'm on your side. Think about it, though. Lately it's been made glamorous since all of these stars are having it done. That's how they sell us everything.

Wendy: Don't worry. That has no real effect on me.

Helena: Maybe not, but still, Wendy, I just hope you know whether you really want a C-section. Ask yourself about the pressures from the media, from your boyfriend, and from other women who have been sold this bill of goods and want to justify themselves. There's a powerful social system constructing women's choices. Giving birth was a hugely empowering achievement for me. C-section is just surgery empowering surgeons.

Wendy: No, it just gives me another option that I can choose or not. I know you want to help me, Helena, but you're mistaken. Nobody is manipulating me. I know what I'm doing.

DEBATE

Clarifying the Case and Identifying Relevant Facts

Patrick: Right off the top we need to be clear about what exactly counts as CSBC. I know some planned C-sections are considered elective even though they are required for good medical reasons.

Warren: That's right, some women may have medical conditions that make C-section a reasonable option, and they may elect in advance to go that route. But CSBC is different. It is defined as "Caesarean delivery in the absence of medical indications."[1] The choice is that of the mother.

> **DEFINITION**
>
> What we are calling CSBC is often referred to as "Caesarean Delivery on Maternal Request" (or CDMR).

Patrick: Does this happen much?

Warren: CSBC is more and more common, although exact figures are hard to come by. What is known is that the percentage of C-sections, in general, has increased over time, and that rates of C-sections vary a lot both between

> **TECHNIQUE**
>
> Note that when examining an issue, it is generally good practice to begin by defining it.

countries and within parts of countries. In Canada, for instance, in 2016, 28 percent of births were C-sections, with British Columbia having the highest rates at 35 percent. The percentages of C-sections in other developed countries range from 15.6 percent in the Netherlands, to 25 percent in England, to 32.9 percent in the United States, to 36 percent in South Korea, to more than 38 percent in Italy.[2] It is unclear what percentage of C-sections are CSBCs, but the American College of Obstetricians and Gynecologists (ACOG) estimates that 2.5 percent of all births in the United States are CSBC.[3] I don't know how reliable the 2.5 percent number is for the United States, and, just as with C-sections generally, the rates of CSBC probably vary a lot from place to place. But it stands to reason that the rates of CSBC will be lower in places where there are policies and social norms against performing them, and where C-sections are in general not encouraged, than in locations where CSBC is permitted and C-sections are more the norm.

Doran: The 2.5 percent figure would add up to a large number. There are approximately 4 million births per year in the United States, so 2.5 percent would mean around 100,000 CSBCs per year. Another report out of the United States says that 25 percent of all C-sections were for low-risk situations, so that would be over 300,000 births per year in the United States, though some of these might have been for medical reasons. So, it seems safe to say the numbers are not small.[4]

Patrick: Well, I suppose this would be of concern only if CSBC is more harmful than vaginal delivery. Both Dr. Tan and Dr. Tabor seem to think it is. Is their view widely shared?

Warren: Yes, although there are no conclusive studies, the consensus among medical experts is that vaginal delivery is safer for mother and baby than CSBC.[5] The International Federation of Gynecology and Obstetrics (FIGO) states, "At present there is no hard evidence on the relative risks and benefits of term Caesarean delivery for non-medical reasons, as compared with vaginal delivery. However, available evidence suggests that normal vaginal delivery is safer in the short and long term for both mother and child."[6] Similarly, the ACOG concludes that vaginal delivery is preferred to C-section for non-medical reasons. They write, "Given the balance of risks and benefits associated with cesarean delivery on maternal request, the Committee on Obstetric Practice offers the following recommendations[:]… In the absence of maternal or fetal indications for cesarean delivery, a plan for vaginal delivery is safe and appropriate and should be recommended."[7] And a 2013 study in Sweden found that outcomes were worse for both mother and child with CSBC versus those who had a planned vaginal delivery.[8]

Doran: I agree with Warren that the consensus view is that vaginal delivery is generally safer than CSBC for both mother and child, but there are physicians that are not so sure. In part, this is because there is a lack of strong studies comparing vaginal delivery to CSBC.[9] Most analyses of the data compare vaginal delivery to C-sections in general, not just to CSBCs. But this might make CSBC look riskier than it in fact is, since higher-risk pregnancies and emergency C-sections can be expected to have more problems than a planned C-section for non-medical reasons. Other reasons that make it difficult to compare the risks of CSBC and vaginal delivery are that the risks of each procedure are so different. For instance, in a vaginal delivery there are higher risks of maternal bleeding and pelvic floor problems, whereas in C-section there is risk of infection from abdominal surgery and from longer hospital stays, plus it increases the likelihood of **hysterectomy**; and for infants there is greater risk of umbilical cord problems and infection from premature membrane rupture through vaginal delivery, but babies born via CSBC are at risk of laceration, have higher rates of respiratory problems, and, it appears, obesity later in life.[10] Babies born via C-section also lack contact with what appear to be beneficial microorganisms in the vaginal canal, although there is a small study generating the hypothesis that this loss can be overcome by swabbing the newborn in vaginal fluid.[11] And this is just a partial list of the different risks of these two forms of giving birth.

Patrick: So, it's fair to say that this is very complicated. Neither mode of delivery is risk-free, and the sorts of risks faced by each mode of delivery are very different. Things are further complicated by the fact that a significant percentage of planned vaginal deliveries end up being emergency C-sections, where presumably the risks of emergency C-sections are greater than planned CSBCs. I read that while up to 95 percent of women in the United Kingdom want to have a vaginal birth in their first pregnancy, only around 75 percent do. Some 21 percent have an emergency Caesarean section during labour, which is not as safe as a planned one.[12]

Doran: Yes. Some medical societies don't take a stance on which is safer, vaginal delivery or CSBC, though there is much stronger agreement that CSBC is not recommended if the mother wants to have more than one pregnancy. However, when all is said and done, I agree with Warren that most experts think vaginal delivery is the safer path than a CSBC for most women. And presumably, this would be especially true in Wendy's case. Wendy, as a personal trainer, could be expected to have a very successful vaginal delivery, whereas a CSBC is a major surgery that would involve a longer hospital stay, a longer recovery period, and greater risk of infection.

BACKGROUND

"Pivotal in the decision-analysis for many women should be the intended future family size. With rising caesarean section rates, placenta accreta becomes increasingly common.... Placenta accreta and percreta may be associated with significant maternal mortality and **morbidity** including massive haemorrhage requiring emergency hysterectomy." (emphasis added)

Source: Royal Australian and New Zealand College of Obstetricians and Gynaecologists, *Caesarean Delivery on Maternal Request (CDMR)* (Melbourne: RANZCOG, 2013), 5, https://www.ranzcog.edu.au/RANZCOG_SITE/media/RANZCOG-MEDIA/Women%27s%20Health/Statement%20and%20guidelines/Clinical-Obstetrics/Caesarean-Delivery-on-Maternal-Request-(C-Obs-39)-Review-Nov13.pdf?ext=.pdf.

There is also evidence that there are greater difficulties in conceiving and higher incidences of miscarriage and stillbirth in subsequent pregnancies after a C-section.

TECHNIQUE

Sound ethical reasoning requires not only a careful use of moral principles but also sensitivity to relevant empirical matters. Deciding whether CSBC is morally permissible will involve consideration of how safe or harmful it is thought to be. This turns out to be a question that experts do not answer with one voice. We must, therefore, ask what is morally required under conditions of uncertainty.

BACKGROUND

A large study in China of women giving birth for the first time compared those who tried vaginal delivery to women who underwent CDMR (Caesarean delivery at maternal request). It found that those who had a CDMR had "similar short-term maternal outcomes with some neonatal *benefit*" (Liu et al., 2015, emphasis added). However, this is just one study, and it compared only the short-term risks of these modes of delivery. And a 2013 Swedish study observed the opposite outcomes (see note 8).

Source: Xiaohua Liu, Mark B. Landon, Weiwei Cheng, and Yan Chen, "Cesarean Delivery on Maternal Request in China: What Are the Risks and Benefits?" *American Journal of Obstetrics and Gynecology* 212, no. 6 (2015): 817e1–9, https://www.ncbi.nlm.nih.gov/pubmed/25640048.

Patrick: Okay, so the prevailing view among medical experts seems to be that vaginal delivery is generally safer than CSBC for most young, healthy women in developed countries. Is there a similar consensus on whether CSBC is unethical?

Warren: No, not really. International organizations like FIGO say, "At present, because hard evidence of net benefit does not exist, performing Caesarean section for non-medical reasons is ethically not justified."[13] And the Society of Obstetricians and Gynaecologists of Canada and organizations representing other Canadian maternity health care providers have published a joint policy statement on normal childbirth that states, "Caesarean section should be reserved for pregnancies in which there is a threat to the health of the mother and/or baby."[14] In Canada, where vaginal birth is so safe for young, healthy women, changing to surgery might look much more dangerous than in some other countries.

But professional associations in the United States, United Kingdom, Australia, and New Zealand don't rule out CSBC as unethical.[15] As a case in point, here are the current guidelines for CSBC in the United Kingdom by the National Institute for Health and Care Excellence (NICE):

1.2.9 Maternal request for CS
1.2.9.1 When a woman requests a CS explore, discuss and record the specific reasons for the request. **[new 2011]**

TECHNIQUE

Notice how the discussion proceeds in a logical manner. First, we define CSBC; then we identify what are believed to be the risks of CSBC compared to vaginal delivery; then we ask whether medical societies view CSBC as an ethically acceptable option. Once these background conditions are clarified, we will be in a better position to determine whether CSBC is morally permissible and what the medical communities' policies ought to be.

1.2.9.2 If a woman requests a CS when there is no other indication, discuss the overall risks and benefits of CS compared with vaginal birth and record that this discussion has taken place.... Include a discussion with other members of the obstetric team (including the obstetrician, midwife and anaesthetist) if necessary to explore the reasons for the request, and ensure the woman has accurate information. **[new 2011]**

1.2.9.3 When a woman requests a CS because she has anxiety about childbirth, offer referral to a healthcare professional with expertise in providing perinatal mental health support to help her address her anxiety in a supportive manner. **[new 2011]**

1.2.9.4 Ensure the healthcare professional providing perinatal mental health support has access to the planned place of birth during the antenatal period in order to provide care. **[new 2011]**

1.2.9.5 For women requesting a CS, if after discussion and offer of support (including perinatal mental health support for women with anxiety about childbirth), a vaginal birth is still not an acceptable option, offer a planned CS. **[new 2011]**

1.2.9.6 An obstetrician unwilling to perform a CS should refer the woman to an obstetrician who will carry out the CS. **[new 2011]**[16]

Patrick: It appears that what's going on here is that some professional organizations are adopting a sort of precautionary principle that says not to introduce surgeries without clear medical benefit, while other organizations are favouring a principle that says when the medical evidence is not clear, inform the patient of the believed risks of each form of delivery and then respect the patient's choice.

Warren: I think those may be the motivations. Take Wendy's case: there are all sorts of reasons to believe that a vaginal delivery would be safe for her and her baby, and it just seems reckless to do a surgery that introduces possibly catastrophic harms when there is no medical reason to do so. In contrast, defenders of CSBC will claim that because there are risks in both modes of delivery, we should inform the patient that we do not have real knowledge of the comparative risks, tell her what long- and short-term risks we do know of in each mode of delivery, and let her decide in light of that information and her values.

Patrick: I have another question. So far, we have been considering the relative risks to mother and baby of vaginal delivery versus CSBC, but something else to consider are the economic costs of each form of delivery. What do we know, for instance, about the costs of CSBC in comparison to vaginal delivery?

Warren: Here there is widespread agreement that vaginal delivery is less expensive than CSBC, as hospital stays are shorter and there is usually no need to use an operating room.

Doran: But, again, things may be more complicated than they first appear. Planned vaginal deliveries sometimes end up as emergency C-sections. This presumably is a lot more expensive than if a C-section was scheduled in the first place. Nevertheless,

I do agree with Warren that CSBC is likely more expensive than planned vaginal delivery. According to a report by the BBC, "the cost of a planned Caesarean section was estimated at £2,369, with a planned vaginal birth costing £1,665."[17]

Patrick: Okay, to summarize:

1. CSBC is a C-section for non-medical reasons, performed at the request of the mother.
2. The prevailing view among experts is that CSBC in a case like Wendy's is probably less safe than vaginal delivery for both her and her baby, and that CSBC is probably more expensive than a planned vaginal delivery.
3. Medical associations disagree about the ethics of performing CSBC. Some medical associations say they are unethical to perform, while others say that they may be ethically performed, under certain conditions.

With all of this in mind, what ethical question should we debate?

MORAL ISSUES RAISED BY THE CASE

Doran: The drama certainly raises a lot of thorny moral problems related to CSBC. There are questions about the ethics of Wendy's particular decision to choose a C-section; there are questions of professional ethics, such as whether it is unethical for a health care professional to grant Wendy's request for CSBC; further still, one might wonder whether the medical system should provide (and pay for) Wendy's CSBC given that it is not medically indicated and health care resources are scarce.

And, of course, beyond the specifics of Wendy's case, one should consider whether CSBC is, *in general*, a morally permissible choice for women to make, for health care professionals to accede to, and for the health care system to provide.

Warren: Further to this last point, there are concerns about the ills attendant on CSBC as a social policy—a policy that might harm women as a group.

Patrick: Well, we obviously cannot consider all of these questions, so let's proceed systematically and focus on the more central questions. *I propose that we begin by considering the moral permissibility of Wendy's decision to opt for CSBC, and the permissibility of CSBC more generally.* Later, we can turn to other moral questions if time permits.

Warren: Okay, let's get started. Doran, why don't you begin by stating your view about the moral permissibility of Wendy's having a CSBC?

Stating Our Positions

Doran: This is a tough case, and I am not sure what to think. Perhaps the easiest thing to argue would be that Wendy's decision to go for CSBC is wrong, given that the

> **THEORY**
>
> Feminist author Carol Gilligan might find the whole discussion here misguided. Instead of trying to arrive "at an objectively fair or just resolution to which all rational persons could agree, the responsibility conception focuses instead on the limitations of any particular resolution and describes the conflicts that remain" (21–22). Moral judgments will be more contextual and dependent on relationships, according to an ethics of care. A care-based approach would be reluctant to consider the morality of CSBC in general. Instead, each individual case of CSBC needs to be considered on its own terms, and solutions need to be arrived at by bringing together the interested parties.
>
> So-called "radical" feminists might oppose CSBC by asking who the practice serves: is it catering to the preferences of male partners or to the schedules of obstetricians who can then control the timing of births? Some so-called "liberal" feminists might support CSBC on the grounds that it honours the woman's choice, while others may question the autonomy of a woman's choice for CSBC.
>
> *Source: Carol Gilligan,* In a Different Voice: Psychological Theory and Women's Development *(Cambridge, MA: Harvard University Press, 2003), 6–22.*

risks to self and baby appear to be greater with C-section than vaginal delivery, and given that the reasons Wendy has for opting for CSBC seem less than compelling. But I want to try to argue for a different conclusion. Thus, my tentative conclusion will be that while Wendy's is not the best decision, it is not morally wrong, either. From my deontological pluralist view, respect for individual liberty, and the absence of clear, conclusive evidence of serious enough harm to others, incline me to view her choice as morally permissible.

Patrick: I agree with you, Doran, that we ought, in general, to respect autonomy. And this entails that we should often permit people to make choices and act in ways that are not best, provided that the risk of harm (to others, in particular) is not too great.

Though we don't know for certain, the available evidence does suggest that CSBC *may* put mother and child at greater risk of serious harm than vaginal delivery. The risk, in absolute terms, may be relatively small, but the possible harms are serious. Given this, I believe it would be rather foolish, reckless, and irresponsible to opt for CSBC unless one has good reasons for having one. When we look at Wendy's situation, I'm not convinced that her reasons are good enough to justify CSBC. So, all things considered, I think CSBC is wrong in Wendy's case.

Warren: This is a vexed issue, all right. I find it very troubling to sort out my views, but I will side with Patrick here. Although a very strong right to autonomy would be supported in the original position, even if Wendy's decision is autonomous it would be a morally wrong decision. Her choosing C-section is wrong because she is needlessly taking unknown risks for no clear benefit. She is gambling with her child's life and health as well as with her own life and well-being. As parents we ought not to take such chances with ourselves for our dependents' sake, and we certainly shouldn't risk harming our kids for no good reason.

At the same time, however, I recognize that women's rights to control their own bodies with respect to reproduction are often wrongly restricted. Those who oppose these rights often assert instead the rights of the unborn child. I wish to strongly differentiate my view from the position of, for instance, the anti-choice movement in the abortion debate. Here I am concerned with possible harms to a wanted, born child.

Patrick: Nice point, Warren. I, too, would differentiate my view about this case from an anti-choice position regarding abortion. Although I believe that Wendy's having a CSBC is wrong, I'm not arguing that the alleged rights of the unborn child trump a woman's right to have a CSBC or an abortion.[18]

Warren: Doran, why don't you give us your argument for thinking CSBC is a permissible choice for Wendy, and see if you can get Patrick and me to change our minds?

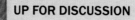
UP FOR DISCUSSION

What are your initial thoughts about the moral permissibility of Wendy's CSBC? Explain your reasons.

DORAN'S ARGUMENT FOR WHY WENDY'S DECISION IS MORALLY PERMISSIBLE

Doran: I'll give it a shot, with the reminder that I am not at all sure that my view is the correct one. I am prepared to advance an argument for my view, but it may well be the case that you guys end up showing me the error of my ways.

Let me begin by outlining my reasoning. The details can be filled in later as we debate.

TECHNIQUE

Notice how philosophy differs from what is commonly known as "debate." In a debate, one typically takes a position and then defends it at all costs, regardless of whether one agrees with the position defended. However, in philosophy the goal is to find the truth through the careful use of reason. Accordingly, if it turns out that the arguments against are stronger than the arguments for, then one should be willing to revise or jettison one's original views and embrace the strongest arguments.

---

(1)   The autonomous decisions of competent patients are, **presumptively, morally permissible**.

(2)   Wendy is a competent patient who exercises her right to autonomy when she opts for CSBC.

(3)   Therefore, Wendy's decision for CSBC is, presumptively, morally permissible.

(4)   This presumption ought to be respected unless it is seriously wrong in other respects—e.g., it seriously harms others, or is unfair, or violates the rights of others.

(5)   Wendy's choice is not seriously wrong in these other respects.

(6)   Therefore, her CSBC is morally permissible.

Many of these premises will require a detailed defence—but that is an outline of the argument that I hope to show is sound.

> **TECHNIQUE**
>
> Doran puts his argument in **standard form**, numbering the premises and conclusion and stripping the argument down to the essentials. This allows easy reference to individual premises. It also enhances the clarity of the argument and allows readers to focus their evaluation.

Warren: Well, I don't think you will have to do much to defend premise (1), since it is not controversial as long as you mean that the right to autonomy should, other things being equal, be respected in patients' decisions that affect mainly themselves, or other competent persons with their consent. Of course, Wendy's is not one of those cases where other things are equal. Others are seriously affected in Wendy's case. I accept your premise (1) on my interpretation, and I will bring up considerations about people other than Wendy later.

For the sake of argument, let us accept premise (2) as well. Like Wendy's friend Helena, I have some concerns about subtle social coercion or coercion from her partner undermining Wendy's autonomy, but we do not really know enough about these things in Wendy's case to know whether she is being coerced. Let's focus, then, on the question of harm to the child and mother.

Patrick: I too have concerns about Wendy's autonomy. She is informed, in the sense that her doctor tells her about the risks and the uncertainty surrounding CSBC, but she stubbornly refuses to accept what her doctor is saying. Wendy's tone throughout the drama suggests to me that she has already decided to have a CSBC, and

> **TECHNIQUE**
>
> To accept a premise for the sake of argument is not to accept it as true. It is just to accept it for the present purposes to focus on a different part of the argument. The premise may still be rejected later on.

that she could not be persuaded otherwise. This leads me to have some doubt about her ability to make an informed and, hence, autonomous choice. I'm willing to go along, however, with the assumption that she is autonomous and focus on the question of harm.

UP FOR DISCUSSION

Given the concerns expressed by Warren and Patrick, do you think that Wendy's choice is autonomous? Why or why not? (For a more involved discussion of the concept of autonomy, see chapter 4.)

DO POTENTIAL HARMS MAKE WENDY'S AUTONOMOUS CHOICE WRONG?

Patrick: Let's see, Doran, whether you can give a sound argument for your claim in premise (5), that the possibly harmful effects of Wendy's (autonomous) choice are not sufficient to show that her freely chosen act is wrong. This is probably the most controversial premise of your argument, and so it is the one on which we should focus most of our attention.

Warren: Yes, I must say that this premise surprised me, since most experts agree that CSBC puts one's baby at greater risk of respiratory problems and of not gaining the benefits of breastfeeding. Much worse, but much less common, things can happen as well, like serious accidental surgical cuts to the baby or even the death of the baby. Surely it is wrong to assume these greater risks of unknown probability, risks of harms to others, without a good reason to do so. Also, CSBC might wrong others in more insidious ways. For instance, CSBC might strain the medical system, or unfairly use up scarce medical resources. Also, there is the concern that CSBC will needlessly **medicalize** what is a safe natural process, significantly changing the culture of birth for the worse. CSBC, if accepted, would needlessly give the medical establishment effective control over birth. These harms would affect everyone, but especially women.

DEFINITION

To **medicalize** an event in a patient's life is to intervene to a great extent medically rather than letting the event proceed naturally. There is much debate, however, about what it means for an event to proceed naturally.

Patrick: I am inclined to agree with you, Warren, that Doran's premise (5) is false. However, I am not sure that CSBC is likely to have all of the insidious harms that you suggest. I'm also rather skeptical of the idea that CSBC medicalizes an otherwise natural process. After all, some uncomplicated vaginal births in hospitals are highly medicalized procedures and so not very natural.

UP FOR DISCUSSION

What is a "natural" birth? Are "natural" births always morally better than "unnatural" births? Explain your answer.

Harms to the Baby

Doran: Okay, let's start with a discussion of possible harms to the child, and then later we can consider whether CSBC harms others besides the child.

Warren: Doran, in general, do you agree that CSBC is worse for the baby than vaginal delivery? And do you accept that vaginal delivery is medically the best choice for Wendy's baby?

Doran: In deciding this issue, things are complicated by our limited knowledge about the risks of CSBC to the baby when compared to vaginal delivery. I'm not sure I agree that all of these risks are relevant, because of their extreme rarity, and because there are horror stories with respect to vaginal delivery as well. I am willing to grant that the evidence appears to be quite clear that CSBC probably poses some greater risks to the baby than vaginal delivery poses, at least in standard cases. (Respiratory issues are probably the biggest concern.) Other things being equal, therefore, I am willing to grant that it would be *better* for the baby if mothers in general, and Wendy in this instance, opted for vaginal birth over CSBC. But the question is whether it would be *wrong* for her to opt for CSBC.

Warren: I think it would be wrong. People in the original position would bias their decisions in favour of protecting the vulnerable. This is because they realize that they may themselves be vulnerable in the real world, at some point. Further, people in the original position are going to want to protect themselves from needless, serious harm. Thus, they will adopt a principle that says, "Do not take unnecessary risks of seriously harming others unless there is a good reason." We can call this latter principle the *good reason requirement*. Now, Wendy's CSBC violates this principle, since she does not have a good reason to expose her baby to the needless, serious harm posed by C-section, at least she has not expressed a good reason. There is no business advantage, in spite of what Wendy argues, since it is a medical fact that it will take her much longer to heal from a C-section. Being unable to conduct one's business tends to be a very serious business disadvantage which is hard to outweigh. She appears in the case to be mistakenly assuming that recovery from C-section is quicker. There is, moreover, no medical reason to expect a difference in the appearance of Wendy's body either, except that Wendy will have a scar. C-sections do not prevent stretch marks, as is sometimes supposed. Therefore, it is hard to understand the supposed aesthetic superiority of a C-section in Wendy's view. There is a great deal of pain associated with recovering from major abdominal surgery, while the pain of labour Wendy wishes to avoid can be minimized with medical pain control. She will have learned that sexual function is not improved with C-section and neither stress-incontinence nor prolapse is a necessary consequence of vaginal birth. Wendy becomes informed about the realities by the time she visits Dr. Tabor. Following the good reason requirement, Wendy should not take even low risks of serious harm to her child.

Doran: Can you say a little bit more about what a good reason is in this context?

Warren: We want people to be able to have reasons that would justify taking risks. Presumably, the greater the risks, the stronger the reasons one will require. There will, of course, be disputes about what will count as a good enough reason. For me the idea would be that a good enough reason would be one that justifies the risks even if the worst harms were to come to pass.

Patrick: I suppose I agree with the good reason requirement, at least insofar as we're talking about parents and their children. But even then, there may be exceptions. In general, though, it does seem reckless and irresponsible for parents to put their children at risk of very serious harm, even if the harms are improbable, unless they have good reason to do so. And, as Warren just noted, Wendy does not seem to have good reasons for wanting a CSBC.

Doran: I don't agree with the good reason requirement. People do not need to justify their choices with "good" reasons when those choices are very unlikely to harm others. Since the probability of Wendy's CSBC harming others is extremely low, she does not need to have good reasons for a CSBC. Alternatively, I suppose I could agree with the good reason requirement and still hold that Wendy's reasons for having a CSBC are good enough. In that case, the good reason requirement would be trivially true, since virtually any reason would count as good enough when the probability of harming others is really low.

> **UP FOR DISCUSSION**
>
> Notice that Warren and Patrick do not claim that CSBC is always morally wrong. In their view, CSBC can be morally permissible if there is a good reason for it. Do you agree with the good reason requirement? Given the risks to the baby involved in Wendy's CSBC, does she have a good enough reason for a CSBC? Can you think of a case of CSBC that would more clearly satisfy the good reason requirement?

I believe I can show, moreover, that Wendy's CSBC is morally permissible, and that the good reason requirement is therefore false (or trivially true), by comparing it to other cases where parents act permissibly when they needlessly take real but somewhat unknown risks of harm with their children for not very good reasons. Consistency requires that if we view these parental decisions as morally permissible, then we should not condemn CSBC on the grounds of the risk of harm it exposes the baby to. Let's start with this case. Consider parents who for reasons of convenience visit fast food restaurants to purchase cheeseburgers, soft drinks, and fries for their kids on a regular basis—say two times per week.

Doran is attempting to defend his view by using an argument by analogy. To prove that Wendy's CSBC is not wrong because of the risk of harm it poses to her infant, he creates scenarios (analogous cases) that are claimed to be relevantly similar to Wendy's CSBC in that they too involve risks of serious injury to a child for no good reason. He then claims that the actions in the analogous cases are not morally wrong, and so, by analogy, the risk of injury to the infant posed by Wendy's CSBC is also not sufficient to make her CSBC morally wrong.

These analogies, if successful, have a secondary function. They will either serve as counterexamples to the good reason requirement—the requirement that prohibits taking unnecessary risks of serious harm to others without a good reason—or they will show that when taking remote risks of serious harms to others, almost any reason will count as a good enough reason.

Warren: I don't think that this is a good analogy. Are the risks of obesity comparable to the risks Wendy is running for her child? We just don't know, but I suspect that the risks of CSBC could be much worse if planned C-section is any indication.[19] Further, obesity and other ill effects from a poor diet are things a child can overcome with help. CSBC can cause problems to both the mother and the baby which cannot be eradicated.

Patrick: I also have doubts about whether this is a good analogy. In any case, even if it is a good analogy, I don't think it will help your argument, Doran, because it is surely wrong for parents to feed their children junk food on a regular basis, assuming more healthful foods are available. The virtuous parent would obviously show an appropriate level of concern for the health and well-being of their children. Giving your child fast food twice a week is rather irresponsible, given the long-term harms, if other options are available. A good parent would not regularly put convenience ahead of the child's health.

Warren: I too think it is wrong of a parent to induce obesity and risk diseases associated with obesity in a child just because it is convenient.

Doran: Well, then, consider a different analogy, one that clearly involves

TECHNIQUE

Here Warren and Patrick illustrate the two ways one can reject an argument by analogy. One can argue, as Warren does, that there are relevant differences between the analogy (eating too much fast food) and the case under consideration (CSBC). Or, one can argue, as Patrick does, that even if the analogy is relevantly similar to the case under consideration, both are objectionable in the same way. Doran intends the fast food analogy to illustrate a case of permissible behaviour, but Patrick thinks that such behaviour is, in fact, impermissible.

taking risks of possible harms to the parent and the child that are serious and possibly permanent. Parents routinely drive their children a kilometre or two to elementary school when they could have walked instead. Let's suppose evidence suggests that the risks of injury when driving are greater than when one walks to school. Would it be morally wrong to drive merely because of the increased risk it poses to the child?

UP FOR DISCUSSION

Do you think it is morally wrong for parents, for convenience, to take their kids for junk food a couple of times per week, given that this risks inducing obesity? If you think this is not wrong, do you think this example disproves the good reason requirement? Is this case analogous to the risks posed by CSBC?

Warren: That's a more persuasive example since, as you pointed out, driving, like CSBC, can result in death and injury immediately both to the child and the parent. I would say driving is wrong for parents who have a good alternative, though I suspect that many would not. For example, if I chose to drive my child to school just because I prefer not to walk, I would consider myself in the wrong. I would be needlessly endangering the vulnerable child in my care, on your assumption that driving really is more dangerous.

Patrick: Yes, this is a better analogy, but again, I'm not sure it helps your case, Doran. Most parents, or at least many of them, have a good reason for driving their children to school. In most or many cases, it may be the only way to get their children to school in a timely manner. But if walking is a genuine option, and it's less risky than driving, then surely that is what parents ought to do.

UP FOR DISCUSSION

Do you agree with Patrick's claims that "most parents, or at least many of them, have a good reason for driving their children to school" and that "if walking is a genuine option, and it's less risky than driving, then surely that is what parents ought to do"? Why or why not?

Doran: Well, you two may have that reaction, but I bet many of our readers won't. Common sense, they might argue, suggests that it is not morally wrong to drive one's kid to school, even if walking would be better. I side with common sense on this point.

Warren: I too would bet that many readers won't think driving is wrong, but that is because they do not accept the hypothesis of the case. They believe their children are safer in their SUV than they are when crossing the road in front of somebody else's. SUVs have been successfully advertised as bastions of security. Actually, almost any car encases us in metal and gives us a sense of being well protected. If parents were really convinced that walking was safer, the psychological reaction might be different.

Patrick: I'm not so sure about that, Warren. Unfortunately, I think many parents, in their day-to-day choices, put greater weight on convenience than the health and safety of their children. We all seem to do this to a greater or lesser extent, even when we recognize that it is wrong.

Doran: People in our society do things routinely in their automobiles when they could have easily walked instead—driving to a new restaurant rather than going to one closer to home, driving to the store instead of walking or ordering something on-line, driving to church rather than walking, and so on. Perhaps such needless automobile trips are wrong because of the environmental damage they cause. But that's not relevant to the issue we are debating. Our present concern is with the level of permissible risk. And I believe that common sense tells us both that such automobile trips are riskier than walking, and that the added risk to the car's occupants is such that it is not enough to make such car trips wrong.

Patrick: The added risk to the occupants of the car does not by itself make these various car trips wrong. But the added risk and the absence of good reasons for taking the risk do make the car trips wrong. It is surely irresponsible, selfish, and reckless to put others at risk of serious harm when one has no good reason for doing so. If common sense disagrees, as you suggest, Doran, then so much the worse for common sense.

Doran: Let's move on and see whether this next case will persuade you. This case may be the most analogous to CSBC since it too involves decisions surrounding childbirth. Let's suppose we had a parent who favoured home birth (because her peers are doing it, she likes the idea, and so on), and let's stipulate—though I am not saying this is true—that the risks to the child of home birth are unclear but appear to be slightly greater than the risks of birth in a hospital. Let's also say that some physicians are comfortable with the idea of home births, though the majority of physicians oppose it. I guess your view would be that you don't think it would be morally permissible for the mom to choose home birth, but that is not my reaction. I believe that if it can be shown that home births are safe in the vast majority of cases, then women should have that option, even if it is not the safest choice.

 UP FOR DISCUSSION

Consider the case of a mother who chooses not to breastfeed her newborn. Suppose that her reasons for not breastfeeding are roughly similar to Wendy's reasons for not wanting to undergo vaginal birth. Also, suppose that breastfeeding is generally believed to be best for the baby. Do you think that it would be morally wrong for this mother not to breastfeed? In what ways is this similar to CSBC? In what ways is this different? Do these similarities and differences affect moral permissibility?

Patrick: If the risks of a home birth are comparable to those of CSBC, and if a woman's reasons for wanting a home birth are as shallow as Wendy's appear to be for wanting a CSBC, then I would also say that the home birth is wrong. I suspect that in many cases, however, the reasons behind home birth are much better. A hospital birth might genuinely conflict with deeply held values. In that case, the risks may be permissible.

Warren: This home birth example is a good challenge. I agree with Patrick: if the features of home birth were similar to CSBC, then I would count home birth as wrong. Some unsafe home birth practices *are* wrong. If, however, one has a registered midwife with proper equipment and backup, the features are rather different from CSBC. There can be considerable safety and signal advantages. In those cases, the parents are not taking an unknown risk with terrible worst-case scenarios for little reason. I do not see a strong enough analogy here, since the reasons for home birth are, as Patrick pointed out, likely to be better than Wendy's reasons for CSBC.

 UP FOR DISCUSSION

What is your reaction to the home birth analogy? Is it sufficiently analogous to influence your views about CSBC? How?

 UP FOR DISCUSSION

See if you can come up with a case that is analogous to Wendy's CSBC. What does this analogy reveal about the moral permissibility of Wendy's CSBC?

Doran: Well, it seems to me, though not to you two, that these analogies suggest that there are lots of situations where parents put their children at some small increased risk of serious harm for reasons that are not always very compelling, and where most people would not think that these parents are doing wrong. And if that is so, then most people should not oppose Wendy's CSBC on the grounds that it puts her child at some small increased risk of serious harm.

Further, and beyond an appeal to consistency, what I chiefly think is motivating my position is the belief that we ought to allow people freedom, and to limit it only when there is clear evidence that their actions pose a substantially greater risk of seriously harming or significantly wronging others. In cases where the increased risks of significant harm to others are really small, I think it is mistaken to condemn such choices as morally wrong. The fact of the matter is that in Canada, the actual risk of serious harms to infants in healthy pregnancies is very small, both for vaginal delivery *and* for CSBC. Infant mortality rates in Canada, while higher than many industrialized nations, are still low—and a lot of infant mortality that does exist is attributable to poverty, low birth weight, and congenital problems—but these are not relevant to the issue under consideration.[20] A general respect for liberty should therefore permit these choices, given that the likelihood of significant harm is so small. If we respect liberty, we must not require people to choose the very best.

So, what does this tell us about your good reason requirement, Warren? Again, it could be that the good reason requirement is true, but in cases like these, where risks of serious harms are really small, almost anything counts as a good enough reason to justify the action. But what I'm more inclined to say is that the requirement to have a good reason whenever one puts someone else at greater than necessary risk of serious harm is false, and that this good reason requirement should only come into play when risks of significant harm to others become sufficiently likely. I believe this because

I think respect for people's freedom means that we should not constantly require of them that they have good reasons for their choices, when those choices carry little real risk of harm to others.

Warren: Common sense does not approve taking risks of catastrophe without a good reason. I do not think your examples show otherwise. Note, moreover, that it is not enough that the increased risk of harm to others be low to make it reasonable to take the risk. A reasonable person would not take unnecessary risks that include utterly unacceptable consequences of unknown probability for little benefit. When we justify choices on the basis of liberty, they must be choices that exercise a reasonable standard of care. This is especially the case when we are dealing with the most vulnerable in our society, like children. In Wendy's case, CSBC does not demonstrate a reasonable standard of care, and thus is ruled out by the good reason requirement.

 UP FOR DISCUSSION

Suppose a slightly intoxicated parent runs an errand in his automobile with his child in the back seat. Given that his route has very little traffic, and given that he is only slightly impaired, he knows that his risk of crashing and significantly harming others is very low. What are the similarities and differences of this to CSBC? How do these affect permissibility?

Patrick: I agree, Warren, insofar as we are talking about parents taking risks with their children. It seems intuitively clear that virtuous parents would not put their child at risk of serious harm, even when the probability of harm is low, without having a sufficiently good reason for taking this risk. Wendy's reasons for wanting a CSBC are not strong enough to justify the possible harms to her child. So, her choice to have a C-section is wrong—it's irresponsible, selfish, shallow, reckless, and so forth.

What Doran's analogies suggest, then, is not that Wendy's CSBC is permissible; rather, they suggest that many other choices that parents make might also be wrong. In all of these cases, parents are behaving recklessly and irresponsibly: they are putting their children at a small risk of great harm for no good reason.

Doran: As I have tried to explain, I believe that the right to autonomy will not be sufficiently respected if we accept Warren's principle that people should not take unnecessary risks of serious harm affecting others without a good reason. Too many things that we routinely choose for trivial reasons would fall into your category of putting others at greater risk of unknown harm, and so would be rendered immoral on your principle.

Patrick: But that, of course, doesn't show that the principle is false. It may be, as I've suggested, that many things that parents routinely do are in fact morally wrong.

Doran: That's true, Patrick. Interestingly, though, it does show that it may be wrong for people to condemn Wendy for CSBC and not to condemn other much more common behaviours. So, even if my arguments fail to persuade people of the permissibility of CSBC, they may persuade people to re-evaluate the permissibility of other actions where parents put their children at risk for unknown benefit.

UP FOR DISCUSSION

Do you accept the good reason requirement? If the probability of harm is low, what would count as a good reason for putting one's child at slightly increased risk? Did Wendy have a good enough reason for CSBC to justify the possible harms to her child?

Harms to the Mother

Patrick: Thus far we have considered whether Wendy's CSBC is wrong because of the risks it poses to her baby, but we also should consider the related issue of whether Wendy is wrong to choose a CSBC because of the increased risks of harm to herself posed by the procedure.

Warren: Yes, let's consider those risks. While there is no study that tells us exactly what we want to know about the risks of CSBC, there's a major Canadian cohort study of planned primary Caesarean section for **breech presentation**. The women in this study are healthy. They have no special risks aside from breech. This low-risk population showed a risk three times greater than women giving birth vaginally of serious problems like cardiac arrest, major infection, anaesthetic complications, venous **thromboembolism**, and bleeding that required hysterectomy.[21]

DEFINITION

Breech means buttocks, and **breech presentation** is the presentation of the buttocks or feet in labour, which entails more risk than presentation of the head. A **thromboembolism** is the obstruction of a blood vessel with particles carried by the blood from another site.

Doran: It's noteworthy that the maternal mortality was the same for this group as for the vaginal group, and the rate is *extremely low* in Canada for all births.[22]

Warren: That's right. Data from maternal registries in Britain and the United States, however, do show a higher rate for C-section generally than for vaginal birth generally.[23]

Patrick: But here in Canada risks to the mother of this procedure are generally low in absolute terms, are they not?

Warren: Yes, in Canada we are blessed with such rarity of maternal mortality that the absolute risk is slight. Still, I have a report here that says, "Although the absolute difference is small, the risks of severe maternal morbidity associated with planned Cesarean delivery are higher than those associated with planned vaginal delivery. These risks should be considered by women contemplating an elective Cesarean delivery and by their physicians."[24] We also have to consider risks to the mother incurred in future pregnancies. Risks go up with the number of C-sections, and vaginal birth after C-section presents its own difficulties for the mother as well.

Doran: Well, I will grant that there may be increased risks to the mother from CSBC. Choosing CSBC may, therefore, be imprudent, but is it morally wrong for a woman to make this choice? Is there a duty to oneself that is sufficiently strong that it should outweigh a woman's freedom of choice?

Patrick: I would say there are duties to oneself, since living virtuously—living a flourishing life—requires that one show appropriate concern for one's mental and physical health. A virtuous person is not only courageous, honest, and trustworthy, for instance; they are also not reckless, intemperate, and gluttonous. But I want to tread carefully here, to avoid saying that people must be saints. A virtuous person would take appropriate care of her body, but this doesn't mean she can never indulge herself or take risks. Again, I don't think there's a general rule that would correctly state the appropriate level of concern for oneself; instead, it must be addressed on a case-by-case basis. I doubt that the risk to self in this case is weighty enough on its own to show that Wendy's CSBC is wrong. But the risks to self, when added to the risks to the baby (and perhaps others), give us good reason, I think, for holding that Wendy's CSBC is wrong.

Doran: I am inclined to agree with you that there are moral duties to self—what we often call *self-regarding duties*—though I would tend to follow Kant and say that there are certain things that one ought not to do to oneself because they would fail to show proper respect for one's own rational or autonomous nature. For example, I think a case could be made that sniffing glue or taking crack cocaine is not only imprudent, it is also immoral, since it directly assaults one's ability to operate as an autonomous being. But I doubt that merely taking risks that are involved in CSBC are sufficient to make the act a violation of a self-regarding duty. The parent is still, almost certainly, likely to recover and to be able to function autonomously. So, while the choice may be rather foolish from the perspective of health, I tend not to think it is wrong on grounds of harm to self.

Warren: Whatever duties are accepted in the original position would have to be duties that will serve our interests in the real world. Certainly something like W. D. Ross's duty of self-improvement, a duty to make ourselves better in respect of knowledge, virtue, and happiness, is in our interest.[25] This must, nonetheless, be balanced against a strong right to autonomy which is crucial to our self-interest. I think that the risks of CSBC might be small enough to justify the mother's taking them on the grounds that the right to autonomy

> **THEORY**
>
> W. D. Ross is a pre-eminent ethical intuitionist. Although Warren is a contractarian and not an intuitionist, he thinks some of Ross's rules would appeal to a majority in the original position.

> **UP FOR DISCUSSION**
>
> Can people have duties to themselves? What duties would they include? Would they count as reasons against Wendy's CSBC?

would outweigh the duty of self-improvement if the mother alone were seriously affected by CSBC. That, however, is impossible, since if the mother is harmed by CSBC, then almost certainly so will her baby be harmed, and all others who care about them.

Patrick: So, it seems we all agree that the harms to Wendy herself are not, by themselves, sufficiently weighty to show that choosing CSBC is wrong. The wrongness depends importantly on other factors, in particular on harms to the baby.

Warren: And to others.

Doran: What harms to others do you have in mind, Warren?

Harms to Others besides the Baby and the Mother

Warren: CSBC may cause various sorts of harms to others besides the mother and the infant. These harms are more at the level of a policy that allows for CSBC than for any individual CSBC. Let's focus on that.

Patrick: Okay, what harms to others do you see resulting from a policy that allows women the option of CSBC?

 UP FOR DISCUSSION

A Brazilian study claims that three-quarters of CSBC mothers surveyed said that the choice was not really theirs but that of their doctors or their partners. In a society where there is evidence that CSBC undermines women's autonomy, should CSBC be allowed? Does this affect the permissibility of CSBC in other societies? How, in general, do strong social pressures to accept medically unnecessary procedures affect their permissibility?

Source: See D. P. Béhague, C. G. Victora, and F. C. Barros, "Consumer Demand for Caesarean Sections in Brazil: Informed Decision Making, Patient Choice, or Social Inequality? A Population Based Birth Cohort Study Linking Ethnographic and Epidemiological Methods," *British Medical Journal* 324, no. 7343 (2002): 942–45. See also, Olga Khazan, "Why Most Brazilian Women Get C-Sections," *The Atlantic*, April 14, 2014.

 UP FOR DISCUSSION

In opposing the position that CSBC enhances women's autonomy, Véronique Bergeron claims that informed consent cannot be meaningfully exercised unless women are made aware of the sexist underpinnings of the medical model of childbirth and its influence on the ethical reasoning of the American College of Obstetricians and Gynecologists. Are there moral implications of such a position for Wendy's CSBC? What, if any, evidence of harms to women's autonomy generally would be sufficient to deny the permissibility of CSBC as a policy?

Source: See Véronique Bergeron, "The Ethics of Cesarean Section on Maternal Request: A Feminist Critique of the American College of Obstetricians and Gynecologists' Position on Patient-Choice Surgery," *Bioethics* 21, no. 9 (2007): 478–87.

Patrick: Do you have in mind financial burdens to our medical system that could result if we had a policy permitting CSBC?

Warren: Yes. I have here a recent study that says that Caesarean delivery costs much more than vaginal birth. In Canada, for instance, a 2016 report estimates the costs for the typical vaginal delivery to be $3,195 and for a C-section to be $5,980, and a 2008 report claims that $36,640,000 could be saved each year in Canada just by reducing Caesarean delivery from 26 percent to 20 percent of live births.[26] In a public health care system that is strapped for cash, this is an unjustified expense for a medically unnecessary procedure. That money could be used, for instance, to lessen the excessive wait times for some medically necessary procedures.

Doran: There seems to be something right about your point that we should not burden an already stressed public medical system with unnecessary, costly medical procedures, although I wonder whether our public system offers other unnecessary, costly medical procedures. If so, then there may be a fairness requirement that allows for publicly funded CSBC as well.

Patrick: Right. It's not at all clear to me that a publicly funded system of health care should provide only medically necessary procedures. And I wonder whether we can sharply distinguish procedures that are medically necessary from those that are not. Intuitively, the distinction seems clear. But suppose, for instance, that a pregnant woman prefers a home birth to a hospital birth because the latter conflicts with deeply held religious beliefs or values. Would the possible psychological harms of a hospital birth make the home birth medically necessary? If not, should it still be funded in a public system like the one we have in Canada?

Doran: Those are good questions, but we cannot adequately address them in the remaining time. So, I suggest we set them aside, and focus on Warren's claim that a policy permitting CSBC would add an additional, and unnecessary, burden to our health care system.

Patrick: That's fine by me.

UP FOR DISCUSSION

What counts as an unnecessary, costly medical procedure? Can you think of unnecessary, costly medical procedures that our public health care system provides? Consider these procedures: vasectomies; providing "artificial blood" or "bloodless surgery" to replace blood transfusions for Jehovah's Witnesses; using obstetricians for births that could be safely delivered by less costly midwives. Are any of these procedures medically unnecessary? If the public health care system provides these procedures, does that mean we should offer CSBC, too? If we decide not to offer CSBC as part of publicly funded health care, then should we decide not to offer similarly costly and unnecessary procedures?

Doran: Even if you are right, Warren, that we should not burden an already stressed public medical system with unnecessary, costly medical procedures, I am not sure we can apply the dollar amounts you just cited to CSBC, for surely some of the reasons that make C-section more expensive do not apply to CSBC. For instance, C-section in general is probably done on women who have more health problems than women who deliver vaginally, but that factor would not apply to CSBC. Also, there are undoubtedly added costs with emergency C-sections that happen in the middle of the night, but those would not apply to CSBC procedures, since they would be scheduled procedures.

Notice, further, that even if CSBC is more costly than vaginal delivery, this concern can be dealt with without stopping women from having the option of CSBC. There may be a way to fund them privately, for instance, without harming the public health care system.

Patrick: Well, a private system for CSBC might still end up harming the public health care system. Re-hospitalization is more common for C-section than for natural birth, and so complications arising from these private instances of CSBC may eventually cut into the public system.

Doran: That's true. I grant that it may take some work to get a system including CSBC that would not harm the public health care system, but I think we can see that it is at least a live possibility. Costs do not provide a reason, in principle, for the impermissibility of CSBC as a practice. But they may provide a reason against providing CSBC in the public system, if it turns out to be more costly than vaginal delivery.

> **UP FOR DISCUSSION**
>
> If, in the future, or in some parts of the world, home birth becomes less expensive and as safe as hospital births, would it be wrong to provide women with the choice of hospital births? If C-section becomes safer (for mother and baby) and less expensive than vaginal delivery, would it be wrong for women to have the option of vaginal delivery?

Patrick: The issue of allowing private CSBC gets tricky. There would be concerns about allowing access to CSBC only to the relatively wealthy, for instance, and that, of course, raises questions of fairness.

Doran: Good point, Patrick. Whether it would be unfair or not to offer CSBC only on a private-payer basis raises the whole complicated issue of the morality of offering private health care alongside a public health care system. This is a very interesting topic, but is best saved for a separate debate.[27]

Patrick: Agreed.

Warren: Well, it looks as though you two aren't convinced either that CSBC is more expensive than vaginal delivery, or that it would be wrong to adopt a policy permitting CSBC even if it could be shown that it is more expensive. I have more arguments up my sleeve, but they'll have to wait for another day.

UP FOR DISCUSSION

In the final analysis, do you think that Wendy's CSBC is morally wrong? In general, is CSBC wrong? Why or why not? Have your views or reasons changed in the light of this debate? If so, how?

SUMMARY

Here is a summary of the main questions, concepts, and arguments covered in this chapter:

- The main questions explored are: Is it morally permissible for Wendy to have a CSBC? Is it morally permissible for women in general to have CSBCs?
- CSBC is defined as a C-section that is not medically necessary, but rather chosen by the mother for non-medical reasons.
- *Autonomy* is defined as self-determination. The right to autonomy refers to a person's right to make her own decisions, including the right to choose her course of care without undue interference.
- The available evidence suggests that CSBC may carry greater risk to the child and mother than planned vaginal births; however, the data regarding the risks and benefits of CSBC are not conclusive, and the correct interpretation is a matter of some dispute.
- Doran argues for a strong presumption in favour of respecting the autonomous choices of patients. This presumption ought to be respected unless it is seriously wrong in other respects. Doran argues that Wendy's CSBC was autonomously chosen and was not seriously wrong in other respects. Although he admits that CSBC poses greater risks to the mother and baby than vaginal birth, he does not think these risks are great enough to override a woman's right to autonomy. He concludes, therefore, that it was morally permissible for Wendy to have a CSBC.
- Patrick argues that CSBC is permissible in some cases, but given the possible risk of very serious harms to the child, it is permissible only in cases where one has sufficiently good non-medical reasons for choosing a C-section delivery. Wendy does not have sufficiently good reason; her choice for a C-section manifests various vices and is therefore morally wrong.
- Warren agrees with Patrick's conclusion that Wendy's CSBC is morally wrong, but he agrees for different reasons. Persons in the original position would support a strong right to autonomy; at the same time, however, they would not approve of parents subjecting their children to serious risk without any clear benefit. Since Wendy's having a CSBC would put her child at risk of serious harms, CSBC is wrong in her case.

- The questions of whether a policy that permits CSBC would be justified in a public system of health care like the one we have in Canada, and the permissibility of CSBC if it is performed and paid for privately, are briefly considered.

REVIEW QUESTIONS

1. What does *autonomy* mean?
2. What are the possible benefits and risks of CSBC?
3. Why is the ethical debate over CSBC complicated by the fact that experts disagree about the benefits and risks of CSBC?
4. What is Doran's autonomy-based argument for the permissibility of CSBC?
5. Why do Warren and Patrick hold that Doran's argument is unsound?
6. Explain Warren's *good reason requirement.* What does he think it implies regarding the permissibility of Wendy's CSBC and CSBC in general?
7. Why does Doran reject the good reason requirement?
8. Patrick contends that it would be morally wrong for Wendy to have a CSBC. Why? Does he believe that CSBC is always wrong? Why or why not?
9. Why does Doran reject Warren's and Patrick's arguments that CSBC is wrong in Wendy's case?
10. Why might a general policy that permits CSBC be wrong, even if Wendy's CSBC is not wrong?

NOTES

1. Jan E. Christilaw, "Cesarean Section by Choice: Constructing a Reproductive Rights Framework for the Debate," *International Journal of Gynecology and Obstetrics* 94, no. 3 (2006): 262–68. Readers may be interested to know that Dr. Christilaw is married to Warren. Dr. Christilaw has not, however, reviewed this debate, nor are the opinions and arguments expressed by Warren necessarily shared by her.
2. Ana Pilar Betrán, Jianfeng Ye, Anne-Beth Moller, Jun Zhang, A. Metin Gülmezoglu, and Maria Regina Torloni, "The Increasing Trend in Caesarean Section Rates: Global, Regional and National Estimates, 1990–2014," *PLoS ONE* (2016), doi:10.1371/journal.pone.0148343.
3. See ACOG Committee Opinion No. 761, "Cesarean Delivery on Maternal Request" (2018), https://www.acog.org/Clinical-Guidance-and-Publications/Committee-Opinions/Committee-on-Obstetric-Practice/Cesarean-Delivery-on-Maternal-Request#2.
4. See Joyce A. Martin, Brady E. Hamilton, Michelle J. K. Osterman, Anne K. Driscoll, and T. J. Mathews, "Births: Final Data for 2015," *National Vital Statistics Reports* 66, no. 1 (2017), https://www.cdc.gov/nchs/data/nvsr/nvsr66/nvsr66_01.pdf.
5. Tina Lavender, G. Justus Hofmeyr, James P. Neilson, Carol Kingdon, and Gillian M. L. Gyte, "Caesarean Section for Non-Medical Reasons at Term," *Cochrane Database of Systematic Reviews* 3 (2012), doi:10.1002/14651858.CD004660.pub3.

For a carefully referenced discussion, see British Columbia Perinatal Health Program, *Caesarean Birth Task Force Report 2008* (Vancouver: BCPHP, 2008), 54–55.

6. FIGO Committee for the Ethical Aspects of Reproduction and Women's Health, *Ethical Issues in Obstetrics and Gynecology* (London: FIGO, 2012): 88–89, https://www.figo.org/sites/default/files/uploads/wg-publications/ethics/English%20Ethical%20Issues%20in%20Obstetrics%20and%20Gynecology.pdf.

7. See ACOG Committee Opinion, "Cesarean Delivery on Maternal Request."

8. See Annika Karlstrom, H. Lindgren, and Ingegerd Hildingsson, "Maternal and Infant Outcome after Caesarean Section without Recorded Medical Indication: Findings from a Swedish Case-Control Study," *British Journal of Obstetrics and Gynaecology* 120, no. 4 (2013): 479–86, https://obgyn.onlinelibrary.wiley.com/doi/full/10.1111/1471-0528.12129.

9. "At the National Institutes of Health State-of-the-Science Conference on Cesarean Delivery on Maternal Request in 2006, a panel of experts was charged with reviewing the available literature and expert opinions on the subject. A systematic literature review of 1,406 articles was conducted to evaluate the relevance of existing studies on cesarean delivery on maternal request and the quality of the evidence. The panel concluded that the available information comparing the risks and benefits of cesarean delivery on maternal request and planned vaginal delivery does not provide the basis for a recommendation for either mode of delivery." ACOG Committee Opinion, "Cesarean Delivery on Maternal Request."

   Similarly, the Royal Australian and New Zealand College of Obstetricians and Gynaecologists appears not to take a position on whether vaginal delivery is safer than CSBC; see its *Caesarean Delivery on Maternal Request (CDMR)* (Melbourne: RANZCOG, 2013), https://www.ranzcog.edu.au/RANZCOG_SITE/media/RANZCOG-MEDIA/Women%27s%20Health/Statement%20and%20guidelines/Clinical-Obstetrics/Caesarean-Delivery-on-Maternal-Request-(C-Obs-39)-Review-Nov13.pdf?ext=.pdf.

10. See ACOG Committee Opinion, "Cesarean Delivery on Maternal Request."

11. Maria G. Dominguez-Bello, Kassandra M. De Jesus-Laboy, Nan Shen, Laura M. Cox, Amnon Amir, Antonio Gonzalez, et al., "Partial Restoration of the Microbiota of Cesarean-Born Infants via Vaginal Microbial Transfer," *Nature Medicine* 22, no. 3 (2016): 250–53.

12. Mairead Black, "Vaginal Birth Comes with Risks Too—So Should It Really Be the Default Option?" *The Conversation*, July 26, 2016, https://theconversation.com/vaginal-birth-comes-with-risks-too-so-should-it-really-be-the-default-option-62855. The article goes on to discuss some of the other risks of planned vaginal delivery in the United Kingdom: "A further substantial proportion of women experience important complications of vaginal birth. These include an 8% postpartum haemorrhage rate, 1% blood transfusion rate, and a 5–6% third-degree tear rate (40% suffer some degree of tearing). One in six (15%) women end up having an operative vaginal birth, such as use of forceps, which is associated with faecal incontinence and pelvic organ prolapse in later life. Also, it's important to realise that long labours, complications and interventions are associated with maternal distress, postnatal depression and intense anxiety in future pregnancies."

   The author argues that these risks must be balanced against the risks of planned C-section: "While not risk-free, it appears to be similar to that of a planned vaginal birth in the short term and—with a slightly higher risk of respiratory problems at birth—may be even safer for the baby. However, the scarring from a section will make each future pregnancy more risky as it can affect the development of the placenta, resulting in increased risks for the mother of developing major bleeding and hysterectomy, although this is rare. There is also some concern that babies born by caesarean could be at higher risk of developing asthma."

13. See FIGO Committee for the Study of Ethical Aspects of Human Reproduction and Women's Health, *Ethical Issues in Obstetrics and Gynecology* (London: FIGO, 2012), 89, https://www.figo.org/sites/default/files/uploads/wg-publications/ethics/English%20Ethical%20Issues%20in%20Obstetrics%20and%20Gynecology.pdf.

14. See Daniel Robert Reilly, "Caesarean Section on Maternal Request: How Clear Medical Evidence Fails to Produce Ethical Consensus," *Journal of Obstetrics and Gynaecology Canada* 39, no. 12 (2009): 1176–79, https://www.jogc.com/article/S1701-2163(16)34379-1/pdf.

15. See Royal Australian and New Zealand College of Obstetricians, *Caesarean Delivery on Maternal Request*.

16. See National Institute for Health and Care Excellence, "Caesarean Section" (2011), https://www.nice.org.uk/guidance/cg132/chapter/1-Guidance#planned-cs.

17. James Gallagher, "Women Can Choose Caesarean Birth," *BBC News*, November 23, 2011, https://www.bbc.com/news/health-15840743.

18. We consider the morality of abortion in chapter 6.

19. See, for instance, Hernandez-Dias et al., who mention a sevenfold increase in life-threatening persistent pulmonary hypertension of the newborn (a serious respiratory illness). Sonia Hernandez-Diaz, Linda J. Van Marter, Martha M. Werler, Carol Louik, and Allen A. Mitchell, "Risk Factors for Persistent Pulmonary Hypertension of the Newborn," *Pediatrics* 120, no. 2 (2007): e272–82.

    MacDorman et al. report neonatal mortality rates with no indicated risk at 1.77 per 1,000 live births compared to vaginal births with a rate of 0.62. Marian F. MacDorman, Eugene Declercq, Fay Menaker, and Michael H. Malloy, "Infant and Neonatal Mortality for Primary Cesarean and Vaginal Births to Women with 'No Indicated Risk,' United States, 1998–2001 Birth Cohorts," *Birth* 33, no. 3 (2006): 175–82.

    See also Shiliang Liu, Robert M. Liston, K. S. Joseph, Maureen Heaman, Reg Sauve, and Michael S. Kramer, for the Maternal Health Study Group of the Canadian Perinatal Surveillance System, "Maternal Mortality and Severe Morbidity Associated with Low-Risk Planned Cesarean Delivery versus Planned Vaginal Delivery at Term," *Canadian Medical Association Journal* 176, no. 4 (2007): 455–60.

20. Barbara S. E. Verstraeten, Jane Mijovic-Kondejewski, Jun Takeda, Satomi Tanaka, and David M. Olson, "Canada's Pregnancy-Related Mortality Rates: Doing Well but Room for Improvement," *Clinical and Investigative Medicine* 38, no. 1 (2015): e15–e36, https://cimonline.ca/index.php/cim/article/download/22410/18194.

    See also, "Canada Has the 2nd Highest Rate of 1st-Day Infant Deaths in the Industrialized World: Report," *CTV News*, May 7, 2013, https://www.ctvnews.ca/world/canada-has-2nd-highest-rate-of-1st-day-infant-deaths-in-industrialized-world-report-1.1270425.

21. Liu et al., "Maternal Mortality and Severe Morbidity." See also L. W. M. Impey, D. J. Murphy, M. Griffiths, and L. K. Penna on behalf of the Royal College of Obstetricians and Gynaecologists, "Management of Breech Presentation," *British Journal of Obstetrics and Gynaecology* 124 (2017): e151–e177.

22. Liu et al., "Maternal Mortality and Severe Morbidity." Maternal mortality rates are listed by country in *The World Factbook*, https://www.cia.gov/library/publications/the-world-factbook/fields/2223.html.

23. National Collaborating Centre for Women's and Children's Health, *Caesarean Section* (November 2011), https://www.nice.org.uk/guidance/cg132/evidence/full-guideline-pdf-184810861.

24. Liu et al., "Maternal Mortality and Severe Morbidity."

     See also G. Justus Hofmeyr, Mary Hannah, Theresa A. Lawrie, "Planned Caesarean Section for Term Breech Delivery," *Cochrane Crowd*, July 21, 2015; and Impey et al., "Management of Breech Presentation."

25. W. D. Ross, *The Right and the Good* (Oxford: Oxford University Press, 2002), 21.

26. See British Columbia Perinatal Health Program, *Caesarean Birth Task Force Report 2008*; "The Cost of Childbirth across the Globe," *Coyne College*, December 14, 2016, https://www.coynecollege.edu/news-events/cost-childbirth-across-globe.

     See also "Average Charges for Giving Birth: State Charts," *Transforming Maternity Care*, http://transform.childbirthconnection.org/resources/datacenter/chargeschart/statecharges/.

27. See our discussion of two-tier health care in chapter 8.

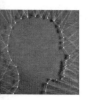

8 TWO-TIER HEALTH CARE

INTRODUCTION

Up until the late 1940s, health care in Canada was paid for privately. Access to medical services was based on one's ability to pay for it. In 1947, however, the government of Saskatchewan introduced the first provincial public health insurance plan that covered hospital services. Other provinces soon followed Saskatchewan's lead, and by the early 1970s, all of the provinces provided universal public health insurance (**universal care**) for both hospital and physician services. Although the administration of these services is the responsibility of the provinces, they receive funding from the federal government. In 1984, Parliament passed the Canada Health Act, which specifies criteria the provinces must meet in order to receive federal funding. Among other requirements, the provinces must provide "comprehensive" and "universal" care to all insured residents.

While Canada's public and universal health care system is the envy of many, it is not without its critics. In recent years, the system has come under fire for increasingly long waits for diagnostic procedures and other services. As we write this chapter, patients requiring **magnetic resonance imaging (MRI)**, for instance, must wait from two to six months. Over the past several years, private medical clinics offering MRI services have been popping up around the country. Those who can afford the roughly $900 fee for a straightforward MRI can now receive one within days in the private sector. Many see this further move toward a more entrenched **blended private/public** or **two-tier health care** system as a positive development, one that will help to take some of the pressure off of the public system and thereby benefit everyone, while others worry that a blended system will erode the public system.

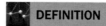

> **DEFINITION**
>
> **MRI** stands for **magnetic resonance imaging**, a technique for scanning for muscle and joint injuries. Both the scans and the machines that perform the scan are referred to as MRIs.

Here we will discuss the problem of queue jumping in the use of private, for-profit care (accessible only to those able to pay high fees) to avoid long wait times for publicly insured health services (accessible to all legal residents of Canada). The two tiers referred to are care accessible to all and care accessible only to those with means. The means may be private insurance, charitable funding, or personal wealth. In any case, some have the money to pay for services that are unaffordable for other residents. To be sure, there are cases of mixed public and private payment for care. While these may blur the public/private distinction for some purposes, we are concerned here only with clear cases of unequal access to care. A two-tier system is any system where such cases exist. The Canadian system is a two-tier system. We will use the term *public health care* to refer to the care universally and completely covered by public insurance, accessible to all lawful residents of Canada. *Private care* is that which is not universally and completely covered, and so is inaccessible to those who lack the means.

> **BACKGROUND**
>
> In British Columbia in 2018, 50 percent of patients were waiting more than 41 days for an MRI and 10 percent of patients more than 199 days.
>
> *Source:* Richard Zussman, "BC Government Promises to Cut MRI Wait Times," *Global News*, March 27, 2018, https://globalnews.ca/news/4108431/b-c-government-mri-wait-times/.

Our drama focuses on Sanders and Ben, two talented high school–aged hockey players who have the potential to achieve their dream of playing in the Juniors, which may lead to the NHL with its promise of riches and fame. Unfortunately, both players are injured and need MRIs to determine the nature of their injuries and the best course of treatment. Sanders is lucky: he comes from a wealthy family that can afford to buy him a private MRI. Ben, however, comes from a family of modest means. His family cannot afford a private MRI. Because Sanders can afford a private MRI and Ben cannot, Sanders can return to the ice much sooner than Ben, and thereby improve his prospects of making it to the next step on the way to the NHL. Ben is stuck in the long queue for publicly funded diagnostics.

The general issue raised by our drama is whether a two-tier system of health care in Canada is morally acceptable. In other words, is it morally permissible, in Canada, for some to be able to use their wealth to access faster or better health care while others who lack the means must wait to access a slower and so, in some respects, inferior health care system? The more specific question we focus on is whether a two-tier system of MRI in Canada is morally acceptable. At the heart of this question is a conflict between liberty, on the one hand, and fairness and equality, on the other hand. Advocates of two-tier MRI argue that people should be free to purchase private medical services if they have the desire and means to do so. Critics argue, however, that it is unfair that the wealthy have access to faster and perhaps better care than the less wealthy. Respect for equality, among other values, requires equal access to care. A further issue raised by our drama, and explored in our debate, is whether it is morally appropriate for people to use the private health care system if the system itself is not permissible.

In this debate, there is significant agreement among Doran, Warren, and Patrick on the question whether two-tier MRI is morally permissible. They agree that it is permissible in Canada, if and only if certain conditions are met. Although there are differences in their views about what the relevant conditions are, there is agreement that private, for-profit MRI, inaccessible to some citizens, is permissible only if it does not undermine the public health care system and the provision of other important social goods (for example, education, social, and economic opportunity). These are *necessary* conditions; the authors argue that further conditions must be met in order to show that private MRI is morally permissible in Canada. Warren, for one, is skeptical of the claim that private MRI in Canada can satisfy these conditions, and so he thinks that private MRI is likely not morally permissible in Canada.

LEARNING OBJECTIVES

After completing this chapter, you should be able to:

- Explain the libertarian argument against taxation to support public health care
- Understand why libertarians think that people should have a right to purchase private health care
- Discuss two egalitarian arguments against two-tier medicine (against adding private to public medicine)
- State objections to these egalitarian arguments
- Describe Warren's, Patrick's, and Doran's views on when two-tier MRI is justified
- Explain why Warren and Patrick think it is permissible for Canadians to access two-tier MRI even if the government should not allow private medicine, and explain Doran's argument to the contrary

---

DRAMA

Please note: This case is based on various true stories, although names, places, and some uncontroversial elements of the case have been changed to preserve anonymity and confidentiality. Discussions of this and similar cases with health care professionals have also informed this fictional case. The drama merely raises issues. The philosophical arguments are to be found in the debate following the drama.

CHARACTERS

Coach: the coach of a high school– aged hockey team

Art: a former player on Coach's team

The scene is a family restaurant where Coach sits looking glum as he eats breakfast. A former player of his, Art, walks in.

Art: Hey, Coach! It's been a long time.

Coach: Art, my man! Where've you been?

Art: Uganda. I've been setting up a computer system for Makerere University on a CIDA project.

Coach: Hell, not much ice time there, I'll bet.

Art: Yeah, hockey is not a concept there. Hell, cold is not a concept. Hey, I hear you're coaching the Arrows now.

Coach: Yeah.

Art: You don't sound overjoyed, Coach. What's up?

Coach: Don't get me wrong. I love the job. It's just player injuries that are weighing on my mind. You see, I've got this line we call the Sandbag Line that has been doing all the scoring. Ben Begin and Sanders Carter are what really make it cook. Sanders is right wing, Ben is left, and they click like magic. Ben sets up the play and Sanders pops it in.

Art: Who got hurt?

Coach: That's the hell of it. Both are hurt. Ben took a bad hit in the last game of this season and his knee is bad, but they don't know for sure what it is. They need to do an MRI. They told him he's got at least a three-month wait for that!

Art: Geez, that's hard. At least he finished the season. But man, three months is a lifetime when you're that age.

Coach: God, yes. A kid like that laid up through the summer. Ouch! So that injury was four weeks ago. The thing is, will he be diagnosed and treated in time to start next season? I'm really pulling for this kid. He's got heart. His family hasn't got two nickels to rub together, and since he's been old enough he's always worked and helped out with the costs. Hockey is expensive. His family scrimped and saved to put him in hockey and keep him there until he was old enough to handle most of the costs by taking part-time jobs. His family can't help any more. They've got younger kids to look after. Ben just keeps plugging away, though. He buys all his gear second hand. He just loves the game. He doesn't let anything stop him. But he may be skewered now.

Art: Let's hope not. What about the other guy?

Coach: Well, Sanders hurt himself hang-gliding just last week. He did something to his shoulder. Talk about a contrast. He gets an MRI the next day 'cause his Dad can plunk down $875 like it was a penny. Carter owns that fancy restaurant, Le Maître, and half a dozen other businesses. It turns out that Sanders's family physician went to med school with the top specialist and Sanders has already had his operation. No chance he won't be starting next season. If you can prime the pump with a few bucks, the government will let the treatment flow. If you can't, you wait.

Art: Yeah, it stinks.

Coach: Don't get me wrong. I'm happy for Sanders, but he's had everything handed to him on a plate. You know, he gets the best of everything, the latest gear. He's not a bad guy, but spoiled and a bit full of himself, of course. He offered to give Ben his old equipment whenever something new comes on the market, but Ben insists on buying it. Still, Ben is better equipped than he could be otherwise, so Ben kind of benefits too from old man Carter's largesse. The thing is, if we don't do something, Sanders will be out there hot-dogging around catching the eye of the scouts while Ben will still be laid up, you know? That could be crucial. That might make a career difference, see?

Art: "Them that's got shall get, them that's not shall lose, so the Bible says, and it still is news."

Coach: That about sums it up. What's that saying from?

Art: The song "God Bless the Child."

Coach: Oh, yeah. Great song.

Art: You know, Coach, it's all relative. Kids I know in Africa see Ben's life as the impossible dream. They'd all give their right arm to be in his shoes.

Coach: Yeah, that puts it in perspective. Life ain't fair, and it's more unfair there than here. But damn it, Artie, this is Canada. At least at home we pride ourselves on being fair to our own.

Art: This is really getting to you, isn't it, Coach?

Coach: Yes, and it's not just the kids, Art. There's seniors in this town hobbling around waiting for knee surgery. Damn it, Art, it's not Africa here. The government should give everybody the medical help they need. In a rich country like this, nobody should have to beg for the essentials.

DEBATE

Clarifying the Case and Identifying Relevant Facts

Patrick: Are these boys still in high school?

Warren: Yes, but they are at the age where the scouts are starting to watch them. They are waiting to be picked to play in the Juniors in towns like Medicine Hat and Swift Current, the first big step toward the NHL.

Patrick: So a concern here is that Ben may have to miss the next season, whereas Sanders won't, and this could hurt Ben's prospects for turning pro.

Warren: Right.

Doran: If Sanders gets his MRI more quickly, then presumably he will get his diagnosis more quickly, but does it also mean he will get treated for the problem sooner?

Warren: Yes.

Doran: Why? Isn't there a backlog for physical therapy, surgery, rehab, and other procedures?

Warren: It depends. Surgeons and physical therapists often have room to treat people. But sometimes there is a backlog there as well, especially to see surgeons. The thing is that you typically cannot get in line to see a surgeon until you have had your MRI to diagnose the problem. Our story takes place in the diagnostic part of the queue, where there is a bottleneck. Sanders gets in line for surgery first, in any case.

Doran: Are private MRIs legal in Canada?

Warren: It's iffy, but they are being done. Private clinics even advertise newer, superior scanners.

Patrick: How are MRIs delivered privately? Are they always done in private clinics?

Warren: Usually. Some hospitals have rented out their machinery to private clinicians after hours, but I think that has been stopped.

Doran: Do you know the cost of an MRI?

Warren: As we speak, depending on how much competition they have from other clinics, they will price it from about $900 for a basic knee scan.[1] This is one of the easy and profitable MRIs to do. The difficult ones may be left for the public system. They'd be a lot more expensive to purchase privately.

Patrick: I suppose if they were not offered in Canada, patients could go down to the States, get an MRI, and then bring back the report to their physician in Canada?

Warren: Yes. Though it is worth mentioning that the out-of-pocket costs for an MRI in the States are typically greater than in a private clinic in Canada. Indeed, it is rather interesting how much MRI costs vary by locale.[2]

Doran: Why doesn't the government buy more of these machines if there is such a shortage? Are the costs that out of line?

Warren: The costs are very high, around $3 million per MRI scanner to purchase, and hundreds of thousands per year to run and maintain.[3]

BACKGROUND

"The rapid growth of private MRI (magnetic resonance imaging) clinics, which permit people to purchase faster service and then use test results to '**jump the queue**' back into the public system for treatment, is a troubling case." (emphasis added)

Source: Roy J. Romanow and the Commission on the Future of Health Care in Canada, *Building on Values: The Future of Health Care in Canada—Final Report* (Saskatoon, SK: Privy Council, 2002), xxi, http://publications.gc.ca/pub?id=237274&sl=0.

There is also a shortage of technicians, and it takes time and money to train them and much more money to pay their salaries. So, adding more MRIs would require more staff to run them. The operational costs are more of a problem than the capital costs of the machines.

Patrick: Is there evidence that shows that allowing private MRI shortens the wait times in the public system?

Doran: Yes, would things be worse in the public system without them?

Warren: There are complaints from some groups that private MRI does not help the public system and, in fact, hurts it. On the other hand, 1 in 10 patients are waiting up to 200 days in the public system in some regions to get MRIs,[4] so private clinics are offering their services to shorten wait times.

Patrick: So, as things are, if someone tears a ligament or something, that person has to wait that long in the public system just to get the scan? Clearly, more diagnostic equipment and technicians are needed.

Warren: Yes, but you can understand governments' reluctance to increase diagnostic procedures. More diagnostics can make for strains on other parts of the system. I have anecdotal evidence that people have needless exploratory operations now because of MRIs done in the States that show a possible problem that turns out to be benign. Before MRI, the apparent problem would never have been noticed. Add to that the lack of clarity about whether the private MRIs really reduce wait times in the public system, and you can see why the system managers avoid just pouring money into this one.[5]

Patrick: Interesting, Warren. Well, if Ben does get an MRI, and if it turns out he needs surgery, I wonder how long it will take to receive the necessary operation. Do you know?

Warren: I think it is pretty quick for the surgery. Weeks in Ben's case, I bet. It depends on the specialty needed, the demand for the needed procedure, availability of appropriate facilities in the area where it's being done, and other factors such as these—factors that commonly affect the responsiveness of a health care system.

Patrick: Some might wonder whether there really is a problem in this case, though. If Ben really is talented and set on a career in the NHL, and an MRI costs (only!) $900, then it seems that it wouldn't be too hard to find a way to pay for it.

Warren: Ben is from a large family. His parents can't help. He is strapped supporting his hockey habit with work after school—$900 is huge in those circumstances. His family is already deeply in debt and unable to take on more, given their meagre salaries.

Patrick: I suppose that's right. For some, $900 is no big deal, but for others it's rent.

Doran: The situation is particularly tough for Ben, since it has already cost him and his family a lot just to equip him and to pay the fees to get him on a team. Indeed, more and more Canadians are unable even to play organized hockey because they cannot afford it. Ben's family has made all those sacrifices to get him to this point, but this last obstacle is too great. Coming up with the extra $900 is simply beyond their means.

Patrick: So Ben's lack of resources puts him, yet again, in a difficult position that Sanders doesn't face.

Warren: And pulling himself out of poverty by getting a shot at the Juniors and ultimately at the NHL makes the opportunity to be scouted for professional teams mean so much more to Ben than to Sanders.

Patrick: Right. If Sanders doesn't make it in hockey, he likely has other lucrative career options. For Ben, it appears that pro hockey is his ticket out of poverty.

> **BACKGROUND**
>
> "The Vital Signs/True Sport Foundation study finds that the rising cost of sports is also a barrier for many families. The most recent data shows that 6 out of 10 children from low-income households are active in sports, compared with 8.5 out of 10 from families with incomes over $80,000."
>
> *Source:* Jamie Strashin, "No More Joiners: Why Kids Are Dropping Out of Sports," *CBC News*, May 10, 2016, https://www.cbc.ca/sports/sports-participation-canada-kids-1.3573955.

Warren: Ben's grades aren't great because he puts it all into hockey, and working part-time doesn't leave him much time to study.

Patrick: I imagine it's not uncommon for young players to get injured and have to miss part or all of a season. Does this really seriously affect their chances?

Warren: At this stage in his hockey development, Ben is likely to suffer huge disadvantages if he misses too much of the coming season. His skills may get rusty, his conditioning will no doubt suffer, he will miss the start of the season, and he will probably be viewed by the scouts as injury prone. As a result, he may not look very good to the scouts in the future if he is off for an extended period. There is a tide in the affairs of a young hockey player, which, taken at the flood, leads on to the NHL. The timing is crucial for Ben. His boat might be left high and dry at low tide after Sanders sails away. If, moreover, Ben does have to wait even the average time for an MRI, he may become more difficult to treat, and treatment may not be as successful. These would be disadvantages for any athlete, but in the fierce competition for the attention of the scouts and for a place in the top rung of the Juniors, this delay can be very significant.

MORAL ISSUES RAISED BY THE CASE

Patrick: Okay, I think we've got the relevant background facts straight. The main moral issues raised by the case are pretty straightforward—they concern the permissibility of two-tier MRI in particular, and two-tier health care in general, given the apparent unfairness this involves.

Doran: Perhaps we should limit ourselves to the more specific question, though. I would be content if we could clarify the simpler question of whether private MRI is morally acceptable in Canada. Clarifying our thoughts on this question would be very helpful since this is a matter of current concern in Canada. Also, if we reach some conclusions about this more limited question, it may serve as a template for thinking about the larger question of whether two-tier health care, in general, is morally appropriate in Canada.

Warren: Yes, given the complexity of the problem, let's just stick to the more limited question of whether private MRI is morally permissible in Canada. A caveat, however, is in order. Whether or not two-tier medicine in Canada can be effectively delivered is largely an empirical question. As philosophers, we have no special insight into such matters. What we can do, however, is try to answer the following question: *Is two-tier MRI ever morally acceptable, even in principle, and if so, under what conditions?*

Patrick: That sounds right. Well, why don't we begin as usual by stating our initial views on this issue?

Stating Our Positions

Doran: The question of two-tier MRI in Canada brings to the fore a host of moral values: front and centre are questions of liberty, equality, fairness, compassion, self-respect, and so on. On the one hand, those who favour liberty as a basic value may defend the permissibility of private MRI as a matter of principle; those who are motivated by compassion or care may also support private MRI if it means their loved ones will get needed care more quickly. On the other hand, fairness, equality, and the value of self-respect seem to speak in favour of a one-tier system that distributes health care on medical grounds alone and does not give special advantages to those who happen to be affluent. I am torn by this difficult issue; however, I believe that two-tier MRI in Canada is morally permissible, but only if certain conditions are met. For me, the most important conditions are (1) two-tier MRI must not threaten the robust social safety net that should be available to all Canadians, and (2) where such a social safety net is lacking, two-tier MRI ought to be allowed only if it is the best means of providing this robust social safety net.

Warren: First of all, let me say that I sympathize with those who seek private MRI, since it is a moral failing of the Canadian government not to support publicly funded MRI adequately. As you say, this issue is extremely difficult. I agree with your first condition given Canada's current wealth, but that could change. From the **original position**, people would require different degrees of strength of the safety net depending on the society's wealth. Given its current wealth, Canada should provide a robust social safety net, but it has failed to do so. Something like your condition (2), substituting "good" for "best" seems acceptable in the original position as well. I suspect, though, that private MRI will drain talent from the public system. Private MRI may also cause other social harms outside the health care system. I think, therefore, that allowing private MRI is not morally permissible in Canada under current conditions. I concur with your conclusion, Doran, though I would justify it differently.

Patrick: Well, it seems unfair that those who happen to be wealthy have better access to such a basic good as medical care; however, I agree that private MRI would be morally permissible if certain conditions were met. If allowing private MRI benefits those in the public system, then I believe it is permissible. Private MRI may also be permissible, I think, even if it doesn't benefit others, provided that it doesn't harm those in the public system. A virtuous society would be a compassionate society, one that ensures that everyone has a reasonable stock of **primary social goods**— that is, goods that everyone (or almost everyone) needs to live well. So, as long as private MRI improves everyone's lot, or at least doesn't worsen things, I believe it is permissible. This is just a rough statement of my current view, but I'll refine it as necessary as we proceed.

> **THEORY**
>
> Some virtue theories speak only to matters of character and moral claims among indi-
> viduals. They have nothing to say about the design of social institutions. Patrick's virtue
> theory incorporates elements of "ideal observer" theories. The right act or policy is the
> one that a virtuous person with full information would see as right. This allows a broader
> application of his virtue theory.

Doran: It looks as if we all agree that two-tier MRI could be morally permissible under
the right sorts of conditions, though we differ somewhat on the conditions that would
need to be in place in order to make two-tier MRI morally acceptable. Now that we
have the rough initial statements of our views, how would you like to proceed?

Patrick: Given the complexity of the problem, and given that each of us claims to support two-tier MRI in some circumstances but not in others, it may be best if we begin with some of the more straightforward and extreme views, such as that private
MRI is always permissible, or that private MRI is never permissible.

Doran: I agree. By understanding why these simpler arguments fail, we may also see
why a more nuanced position with respect to two-tier MRI is best.

Warren: Yes, once we consider these more extreme views, we can turn to our own positions, and see if there are any devils in the details.

A LIBERTARIAN ARGUMENT

Doran: Libertarians would defend the existence of private MRI on the ground that
it would be unjust for the government to prohibit it. The basic thought is that the
government should not interfere with the liberty of its people unless it is necessary
to prevent violence, theft, or fraud. In the marketplace, people should be free to do
what they want provided that it does not violate anyone else's rights.

Patrick: That's right. According to libertarians, if I have justly acquired some wealth, then
I have the right to spend my wealth in any manner that I choose, provided that doing
so does not violate anyone else's rights. If, for instance, Sanders's father wants to purchase an MRI for his son, and if someone else wants to sell him one, then they should
be free to make that exchange, provided that doing so violates no one else's rights.

Doran: So, putting these points together, the libertarian argument as it relates to the
present case can be stated as follows:

(1) If a person freely consents to an action and the action does not violate the
rights of others, then the government is not morally permitted to interfere
with that action.

(2) If a person does not engage in violence, theft, or fraud, then the person
does not violate the rights of others.

(3)   Sanders freely consents to getting a private MRI without engaging in any violence, theft, or fraud.

(4)   Therefore, the government is not morally permitted to interfere with Sanders getting that private MRI.

Patrick: That sounds like a libertarian argument, but the libertarian position, of course, goes well beyond just arguing for the permissibility of private MRI. Libertarians also argue that publicly provided health care is inherently unjust. This is because they contend that the taxation needed to fund a public health care system is inherently unjust. Forcing people to pay for a public system, they claim, violates people's rights.

Doran: That's true, the radical position being considered here maintains that not only should people be free to purchase private health care, but also that taxation to fund a public system violates taxpayers' rights.

Warren: Why should anyone believe such claims? It seems strange to me that one would want to have things like MRI governed by the free market rather than regulated reasonably by government, since the market can leave people like Ben out in the cold through no fault of their own. Why should we think that the taxation needed to fund a public system is unjust, and why should we think that the market should determine who receives health care and under what conditions?

> **THEORY**
>
> "Taxation of earnings from labor is on a par with forced labor.... Taking the earnings of n hours of labor is like taking n hours from the person; it is like forcing the person to work n hours for another's purpose."
>
> *Source:* Robert Nozick, *Anarchy, State, and Utopia* (New York: Basic Books, 1974), 169.

Patrick: I share your concerns, Warren. The premises in this argument seem to depend on an unreasonably narrow conception of rights. In particular, they seem to depend on the idea that the only rights people have are **negative rights**. But why should we accept that? Many of us believe that persons have **positive rights** to basic goods like education, health care, shelter, and so on.

> **THEORY**
>
> Philosophical analyses of rights commonly distinguish **negative rights** from **positive rights**. The former are characterized as rights to non-interference, while the latter are described as rights to be provided with money, goods, services, and so on. Thus, for example, my right not to be physically harmed may be understood as a negative right, as it imposes a duty on others not to do a variety of things. If I also have a right to be assisted by others when I am in need, then I would also have a positive right to aid. A right to health care is understood as a positive right, then, since its satisfaction requires the provision of various goods and services.

The Wilt Chamberlain Example

Doran: It may help to see some of the intuitive pull of the libertarian's premises by looking at a famous example presented by Robert Nozick.[6] It goes like this. Suppose we start with a system that is considered fair by the libertarian's opponents. In this initial distribution everyone has equal wealth (or wealth is distributed according to the **difference principle** or whatever principle you consider a fair distribution principle).

> **THEORY**
>
> The **difference principle** says that a just society should distribute income and wealth equally, unless inequality benefits everyone, especially those in the worst-off group. It is one of the principles of justice favoured by John Rawls. For more on Rawls's theory of justice, see chapter 2.

> **BACKGROUND**
>
> Wilt Chamberlain was an amazing player in days gone by. He once scored 100 points in an NBA game, and still holds dozens of NBA records.

Wilt Chamberlain, an amazing basketball player, then signs a contract with a team that allows him to get 25 cents for every ticket sold. A million people cheerfully go to see Wilt play in a season—they happily drop 25 cents in a box with Wilt's name on it. At the end of the year, Wilt has a lot more money than others in the society—$250,000.

But how can we say that he is not entitled to his money? In the initial distribution, by hypothesis, people were entitled to their wealth. They then gave some of their money to Wilt freely and happily. Now, if the government taxes Wilt's income in order to give to people in need, or to fund health care or other social programs, then it is taking something that properly belongs to Wilt. The government is treating Wilt merely as a means to some other end, and that, says Nozick, is inherently unjust.

Patrick: I think the example does have intuitive pull. The idea is that if people start out with what they are morally entitled to, and if they voluntarily make choices that result in a new economic distribution (with Wilt having more money than others), then that new economic distribution is also just. If the government then steps in to take away some of the money that Wilt was voluntarily given, then that intuitively seems unfair to Wilt, since it violates his right to money he fairly acquired.

Warren: Okay, I see the intuitive pull of this example. And I suppose libertarians claim that this point about Wilt Chamberlain can be generalized so that it applies to cases like the one we're considering.

Doran: That's right. Suppose Sanders's father has played by the rules of society, has worked hard, and has earned a large fortune. It seems unjust that someone should now step in and take away some of his justly acquired wealth. Moreover, if Sanders's father wants to use some of his wealth to buy an MRI for his son, and if some physician who has justly acquired an MRI machine wants to sell him an MRI scan, then it seems that it would be unjust for the government to prohibit that. A system that takes away one's justly acquired holdings, or that prevents one from using one's justly acquired holdings in ways that one wants, does seem unjust.

Patrick: So the Wilt Chamberlain example helps to motivate premises (1) and (2) in the libertarian argument. In support of premise (2), it suggests that Wilt's acquisition of wealth violated no one's rights, since he acquired his money not through violence, theft, or fraud, but through a voluntary exchange of money for services. And given that Wilt did not acquire his money in a way that violated the rights of others, then, in support of (1), the example suggests that it would be wrong for the government to interfere with this voluntary exchange of money for services by imposing a **redistributive taxation** scheme that forced Wilt to give up a certain percentage of the money he's been given.

> **THEORY**
>
> A **redistributive tax** aims at redistributing wealth, typically by taking money via taxation from those who are relatively wealthy with the purpose of benefitting those who are relatively less wealthy (say, through welfare payments, daycare subsidies for the children of poor people, pensions for low-income seniors, etc.), or with the purpose of promoting various social goods (such as the arts, parks, public schools, and public health care). Other taxes are not redistributive—for instance, taxes that are used to punish criminals, prevent crime, and secure the nation's defence. Libertarians oppose redistributive taxation but do not oppose non-redistributive taxation.

Is Redistributive Taxation Inherently Unjust?

Warren: Both of the libertarian's premises are problematic. Let's start by looking more closely at the first premise. Suppose, for now, that Wilt acquires his wealth in a way that does not violate anyone's rights, since he does not use force or fraud. Does it follow from this that it would be wrong for the government to interfere with the exchange of money for services by forcing Wilt to pay taxes on the money he collects in order to fund social programs? More generally, is redistributive taxation inherently unjust?

Patrick: To answer this question, let's see if we can follow the same basic strategy as the libertarian, but present an example that elicits intuitions on the other side—intuitions that support the claim that redistributive taxation is *not* unjust. If we can do this, then we will have less reason to find the original Wilt Chamberlain example persuasive.

Doran: Good, so let's tell a story that parallels the Chamberlain example but elicits different intuitions. We begin with some initial distribution of wealth that is agreed to be fair—say, everyone has an equal amount of wealth. Now, suppose that Mary Andrews is a hard-working young woman just recently graduated from college. She is looking forward to her new career as a preschool teacher. Tragically for Mary, and through no fault of her own, she discovers a lump in her breast. It turns out to be cancer. Mary needs an operation, and she needs chemotherapy and radiation treatment. Though she suffers terribly, Mary is courageous and strong, and she is determined to live and to beat her cancer. So, Mary takes all of her savings and pays for her operation, and her chemotherapy and radiation. During this time, she is very weak and so she must take time off from work, but because of the excellent care of her physicians and nurses, and because of her sheer strength and determination, Mary begins to feel better and she eventually is able to return to work. Unfortunately, at one of her follow-up appointments, she learns that her cancer has returned. She needs more chemotherapy and radiation. With the chemotherapy her odds are 50/50 that she will be cured, but without it she will likely die within the year. Mary is determined to do battle again, but the trouble is, Mary has exhausted her savings and has not had time to replenish them. She simply cannot afford her treatments. She begs her bank for a loan, but it refuses. She is a credit risk—if she dies, the bank won't get its money back. For the same reason, her physicians are unwilling to have her defer payment. They want payment up front. Mary is powerless. She needs the treatments but she cannot afford them. Eventually, Mary realizes that she will die. There is nothing that she can do.

> **TECHNIQUE**
>
> The Wilt Chamberlain example is meant to have intuitive appeal. Doran has weakened that appeal by providing an example that is meant to have intuitive appeal in the opposite direction. Libertarians can give examples that elicit intuitions that support their view, but supporters of redistributive taxation can give other examples that elicit perhaps stronger intuitions that support their view.

Patrick: So here we have an example in which health care is governed by the free market. Since some people, like Mary, can't afford needed care, they must go without. A charity might, of course, step in and help Mary pay for the care she needs. But if she can't afford care, and no charities offer to help, then libertarians would say that this situation is unfortunate, but Mary has no right to the assistance of others.

Doran: Right. But suppose we put the case of Mary Andrews beside the Wilt Chamberlain example, and we realize that there could be a public system that taxed Wilt and others who could afford to pay taxes. This money could then be used to fund a public medical system that could help save the lives of those who, like Mary, are unlucky and who fall ill. Is it still so obvious that it would be wrong to tax Wilt? Or do you have the opposite reaction that it would be unjust not to tax Wilt, if that was what was necessary to save Mary?

Warren: Well, it seems clear to me that it would be better to tax Wilt and save Mary than to not save Mary and let Wilt keep all of his fortune. When you consider not just Wilt, but also Mary, and others like her, the Chamberlain example loses much of its intuitive force.

THEORY

A **utilitarian** would agree with redistributive taxation if and only if it is the best way to maximize happiness, and minimize suffering, for all concerned. Given the **diminishing marginal utility** of money, it is very likely that utility will be maximized by taxing the wealthy like Wilt in order to provide the necessities for those that are very poor, like Mary. The idea of the diminishing marginal utility of money is roughly the idea that an extra bit of income is unlikely to benefit a person above a certain level of wealth as much as someone below a certain level of wealth. For instance, consider whether an extra $50 is likely to provide a greater benefit to a millionaire or to a person struggling to pay her rent.

Patrick: I agree that the Chamberlain example no longer looks that compelling once you begin to consider people like Mary who happen to be unlucky. However, the libertarian might respond to us by saying that even if a system of taxation that funded health care had good consequences, it is still wrong because it treats some (namely, those who are taxed) merely as a means to an end.

TECHNIQUE

Patrick here is anticipating an objection the libertarian is likely to raise. By considering objections, and effectively responding to them, one provides more rational support for one's view.

Doran: Good point. But I wonder whether (a) it is always wrong to treat people merely as a means, and (b) whether people who are taxed really are treated merely as a means.

Kant clearly claims that people should never be treated merely as a means, but one could disagree with Kant. If the interference is relatively minor, and if the benefit is relatively large, one might believe it is *not* wrong to treat someone merely as a means. If Wilt and others who are wealthy are taxed and end up slightly less wealthy but still comfortable, and if doing this saves people who otherwise would have died or been impoverished, then I do not think it would be wrong to do this, even if that is treating some as a mere means. The alternative strikes me as much worse.

THEORY

Immanuel Kant, in *The Groundwork of the Metaphysics of Morals*, writes, "Man, and in general every rational being, exists as an end in himself, not merely as a means for arbitrary use by this or that will: he must in all his actions, whether they are directed to himself or to other rational beings, always be viewed at the same time as an end."

To treat people merely as a means is to treat them in a way to which they do not freely consent. It is to treat them like tools, not like persons. Kant believes it is wrong to treat a person merely as means, because it disrespects a person's rational nature. According to Kant, a person is not a thing to be used, but a rational being whose decision-making capabilities are to be respected. The libertarian's point is that redistributive taxation is wrong because it treats those who are taxed in ways that they do not freely consent to, and hence, as mere means.

Patrick: Agreed. I think it's just plain false that we may *never* use people merely as a means. A compassionate society would ensure that its citizens' basic needs are met whenever feasible. It would not allow the distribution of things like housing, education, and medical care to be entirely up for grabs in a free market. To allow this would amount, in many cases, to rewarding the fortunate for their good fortune—their good genes, home, education, and so forth—and punishing the unfortunate for their bad fortune. If it is necessary to tax people in order to ensure that everyone's basic needs are satisfied, then that's what a virtuous society should do, even if this involves treating some people merely as a means.

Warren: In my view, it is acceptable to sometimes treat people merely as a means. Specifically, when it comes to redistributive taxation, people in the original position would be in favour of it, insofar as it is necessary to provide a strong social safety net. Not knowing their own preferences for risk in the real world, it would be reasonable for people in the original position to avoid extreme libertarian or **egalitarian** policies and to occupy the middle ground with moderate redistribution. That way the choosers of rules in the original position would avoid being at the opposite extreme from where their real interests lie. That hypothetical endorsement, however, does not change the fact that some wealthy people's goals and reasons for them will be ignored in the real world by some kinds of redistributive taxation. Therefore, if we implement such policies in the real world, then some wealthy people will be treated merely as a means, but this is nevertheless the right thing to do, since this policy would be endorsed in the original position.

Doran: While I also agree that it is sometimes permissible to treat people merely as a means, especially when such interferences are relatively minor, and when such interferences are necessary to prevent grave harm, I think it is worth considering whether redistributive taxation really does treat people merely as a means.

THEORY

Warren's version of **contractarianism** differs from John Rawls's theory on this point. According to Rawls, all rational people in the original position would agree to principles of justice that worked to the benefit of the worst-off group in society. Assuming redistributive taxation benefits the worst-off group, all people in the original position would choose it. If everyone agrees to redistributive taxation, then it does not treat anyone merely as a means. Therefore, Rawls would argue that taxation for these purposes does not treat anyone merely as means, since all people would agree to these taxes if they were choosing fairly.

Source: John Rawls, *A Theory of Justice* (Cambridge, MA: Harvard University Press, 1971), 83, 278.

It could be argued that there is a straightforward sense in which redistributive taxation does not treat people merely as a means. Suppose you wanted to make a little extra money so you could take your family on a vacation next spring break. You learn about a part-time job that you could do in your spare time. The pay is $40 per hour, but you also realize that after taxes the pay will work out to $30 per hour. You have to decide whether or not it is still worth it to take the job. You decide it is clearly worth it. You then do 10 hours of work and get your first cheque for $400 gross but only $300 net. It would now be bizarre for you to complain that you have been treated merely as a means because the government took $100 from you without your consent. Since you knew of the taxes, and agreed to pay them, it is not true that you were treated merely as a means when you were taxed. Similarly, when Chamberlain agreed to his lucrative contract, presumably he would have known (or at least he should have known) that he would be taxed, so that his net pay would be more like 18 cents per ticket rather than 25 cents. Nevertheless, he agreed to the contract. It is somewhat disingenuous, therefore, to suggest that Wilt was treated merely as a means when his net pay is "only" $180,000.

UP FOR DISCUSSION

Do you think that redistributive taxation uses people merely as a means? If so, does that make it wrong? Is it always wrong to treat people merely as a means?

Warren: That's a strong argument. I wonder, moreover, if we can't just say to the wealthy that a social safety net would benefit them too should they fall from their high position. There but for fortune go you or I. It could also be said that it benefits the wealthy by making the society more stable. This arguably preserves the conditions of their autonomy and so respects them as persons. And if this is correct, then we seem to have another reason why redistributive taxation needn't merely use people.

Patrick: Yes, these are good points. I think we have done enough to show that redis-tributive taxation may well be permissible. If it is permissible, as we've argued, then premise (1) in the libertarian argument is false, since it implies that redistributive taxation is wrong. Libertarians would no doubt have plenty to say in response to our objections, but let's move on to premise (2) in the libertarian argument. This premise states that if a person does not engage in violence, theft, or fraud, then the person does not violate the rights of others. So, for instance, Sanders's dad doesn't violate anyone's rights when he uses his justly acquired wealth to buy an MRI for his son from someone who freely chooses to sell him this service. It seems that this is at the heart of the most central claim made by those who support private MRI. Unlike pure libertarians, they may not oppose government-provided health care, but what they do oppose is interference with their freedom to purchase private care if they are not violating anyone else's rights.

Doran: Right, most who support private medicine probably do not oppose a public system. What they oppose is preventing people from exercising their freedom to purchase health care if that is what they choose, and if doing so violates no one else's rights.

BACKGROUND

"In a free and democratic society where you can spend money on gambling and alcohol and tobacco ... the state has no business preventing you and me from spending our own money on health care."

Source: Dr. Brian Day, quoted in Clifford Krauss, "As Canada's Slow-Motion Public Health System Falters, Private Medical Care Is Surging," *New York Times*, February 26, 2006, http://www. nytimes. com/2006/02/26/international/americas/26canada.html.

Note: Dr. Day was head of the Canadian Medical Association in 2007–08 and founded the Cambie Surgery Centre, a private health care facility in Vancouver.

The Complicity Objection to the Second Premise

Warren: Well, the libertarian asserts, in the second premise of the argument, that the only way to violate people's rights is by violence, theft, or fraud. And so, the liber-tarian reasons that if purchasing private MRI does not use violence, theft, or fraud, then it does not violate anyone else's rights; however, I do not think we should ac-cept the libertarian premise that violence, theft, or fraud is the only way to violate persons' rights. One may be complicit in a large-scale violation of rights without exercising violence, theft, or fraud.

Patrick: I agree with you, Warren, that violence, theft, or fraud aren't the only ways to violate the rights of others. And I think I get your point about being complicit in large-scale rights violations. But can you say a bit more about this?

Warren: Sure. Private MRI may be one of 10,000 small cuts that bring down a great protector of the public interest, thereby undermining a basic right to health care. While my getting a private MRI may not involve my using violence, theft, or fraud against any particular individual, that private purchase may be something a government legitimately opposes to protect citizens' access to care. If, for example, private procedures will lead to a worsening of the public system—say, because scores of physicians and MRI technicians abandon the public system in favour of the more lucrative private sector—then the government would be justified in opposing these private medical procedures. It is the duty of a government to look after access to health care for all citizens, thereby bringing about a fair balance of the liberty of the individual with the needs of the many. If private MRI erodes this right to basic access or rights to other primary goods, then a politician allowing private MRI, and a person who uses such a service, may well be complicit in large-scale rights violations.

 UP FOR DISCUSSION

Do you think people can violate rights even if they do not engage in any violence, theft, or fraud?

Doran: So you hold that people have a basic right to health care, and that this right may be violated not by any particular individual's having a private MRI, but by a system that allows private MRI when it causes serious detriments to some part of the whole socio-economic system? But, just to clarify, you're not asserting that private MRI necessarily interferes with rights?

Warren: No, it is, of course, an empirical question whether private MRI is a villain in this piece. As long as there is robust universal public access to care in a wealthy society like Canada's, and no serious harm done, private MRI may be permissible. If it interferes with provision of that access or other governmental duties, private MRI is not permissible. In the original position, we would set rules so as to avoid any system in which our health depended on our economic good fortune. Whether or not private MRI interferes with rights to access to care or other primary goods probably depends primarily on the taxation system and on what the government provides for its people using tax money.

The Compassion Objection to the Second Premise

Patrick: I'm quite sympathetic with your conclusion, Warren, that a person's rights can be violated even in the absence of violence, theft, or fraud; however, I would, of course, appeal to the virtues, rather than the original position, to explain why.

Warren: What's the virtue-based explanation, Patrick?

Patrick: Virtue requires that we have compassion for others. A virtuous society is, therefore, one in which the government has compassion for its citizens. This entails, I believe, that the government must ensure that individuals are able to satisfy their basic needs for such things as food, shelter, education, and health care. The provision of health care, and other basic goods, can obviously be undermined in ways that do not involve force or fraud. They can be undermined, for instance, by putting the distribution of basic goods entirely in the hands of a free market. In such cases, it seems quite clear that some will receive the care they need while others will have to go without, as illustrated in the Mary Andrews example we considered earlier.

Doran: Patrick, I am not sure that you can say that a virtuous society is one that must ensure that individuals are able to satisfy their basic needs for such things as food,

shelter, education, and health care. For such a requirement violates the principle that "ought implies can." As stated, your view implies that the government has a duty to provide various things, like food, education, and health care, even when it is impossible for them to provide those things. And that, clearly, cannot be correct.

> **BACKGROUND**
>
> It is generally accepted among philosophers that it makes no sense to say that someone ought to do something, if that person is unable to do the thing in question. That is what is summed up in the saying "ought implies can."

Patrick: Right, Doran. When I said that governments have a duty to ensure that citizens' basic needs are met, I was assuming that governments have the ability to do this.

Doran: Not that I disagree with your concern for those who cannot pay for MRI, Patrick, but wouldn't those proponents of private MRI say that the government should also have compassion for those people who could afford to pay for private MRI? Requiring everyone to wait in a queue for months to receive an MRI is hardly compassionate if there are other options available to them that could get them an MRI virtually immediately.

Patrick: That's true, Doran, and that is why I would not argue that private MRI is necessarily wrong. It depends on what effect private MRI would have on the public system. If, for instance, private MRI actually benefitted everyone concerned, both those who opt out of the public system and those who stay in it, then I agree that compassion, along with other virtues, provides support for private MRI. My point above, however, is just that rights can be violated even if there is no violence, theft, or fraud. A caveat is needed here, though. We're evaluating the libertarian claim that the only way to violate rights is by violence, theft, or

> **THEORY**
>
> Although some virtue theorists avoid rights talk, virtue theorists can (and some do) employ the notion of rights within their theories. They hold, however, that morality cannot be understood entirely in terms of rights, and that virtue terminology therefore plays an important explanatory role in morality.

fraud. I'm trying to show that this claim is mistaken using the terminology on the table; as for my own view, I'm not sure whether I want rights to be a fundamental part of it. The duty to ensure that everyone has adequate food, shelter, health care, and so on, it seems to me, is best grounded in virtues like compassion rather than a right to these things.

Doran: On the main point under discussion, I agree with both of you. Private MRI can be objectionable on the ground that it violates rights, even if it does not involve force or fraud. If allowing private MRIs seriously harms the public health care system, then it violates people's right to health care.

Warren: Well, it looks as if there is considerable agreement among us. But before we examine our views further, why don't we consider the view that is almost the mirror opposite of the libertarian position on private MRI? While libertarians (and others) insist on the right to private MRI so long as there is no force or fraud, some philosophers insist that all private health care, including private MRI, would be inherently unjust. Let's call this the *egalitarian* view, since it asserts that everyone should have the same access to the same type of health care regardless of ability to pay.

AN EGALITARIAN ARGUMENT

Patrick: Many people in Canada maintain that two-tier MRI is unjustified in principle. This is because it violates the idea of respect for the equality of all Canadians. To award some better or faster medical care merely because they can afford it, and to deliver inferior medical care to others merely because they cannot afford it, is deeply offensive to many. Just as we would find a health care system deeply offensive were it to give better care to whites than non-whites, or to the university educated than to those without university educations, we should also find a health care system that favours the wealthy over the poor to be deeply offensive.

Doran: It does seem unfair to give someone like Sanders better health care than Ben just because Sanders's family can afford to pay and Ben's can't.

Patrick: Right, it doesn't seem fair. Although I don't agree with the egalitarian argument, I sympathize with the motivation behind it. Imagine, Doran, that you hurt your knee while training for an upcoming marathon. Your doctor orders an MRI, and so you take your place at the back of the line. Given current wait times, you would likely have to wait several months for the procedure. Then, as you wait in line, you see a rich and famous celebrity—imagine a Canadian Kim Kardashian—waltz right into a private clinic and get an MRI that very day. After that, she gets treatment ahead of you in the public system. This seems intuitively quite unfair.

Warren: Right, but I would say we have to go beyond our intuitions here. What if the best way to get health care for everyone, including those in the public system, was by allowing some private MRIs? If that were the case, and no serious harms were done outside of health care, then I would say that people in the original position might choose private MRI. It would depend, I must emphasize, on how private MRI affected the big picture, not just health care.

Patrick: I believe you're right, Warren. If two-tier medicine were the best way to ensure that all Canadians have reasonable health care, and this wouldn't harm us in other areas of our lives, then it seems the compassionate and responsible thing to do for all involved is to allow private MRI. *If* we can best improve the system by allowing private MRI, so that everyone can wait less and receive better care, then it seems that we should permit private MRI. To opt for an egalitarian system that is best for no one would not be virtuous.

Doran: I agree, though I would put the point as follows: I think it is terribly unfair that some get better health care just because they are richer than others. And, I think that for this reason there is a strong *prima facie* reason to oppose two-tier MRI. But, *if* it is the case that we can improve the situation of everyone by allowing for some private MRIs, and *if* there is no fairer way to provide these benefits, then I'd judge that the great moral good of harm reduction outweighs this unfairness.

Patrick: I might build on my previous point by noting that there are other important goods, like education, where we permit those who can afford it to opt out of the public system and to pay for private, arguably better, education. This doesn't seem unfair, provided that the public education system is good and private education does not harm the public education system, or harm the public in other important ways.

> **TECHNIQUE**
>
> An argument by analogy is being employed here to try to support the point that the unequal provision of some important good (like primary education or health care) is not necessarily wrong, especially if it does not harm anyone concerned. The strength of this argument depends crucially on (1) whether or not the reader agrees that private, unequal primary education is sometimes not wrong, and (2) whether or not the reader agrees that the provision of primary education is relevantly similar to the provision of health care.

Doran: Right, if allowing private schools hurts kids in the public system, then that would be problematic, but if it does not harm anyone, or if it actually benefits all concerned, then it would be extremely difficult to sustain an objection that it is unfair merely on the ground that it is unequal. By analogy, it is very difficult to see how an objection to two-tier MRI could be sustained *if* it makes no one worse off, much less if it benefits all concerned.

Warren: From my perspective, two-tier education would be permissible on the same condition as two-tier medicine. It might work, for example, if private educators are required to give scholarships and fellowships to some who show ability but cannot afford private education. It would depend on the effects on the whole society. If private education brought public education into serious disrepute as second-best education or created a power elite, then that might undo any good that private education

UP FOR DISCUSSION

Do you think that two-tier health care should be opposed because it is unfair to distribute health care on the basis of the ability to pay?

might achieve. It would be unfair. We have to look, as always, at the wide effects on society, not just effects within education.

The Self-Respect Argument

Patrick: Perhaps opponents of two-tier health care can further support their position by noting that not only does two-tier health care violate the moral equality of all Canadians, but also that it is damaging to the self-respect of those Canadians who cannot afford to access private health care.

Doran: How might two-tier MRI damage some people's self-respect?

Patrick: Well, as I take it, the thought is that if some get better health care than others merely because they can afford to pay, then those who get worse health care will be made to feel that they are somehow morally less important—second-class citizens, in effect. Take Ben, for instance. He has already had to struggle so much more than Sanders, but now if Sanders also gets better or faster health care than Ben for a similar condition, then Ben might well feel that his society views him as morally less important than Sanders.

Doran: This argument reminds me of something Martin Luther King, Jr. wrote when discussing the effects of segregation on blacks living in the American South.

> You suddenly feel your tongue twisted and your speech stammering as you seek to explain to your six-year-old daughter why she can't go to the public amusement park that has just been advertised on television, and see tears welling up in her eyes when she is told that *Funtown* is closed to colored children, and see the depressing clouds of inferiority begin to form in her little mental sky.[7]

Although I certainly do not wish to compare the degree of harmfulness of racial segregation to the degree of harmfulness of two-tier MRI, I can still easily imagine Ben feeling that he is somehow inferior to Sanders because he is denied, through no fault of his own, the care that would serve him best while Sanders is not. This would be a bitter pill to have to swallow.

Warren: The concern about self-respect is certainly important. It is something that people in the original position would want very badly to protect. In the original position, people would realize that without self-respect, the enjoyment of other goods is severely limited. Self-respect is, therefore, a primary good. If it is threatened at all, we should be wary. The crucial question though is how great a threat to self-respect is posed by two-tier MRI.

Patrick: That's right. If two-tier MRI made the public system *worse*, then I would say both that people in the public system were not being properly respected by their government, and that this could have a very damaging effect on their self-respect. But if private MRI benefitted those in the public system, or at least did not make them worse off, then this would not obviously be damaging to anyone's self-respect. For it could be explained to those in the public system that two-tier was permitted only on the condition that it did not harm them.

Doran: I agree with that. The crucial distinction here appears to be whether or not two-tier harms those in the public system. If it harms people in the public system, then it may undermine their self-respect too, and for that reason may be unjust. However, if it does not harm those in the public system, then it should not cause a loss of self-respect. In that case, the argument that two-tier is wrong because it harms self-respect fails.

Warren: There is another objection to the simplistic self-respect argument. Some harms may be borne with pride for the sake of others. If, for instance, Ben thought that the difference between himself and Sanders was necessary to help those worse off than Ben, he might bear the unfairness with full self-respect. In Canada today, however, it must be admitted that no such sacrifice should be necessary.

 UP FOR DISCUSSION

Do you think unequal access to health care is wrong if it is damaging to some people's self-respect? Does two-tier health care necessarily undermine self-respect? How should we determine whether a policy undermines self-respect?

Patrick: Agreed.

Doran: This seems like a good place to pause and take stock of the arguments for, and objections to, private MRI that we've considered thus far. We agreed that both the libertarian argument for private MRI and the egalitarian argument against private MRI fail. We rejected the libertarian argument (in part) because it implies that private MRI is justified even if it harms those in the public health care system. And we rejected the egalitarian argument because it implies that private MRI would be wrong even if it brought benefits to everyone in both the private and the public system.

Patrick: That's right. We also just considered the objection that two-tier MRI is impermissible because it undermines the self-respect of those in the public system. But we agreed that there's little reason to fear that private MRI would have this effect, unless it *harmed* those in the public health care system in some other way beyond loss of self-respect; however, it might not do this. So, although the libertarian argument in favour of private MRI is unsound, the egalitarian and self-respect arguments *against* private MRI also seem to be problematic.

Doran: We all seem to agree, as well, that private MRI is permissible, provided that it benefits, or at least doesn't harm, those in the public system.

Warren: That's true as long as we consider the system to be the entire socio-economic system, not just the health care system. There is some merit, moreover, to the self-respect argument. We should be very concerned not to adopt policies that harm self-respect, and so if we are to allow two-tier MRI, we may want to find ways to compensate those who cannot afford to access the private health care system. As this shows, we may find something we can use in the ideas of the egalitarians. Similarly, we may get some help from the libertarians. I do need, however, to find a mean between these extreme positions.

Patrick: Since we all agree that two-tier MRI is permissible, at least under the right sorts of conditions, why don't we now consider what those conditions are? For instance, in order to justify private MRI, is it enough to demonstrate that it harms no one? Or does private MRI have to benefit everyone in order to be justified? And what sorts of harms and benefits are relevant here?

TWO-TIER ARGUMENTS

Is Two-Tier MRI Permissible If It Does Not Harm the Public Health Care System?

Doran: One view is that private MRI is justified provided it does not harm the public health care system. Do you agree, Patrick? Should the government allow private MRI so that people like Sanders can get treatment more quickly, provided that this does not make things worse medically for people like Ben who must wait for their care in the publicly funded system?

Patrick: I would say that this is not enough to justify private MRI. This is because there could be serious non-health-related costs to such a system. For instance, if the rich are able to get faster care than the poor, then those who cannot afford private care could possibly suffer serious setbacks in other areas of life, such as in competing for jobs, succeeding in education, earning income, and so forth. Sanders, for instance, might gain significant advantages over Ben when it comes to competing for a place in the NHL, even if private MRI doesn't make Ben's public health care worse. This seems unfair.

Warren: I agree. As noted earlier, a system that had these effects could be damaging to people's self-respect. Think of Ben. He cannot pursue his main opportunity in life as effectively as Sanders, because he cannot get care as fast. He cannot get care as fast as Sanders because he is less wealthy. On the face of it, this looks unfair.

Patrick: Warren and I appear to agree that in order for private MRI to be permissible, we need to show not merely that it doesn't harm the public health care system, but that it doesn't harm the public provision of other important goods.

Warren: Yes, that's right, Patrick. Wouldn't you also agree, Doran?

Doran: I agree that it is not enough to justify two-tier MRI merely by showing that there are no adverse effects to the health care system. In particular, if for some reason two-tier seriously harmed people in some other area of life, then it may still be unjust.

Is Two-Tier MRI Permissible If It Benefits the Public Health Care System?

Doran: Would your reaction be different if private MRI not only did not make the public health system worse but actually benefitted it?

Warren: Again, it depends on the degree of benefit and effects outside the health care system. A small benefit to the public health care system would not be enough to justify private MRIs if that allowed for large differences in advantages in other vital areas of life. Let's say Sanders had his private MRI virtually the same day it was requested, while Ben's wait time was reduced to 41 days from 188 days. This extent of improvement may not be worth it, given the costs to Ben in terms of opportunities and self-respect. Again, an insufficient justification has been given to show that private MRI is fair.

Patrick: I agree with you, Warren. As mentioned earlier, I think we need to evaluate private MRI from a more global perspective. By that I mean we need to evaluate the permissibility of private MRI by considering not just health-related benefits and costs, but also by considering benefits and costs with respect to other primary goods. So, showing that private MRI would provide health-related benefits for those in the public system is not sufficient to show that private MRI is permissible. What also needs to be shown is that there are benefits, or at least not significant costs, with respect to other goods.

Doran: Again, I agree. If two-tier MRI benefits everyone medically, then that is a strong reason in support of it, but if it ends up having grave non-medical costs as well, then that could make two-tier unjust, all things considered.

> **UP FOR DISCUSSION**
>
> Could there be anything wrong with private medicine if it benefitted the public health care system?

Patrick: Well, why don't we describe the conditions under which two-tier MRI might be justified? Warren, why don't we consider your view first?

Warren's Social Contract View on When Two-Tier MRI Is Justified

Warren: I believe that people in the original position would be especially concerned to avoid a situation that was bad for them if they turned out to be in the worst-off group in the real world. Given this, it would be rational for them to choose a society that protected their basic liberties and opportunities and that provided everyone (if the society could afford it) with an excellent safety net (a basic income, good education, good health care, ample opportunities for self-improvement, and the social conditions needed for self-respect, for example). I believe most people in the original position would accept this rule: *We should bias our decisions about allowing differences so as to provide a robust advantage to the least advantaged.* Call this the **robust advantage principle**. People in the original position would rule out private MRI if it threatened this robust advantage for the least advantaged, an excellent safety net in *wealthy* societies like our own. If private MRI were harmless, it could be allowed without benefit to the disadvantaged; but it is not harmless, and offsetting benefits are needed according to the robust advantage principle. Without significant benefits to offset significant harms, private MRI undermines the robust advantage that a wealthy society usually owes to the least advantaged.

Doran: Why do you think private MRI harms the disadvantaged in Canada?

Warren: First of all, it drains talent, from technicians to physicians, from the public health care system. This hurts members of the worst-off group the most, for they have no choice but to use the public system.

It also harms the disadvantaged with respect to access to other primary goods outside health care, such as equal opportunity and self-respect. The case of Ben and Sanders is to the point here. Sanders gets a shot at the NHL with its promises of fame and riches, while Ben misses his chance of a lifetime. He does not have the same opportunities for self-fulfillment as Sanders and may suffer from considerable loss of self-respect. He is left with the impression that his society views him as a less important person than Sanders.

Doran: So is your view that private MRI necessarily harms the disadvantaged?

Warren: No. Suppose the social safety net were exceptionally generous. Suppose that even the disadvantaged were guaranteed first-rate health care, really good education, meaningful opportunities and, in general, the means to self-respect. In this case, private MRI could be made available as long as it did not damage that social safety net. People like Ben would no longer be harmed even if there were differences brought about by private MRI.

Doran: Why not? Couldn't he still miss his chance to be in the NHL?

Warren: Perhaps, but he would still have multiple opportunities for self-fulfillment. He would not miss his one big chance in life and become an embittered, washed-up

---

BACKGROUND

"Medicare rests on the principle that an individual's financial resources should not determine access to services. In the commission's view, governments have a responsibility to guarantee that the public system has sufficient resources to ensure appropriate access to advanced technology.

"Increased investment within the public system for new diagnostic technology can remove the temptation to 'game' the system by individuals and health care providers through the private purchase of diagnostic tests that could allow them to jump the queue."

Source: Romanow, Building on Values: The Future of Health Care in Canada—Final Report, 8.

---

might-have-been. In the original position, people would allow differences in wealthy societies provided that they were guaranteed real opportunities for an excellent life even if they did not occupy the wealthier class.

Doran: Absent this robust social safety net, could we still justify private MRI if it benefitted the disadvantaged?

Warren: That depends on how much it benefits the disadvantaged. If private MRI could be shown to be necessary to provide really significant benefits to the disadvantaged, then that might be sufficient to overcome its negative effects. Suppose that it generated enough tax revenue to eliminate most homelessness: we might accept it even if it provided differences in opportunities, as long as there was no better way to eliminate homelessness and we could maintain self-respect, indeed take pride, in eliminating it. Of course, for reasons I have mentioned, I think it is extremely unlikely that private MRI could be so justified in Canada.

Doran: Patrick, what do you think? What's your view on when two-tier MRI can be justified?

Patrick's Virtue-Based View on When Two-Tier MRI Is Justified

Patrick: I've suggested that private MRI is permissible, provided that allowing it would benefit those in the public system, or at least not make them worse off. I'll now try to refine and clarify this view. But a warning is in order: the position I sketch below is still rather tentative.

If sufficient resources are available, I believe our government has (and governments in general have) an obligation to ensure that citizens have a reasonable basic level of primary social goods. I'm thinking of primary goods roughly in the Rawlsian sense—goods that everyone (or nearly everyone) needs to live well. This includes such things as food, shelter, education, health care, social and economic opportunity, and income. If everyone has a reasonable basic level of primary goods, then the government should allow private MRI, provided that this does not make those in the public system worse off, all things (i.e., all primary goods) considered, than they would be in a purely public system.

Warren: We really have to consider *all* primary goods, though.

Patrick: Right, Warren, we must look at all primary goods, not just health care.

Doran: What if the government is not meeting its obligation to provide its citizens with a reasonable basic level of primary social goods? Would private MRI then be wrong?

Patrick: There are two different situations we should consider. First, suppose the government does not have the resources to provide everyone with a basic stock of primary social goods. Second, suppose the government has the resources, but is failing to meet its obligation to provide basic primary goods. In either case, I think private MRIs are permissible, but only if this *improves* the situation, all things (i.e., all primary goods) considered, of the general public.

Doran: Why do you believe your position is justified?

Patrick: Well, I think that my view on private MRI can be justified from different moral perspectives, but I'll stick to my preferred virtue theory. As I've mentioned before, a virtuous society would be a compassionate, caring, and responsible society. For this reason, a virtuous society would be one in which the government ensures, insofar as possible, that everyone has a reasonable minimal level of primary goods. Without a basic level of these goods, one cannot live a decent life. If we allowed these goods to be distributed entirely by a free market, it is clear that some would have lots, while many others would have little or none. To allow this—that is, to allow some to prosper while many others suffer—with respect to such basic goods would be rather cruel and callous, among other things.

Suppose that the government is not providing everyone with a reasonable level of primary social goods. There might be two reasons for this: the government does not have the resources to do this, or it does have the resources but is simply not delivering the goods. Then, as I mentioned, private MRI is morally permissible provided that this benefits everyone concerned. In the first case, the government could impose a tax on private MRIs and use the money collected to improve everyone's lot. In the second case, the private sector could set up private MRIs and provide subsidies for those who cannot afford the fee. This would seem to be the virtuous thing to do, all things considered. Allowing private MRI in either case would respect the liberty of the wealthy, for those who are fortunate enough to pay for private MRIs could get them. And the system would also show compassion for the less wealthy, since they would see their situation improved.

Now, if the government has ensured that everyone has a reasonable basic level of primary goods, then it seems it would be rather mean-spirited and unfair to prohibit private MRI, if this doesn't worsen the situation of others. A virtuous society would, of course, be concerned with the interests of both the rich and the poor. If a person has an interest in getting an MRI done quickly, and this person has the good fortune of being able to pay to have one done privately, and allowing private MRI wouldn't hurt others, then on what grounds could one reasonably object? I don't like the idea of the wealthy getting MRIs faster than others simply because they have more money. So there is a sense of unfairness here. But, again, it also seems unfair and mean-spirited to make the wealthy wait in line simply because that's what others must do. That's taking egalitarian ideals too far.

Warren: This raises an interesting question of how far is too far. Suppose there is such a high tax on private MRI that the practice is able to continue, but only just. The taxes are used to minimize wait times for public MRI. Of course, the private entrepreneurs would say this is unfair, but what would a virtuous society do?

Patrick: As I said, I think a virtuous society would be one that looks out for the basic interests of both the rich and the poor. By allowing private MRI, we can let the wealthy avoid waiting for an MRI. And by taxing private MRI, we can improve the lot of those in the public system by helping to reduce their wait times. Of course, some will still complain, but this system looks pretty fair to me, since it balances a concern for all affected.

Doran: Let's bring this back to Ben and Sanders. Suppose they live in a society that provides its citizens with a reasonably decent social safety net. Patrick, I take it that your view is that Sanders should be allowed to purchase a private MRI, provided it does not worsen Ben's condition, all things considered (i.e., all primary goods considered). Further, if they are living in a society that fails to provide a decent minimum, then Sanders should still be allowed to get a private MRI only if this can be used to benefit those who are less fortunate, like Ben (say, by shortening wait times in the public system or by taxing these services and using the proceeds to benefit the public system).

Patrick: Yes, that's the basic idea.

Doran: One question I have for you, Patrick (though it is a question that I might well ask of Warren's view, too), is how you think the idea of a "reasonable basic level of primary social goods" should be understood. Specifically, is this something that should be indexed to the general level of wealth of the society, or is it something that is like a floor that does not move over time? For example, does this reasonable minimum mean that everyone should be ensured merely that their basic survival needs are met, that they have basic health care and education, and that is more or less it, or is it something that is more flexible, so that in an affluent society it would not just be that basic survival needs are met, but also that everyone has access to quality education and health care, comfortable lodgings, opportunities for advancement and leisure, access to technological gains from indoor plumbing to high-speed Internet access, and so on?

Patrick: Good question, Doran. I've been thinking of the reasonable minimum not as fixed, but rather as fluid. What counts as a reasonable minimal or basic level of primary goods is relative to how much wealth there is in society. In lean times, the reasonable minimum may not be much—perhaps just enough to survive. In times of abundance, however, the reasonable minimal level will be more than that. The wealth should be shared so that inequalities between the rich and the poor do not become so great that the rich have an unreasonably large advantage over the poor when it comes to things like education, income, opportunities, and so forth.

Warren: Well, that helps to clarify a concern I had. I was wondering why you suggested that a "compassionate and caring" society would ensure only a "reasonable *minimal level* of primary social goods." That sounds rather stingy to me. I would think that a compassionate and caring society would be a lot more generous than providing a decent minimum. I would think that if it had the resources, a compassionate and caring society would want its citizens to have a very generous social safety net—the kind of social safety net that was the envy of the world. But I see now that that is what you're suggesting.

Patrick: That's right, Warren, I'm proposing that the government has an obligation to ensure that its citizens have a reasonable basic level of primary goods. But as I just noted in response to Doran's question, what counts as a reasonable basic level is relative to how much wealth there is in the society. In good times, where there is an abundance of resources, the reasonable basic minimum will be quite generous.

Notice, moreover, that in order to ensure that others are not made worse off (all things considered) by allowing private MRI, the government would have to ensure that the general public has a rather generous basic level of primary goods. This is because others will in fact be made worse off (all things considered) if the gap between the "haves" and the "have-nots" becomes too great.

Warren: It seems, Patrick, that you and I agree that when deciding on MRI policy we need to take a global view, avoiding the ills of flat egalitarianism on the one hand, and the problems attendant on wide class distinctions on the other. Between these extremes we seek a system that leaves incentives to improve MRI technology and training without its becoming a tool of the elite to enhance its position. That may be a tall order when we have trouble just seeing how it affects wait times, but it has to be seen as part of an overall health care policy which in turn is a cornerstone of social policy. We differ primarily on why we should do this.

Patrick: Right, and I think this helps to strengthen our view. We are arguing for a view that can be supported by your contract theory and my virtue theory.

 UP FOR DISCUSSION

When, if ever, do you think two-tier MRI is morally permissible?

COMMENTS ON CANADA'S CURRENT PUBLIC HEALTH CARE SYSTEM

Doran: There is a large amount of agreement in your two views, though you've approached the question from very different perspectives. But the practical implications are not entirely clear. I think we should wrap up our discussion by returning to the question we began with: Is private MRI permissible in Canada? More specifically, is two-tier MRI permissible in Canada today, given our current health care system, and given the current distribution of primary goods in general?

Warren: In Canada, we have a wealthy society. We would need good reasons to believe that it is likely that the overall effect of private MRI on society would further a robust advantage to the least advantaged. This would require a wide-ranging investigation of private MRI's socio-economic effects. If a convincing argument can be made for private MRI in these terms, which I doubt, the electorate should decide its merits, but private MRI should not have been allowed before it was put to that test.

Patrick: Like Warren, I don't think we can give a simple "yes" or "no" answer to this question, since the answer depends on empirical issues that are a matter of some controversy. A conditional answer will therefore have to do for now. Given the amount of wealth in our country, I think that the public health care system is not at all up to par. The government is not providing a reasonable basic minimum, given the available resources. So my view implies that private MRI is permissible, only if allowing it will help to improve the public system and, of course, not impose significant costs in terms of other basic goods. *If* this can be demonstrated, then I think that private MRI is permissible in Canada.

 UP FOR DISCUSSION

After considering the various arguments for and against, do you think two-tier MRI should be allowed in Canada? Why or why not?

FROM THE POLITICAL TO THE INDIVIDUAL

Doran: If we assume, for the sake of argument, that the use of private MRI is unjustified at present in Canada, then the following interesting question arises: *Do you think Sanders's dad is doing something morally wrong by using the private system to get his son an MRI?* Our earlier discussion of the complicity objection to libertarianism suggests that you guys would object to a person's taking advantage of such a situation. But some may think that this seems rather harsh. One may put the point in the language of virtue theory: Wouldn't a compassionate, responsible father utilize the system of private MRI to benefit his son, even if he wished that the general provision of medicine were more just? What do you think? Here the question is being shifted from the political to the personal. Before we wondered about the just or virtuous society, but now we are asking about the virtuous parent and the actions it is permissible for him to take in a situation of injustice.

Warren: Given the system we have in Canada today, I do not think people do wrong when they seek private MRI for serious medical reasons. It is the politicians who do wrong when they put people in the position of having to seek private MRI. As we were stating our positions, I mentioned that I had sympathy for people seeking private MRI in Canada given the excessive wait times for necessary diagnostics. My sympathy is even greater for a parent seeking MRI for

> **THEORY**
>
> Recall that Warren uses a **sympathy metarule** as part of the conditions under which people in the original position choose rules. This says, "The people in the original position must choose rules that people with ordinary human sympathies could follow." Sympathy is construed broadly. See chapter 3 for more details.

a son or daughter. I doubt that I am alone in this. By my **sympathy metarule**, any strict rule against complicity that required us to ignore such sympathies would be rejected or modified in the original position.

Doran: So people with wealth can just enjoy their privilege without compunction, according to rules chosen in the original position?

Warren: No, it's not that simple. People in the original position would accept rules governing social policy that indict the inadequate system we now have in Canada where private MRI is concerned. Politicians would still have a strong moral duty to tie private MRI to the public good if they allowed it at all. All citizens, including Sanders's dad, have, moreover, a duty to hold politicians to account for the injustice to people like Ben and to demand an adequate public diagnostic system as part of a fair social system generally. In my view, the wealthy are not required to join the poor in their misery, but they are not permitted to ignore that misery.

Doran: Well and good, but what social contract rules are we talking about here that underlie these duties, in your view?

Warren: Well, generally speaking, our current MRI policies contravene the robust advantage principle of which I spoke earlier: *We should bias our decisions about allowing differences so as to provide a robust advantage to the least advantaged.* Sanders's dad, however, is not one who is directly allowing the differences. Politicians are. The duty of Sanders's dad, as a man of wealth and thus of some political influence or potential influence, is to shake up the politicians to get them to abide by the robust advantage principle. It's the duty of the whole electorate, really, to demand a fair system of health care from our elected representatives.

Patrick: Though I don't agree with the theory supporting Warren's view, I largely agree with his view on this issue. If Sanders's father happens to have the resources to pay for an MRI for his son, then it is quite understandable that he would take advantage of his good fortune. In fact, it would seem rather callous and irresponsible if Sanders's father made his son suffer and wait for an MRI when he has the means to get him one right away. But those who have the good fortune of being wealthy enough to afford private care should use whatever influence and resources they have to help ensure adequate care for those in the public system. It would be selfish and insensitive of the wealthy to simply ignore the suffering others must endure due to a lack of adequate public health care. As Warren noted, the moral failing here lies not with Sanders or his father, but with governments in Canada. They are simply not meeting their obligations to ensure that residents of this country have reasonable health care. I believe there's an additional moral failing on the part of those who own and operate private MRI clinics. They might show more compassion toward those in the public system by using some of their profits to help improve the public system. One way to do this, for instance, would be to offer free or heavily subsidized MRI for the poor.

CLOSING ARGUMENTS

Warren: I believe it is very likely that two-tier MRI is not justified in Canada today. This is because such unequal access to medical diagnostics ignores the robust advantage principle: *We should bias our decisions about allowing differences so as to provide a robust advantage to the least advantaged.* I have argued that a decision in favour of two-tier MRI appears to ignore this required bias.

The robust advantage principle does not require us to always favour the least advantaged as an excessively egalitarian society might do. We are not required, for instance, to make everyone else radically worse off just to bring about a small advantage to those on the bottom. We should avoid that egalitarian extreme.

By the same token we should avoid the libertarian extreme. While the robust advantage principle does not require us to always put the disadvantaged first, it does not let us ignore them, either. In wealthy societies, at least, we can afford to make sure that everyone has both necessities and opportunities.

The robust advantage principle could, nonetheless, justify inequalities in access to medical care under a variety of circumstances. Here are some examples: (1) a robust social safety net is in place, and the effects of having two-tier care do not worsen the condition of the worst-off members of society; or (2) a robust social safety net is in place, and introducing two-tier care worsens the condition of the worst-off members of society but not to the point where they slip through the net, and two-tier care greatly improves the condition of the vast majority; or (3) a robust social safety net is not in place, and two-tier care is a good way to help bring about these robust advantages for the worst off; or (4) a robust social safety net is not in place, and two-tier care is the only way to save the society from disastrous consequences.

The situations in the first two examples are not like ours in Canada today, since our government has not provided a sufficiently generous social safety net. And I believe we are not in the third or fourth situations either, since I see no credible evidence that allowing for two-tier MRI is a good way to enhance the advantages of the worst-off group, or is necessary to ward off disaster.

Patrick: I agree with most of your conclusions, Warren; however, I am less certain about whether a system of two-tier MRI (or two-tier health care, generally) is justified in Canada today. Specifically, it *might* be the case that carefully regulated two-tier MRI could work to increase the primary goods available to all Canadians. Carefully regulated two-tier MRI *could perhaps* improve the lot of poorer Canadians by shortening queues in the public health care system, increasing the amount of dollars available for each patient in the public system, and benefitting the social system in other ways by taxing private clinics. As you noted, this is largely an empirical question, and I am not sure where the facts lie.

TECHNIQUE

It may seem strange that the debate ignores the presence, next to Canada, of the United States, a bastion of two-tier health care and two-tier education available to many Canadians. Since private health care and education are easily accessible in the United States for most of the wealthy in Canada, there is no effective way for Canadian governments to enforce a one-tier policy. It is, nonetheless, important to discuss Canada as if it were isolated to see what the moral status of two-tier medicine would be under ideal conditions. When we see what our ideal system is, we will see how to ameliorate the injustices in the systems we must accept. As things change in the United States, our health care system will have to respond. If current US policies or new medical technologies create injustice in our health care delivery, we will learn from consulting our ideal system what we must do to our actual system to make it resemble that ideal as much as possible.

Doran: Well, for much of this debate I have been content to listen and to ask questions; however, earlier I argued along with both of you that the libertarian reasons in support of a right to private health care are not compelling, and that the egalitarian arguments against private health care are not necessarily decisive, and can be defeated, at least in principle.

I also think I agree with your views on when two-tier MRI can be justified. For example, it can be justified if a robust social safety net is in place, provided that it does not harm that social safety net, and it can be justified if a robust social safety net is not in place, provided that it improves the condition (broadly construed) of the worst off. In addition to the contractarian and virtue-based arguments developed by you two, I find the arguments by analogy with private primary education to be helpful on this point. I think that, on reflection, most of us would think there was something wrong with a policy that allowed for private education to the detriment of the public education system. And I think most of us would be willing to support a policy allowing private primary education, provided that the public education system was of high quality and that people in it were not made worse off by the existence of a private tier.

Like Patrick, I remain very uncertain about the benefits and costs of two-tier MRI (and two-tier health care generally). It may well be the case that carefully regulated two-tier care could actually work to the significant benefit of the least advantaged by shortening queues, making more public money available per patient, generating greater revenues by taxing the private system, and so on. I just don't know.

Finally, I am not yet persuaded about the permissibility of parents taking advantage of private health care for their children, if it turns out that this private system itself is unjust. In general, I think it is wrong to support unjust institutions, even if such institutions benefit oneself or one's loved ones. And I am quite reluctant to give up that principle. Of course, I think it is understandable if a parent avails herself of the best care possible for her child, even if that care morally ought not to have been available in the first place. I wonder, though, if such behaviour is in fact morally permissible, or if it is merely **excusable**. This is a particularly tough question, since it raises one of the most difficult problems in moral philosophy—how to reconcile (1) the belief that we ought to respect the moral equality of all persons, and so reject institutions that violate this principle, with (2) the belief that a morally decent person is properly partial toward their loved ones.

 UP FOR DISCUSSION

If two-tier MRI should not be permitted, do you think it is wrong for parents to use it to benefit their children? Why or why not?

SUMMARY

Here is a summary of the main questions, concepts, and arguments covered in this chapter:

- Magnetic resonance imaging (MRI) is a technique for scanning for muscle and joint injuries. Both the scans and the machines that scan are referred to as MRIs.
- A two-tier system of health care is a system in which one tier, or level, is publicly funded and one tier is privately funded. The idea is that those who can afford the additional private care can access a higher level of care.
- The main question explored is whether private MRI is morally acceptable in Canada. This is part of the larger question of whether two-tier health care is justified in Canada. Subordinate questions include the following: Is

two-tier MRI permissible if it does not harm the public health care system? Is two-tier MRI permissible if it benefits the public health care system? Is it permissible for a patient to use private MRI in Canada, even if private MRI in Canada is unjust?

- Although the debate is largely restricted to specific questions, it takes place against the backdrop of the national debate in Canada over the permissibility of a two-tier system of medical care. Some tentative ideas are ventured in this regard. Conclusions in the debate are conditional, depending on the empirical question of the effects of two-tier access to MRI on the public health care system.

- Libertarian arguments against redistributive taxation and in favour of a right to private health care are considered and found to be ultimately unpersuasive.

- Egalitarian arguments against private MRI are then considered and are also found to be ultimately unpersuasive.

- Warren, Patrick, and Doran argue that two-tier MRI can be justified under certain circumstances. Given certain empirical assumptions, Warren doubts that those circumstances apply in Canada today. Patrick and Doran are somewhat more cautious about the empirical assumptions.

- Under the assumption that two-tier MRI is unjust in Canada, Patrick and Warren agree that it would, nonetheless, be permissible for a patient to use private MRI. Doran is not yet convinced.

REVIEW QUESTIONS

1. Why do libertarians oppose redistributive taxation?
2. What is the Wilt Chamberlain example, and what is its point?
3. Why is this argument rejected?
4. Why is the argument that people should have a right to use their justly earned wealth to freely purchase private MRI rejected?
5. What two arguments do egalitarians give to oppose two-tier MRI?
6. How do Warren, Patrick, and Doran respond to these two arguments?
7. When do Warren, Patrick, and Doran think two-tier MRI is justified?
8. What arguments do Warren, Patrick, and Doran give for this view?
9. Why does Warren think two-tier MRI in Canada is probably unjust?
10. Why do Warren and Patrick think it is permissible for a patient to use private MRI in Canada, even if private MRI in Canada is unjust? Why is Doran unconvinced?

NOTES

1. See examples of current advertised prices in British Columbia, Canada, at http://www. imageonemri.ca/pricing/.

2. See, for example, average prices of MRI in various countries at https://www.statista.com/ statistics/312020/price-of-mri-diagnostics-by-country/.

3. "MRI Machine Cost and Price Guide," *Block Imaging*, https://info.blockimaging.com/bid/92623/ MRI-Machine-Cost-and-Price-Guide.

4. Edith MacHattie and Rick Turner, "Opinion: MRI Plan a Welcome New Direction for BC Diagnostics," *Vancouver Sun*, April 2, 2018, http://vancouversun.com/opinion/op-ed/edith-machattie-and-rick-turner-mri-plan-a-welcome-new-direction-for-b-c-diagnostics. Rick Turner and Edith MacHattie are with the BC Health Coalition. In this opinion piece, they describe a government plan to improve wait times for MRI.

5. Private MRI clinics have been shown to do scans more often than hospitals, which raises a concern about unnecessary scans. See Jean M. Mitchell and Jonathan H. Sunshine, "Consequences of Physicians' Ownership of Health Care Facilities—Joint Ventures in Radiation Therapy," *New England Journal of Medicine* 327, no. 21 (1992): 1497–1501.

6. Robert Nozick, *Anarchy, State, and Utopia* (New York: Basic Books, 1974), 160–64.

7. Martin Luther King, Jr., "Letter from Birmingham Jail," reprinted in *The Right Thing to Do*, ed. James Rachels and Stuart Rachels, 4th ed. (New York: McGraw-Hill, 2007), 293.

9

MICROALLOCATION OF SCARCE RESOURCES

INTRODUCTION

In this chapter, we will be discussing disaster scenarios in which all medical professionals in the area are required to drop all non-emergency care and come in to the hospital to help. The case used in this chapter to motivate discussion concerns an emergency room in a small town overwhelmed by many injured incoming patients from a vehicle accident. There are insufficient resources to treat everyone immediately. The more serious patients cannot be transferred to other hospitals because they will not survive the journey. The number of critically ill patients exceeds resources to treat them. A **triage** nurse faces extraordinarily difficult ethical decisions about whom, among equally urgent patients, to direct first to the lone physician on duty. Such rare cases test existing triage principles and stimulate discussion on the appropriate treatment priorities in emergency situations.

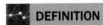

> **DEFINITION**
>
> **Triage:** from the French *trier*, "to sort." It is defined as "the process of determining the order in which a large number of injured or ill patients will receive medical treatment, with priority usually given to those patients with the most severe ailments or the greatest chance of survival" (*Canadian Oxford Dictionary*, 1998).

Some health care professionals may find our interest in such cases puzzling because these cases seem too rare to bother with. In fact, though, they are just what is needed to put great stress on the principles we use every day, stress that will test our commitment to and understanding of those principles. It can be argued, moreover, that a discussion of disaster scenarios is of great practical importance. Emergencies that stretch resources to this degree are rare in our society, but they are, tragically, not rare in many other societies.[1] Further, it is virtually certain that such emergencies will, at some time, occur in Canada. Witness the often-voiced concern about the rapid spread of epidemics like bird or swine flu, the possible dire predictions of terrorist attacks, earthquakes, environmental disasters, and so forth. We need to have a clear understanding of the rules we should follow to handle such crises.[2] Clarity about how to handle admission of equally urgent patients fairly in these crises may also guide us in other more common situations where patients must be triaged in emergency and non-emergency situations.[3]

Warren will use his social contract method to arrive at a set of principles to prioritize patients in emergency situations. Doran and Patrick will challenge Warren's argument and will work with him to begin to develop a set of fair rules. In the end, Doran argues that triage nurses should follow principles that are largely limited to certain medical considerations. Warren and Patrick go further and argue that a greater number of non-medical considerations should sometimes influence who should receive care first.

LEARNING OBJECTIVES

After completing this chapter, you should be able to:

- Define *microallocation* and distinguish it from other types of allocation in health care
- Explain the CTAS guidelines, and discuss why these guidelines are too simple to deal adequately with all triage scenarios
- State Warren's, Doran's, and Patrick's views on whether Alice acted permissibly in caring for her Aunt Lena ahead of Terence
- Discuss the role impartiality should play in the treatment of patients, and how impartiality is limited by the sympathy metarule in Warren's view
- Explain and discuss the rules "worst first," "first come, first served," and "hopeless second"
- Distinguish between *excuse*, *mitigation*, and *justification*, and explain how the sympathy metarule helps identify whether a particular act is excused, mitigated, or justified
- Describe Patrick's and Doran's objections to the sympathy metarule
- Understand why minimize YPLL (years of potential life lost) evolved into substantial benefit under the force of objections
- State some of the challenges for substantial benefit
- Explain the fair turn and innocents first rules
- Discuss whether a person's moral responsibility should ever affect triage decisions
- Describe some relevant third-party interests that may affect the proper order of care in an emergency situation

---

DRAMA

Please note: This case is based on various true stories, although names, places, and some uncontroversial elements of the case have been changed to preserve anonymity and confidentiality. Discussions of this and similar cases with health care professionals have also informed this fictional case. The drama merely raises issues. The philosophical arguments are to be found in the debate following the drama.

CHARACTERS

Alice: a triage nurse for 20 years

Gurpreet: a nurse training with Alice to serve as a triage nurse

---

The scene is set in a small town in southern Ontario.

Alice: Now, Mr. Bains we called a level 1, and sent him in right away. Why was that?

Gurpreet: Well, to tell you the truth, I was a bit surprised at that. He did not seem like a likely candidate for an **MI**. He kept saying it was probably just heartburn, but he wanted to check.

Alice: That's the thing, you just can't tell. You know you might see somebody who is fit like Bains and dismissive of his pain, but it's tricky. If they have unexplained chest pain, send them in.

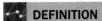

> **DEFINITION**
>
> Level 1 is a category triage nurses use for patients who need a physician's care immediately.

> **DEFINITION**
>
> MI stands for myocardial infarction, a heart attack.

Gurpreet: My goodness! Was that woman with the broken wrist ever ticked when Bains went in ahead of her. Oh, my! Alice, I thought she would…

Alice: Get used to it, Gurpreet. People are always angry. They always think they should go first. Parents with kids get outraged sometimes when you treat somebody ahead of their kid. You just have to do your best. You're always triaging in your head. There's this constant assessment and reassessment of your patients. People come in, sit down, get worse, get better. You have to be watching everybody all the time.

Gurpreet: What happens when you have a couple of people at the same level at the same time? I mean, suppose you have someone like Bains, and then someone like that young woman with the type 2 diabetes … you know the one?

Alice: Yeah, I think I see where you're going with this.

Gurpreet: So she came in first because of numbness in her foot but doesn't have chest pains at first, then in comes Bains and she starts having the pains. Now you've got the two of them both at level 1. Today we have Dr. Anderson and Dr. Horst both in, but suppose one of them was out of town? I would take that young woman first.

Alice: Yes, Ashley—she's the woman with diabetes. She would probably be more urgent than Bains in that case, so sure, you do have to make decisions about who goes first even within levels. And in some kinds of cases you can take a couple of people at once. Dr. Anderson is a good multi-tasker. Dr. Horst is not, though. Anyway, sometimes you just have to choose. It's not often that you can't call in extra help or get a nurse to hold the fort until Dr. Anderson or Dr. Horst can get to it. But when you do get these tough choices, it can be really hairy. I mean, suppose Bains came in kind of grey with left-side weakness. It might be tough to say whether he was more urgent than Ashley. What would you do then?

Gurpreet: Well, I guess to be fair, I'd just take them in the order they came.

Alice: Of course, if it's like you say, Ashley was there first, but for something else, and they both get into real trouble at the same time, then it isn't so clear what's fair. I'll tell you though, the people who work here are really good people. They might look at it and say, "Well, here's Ashley with nothing, living in the shelter, never had a break. And there's Bains, the wealthy dentist, all the advantages." You know, I think we tend to give the people who are the most vulnerable the edge when it comes to a tie. You might have noticed that indigent people get royal treatment here.

Gurpreet: It seems like a kind of reverse discrimination.

Alice: Yeah, maybe.

Gurpreet: But what if you thought Ashley was unable to recover because of her other conditions, but you thought you might be able to save Bains?

Alice: Well, sometimes a patient really has no hope of recovery, but we can't know that. I guess if it seemed really obvious that one person was a candidate for comforts only but the other could have a long life, then the one who had a real chance should go in first. But look, I've been on the job 20 years, and I've never had a decision like that.

Gurpreet: I need to ask about these what-ifs because, you know, you never had a day like last Thursday in your whole career before, either. You had to make tough choices like you'd never made before. I don't know what I'll face in my career. I need to be ready, Alice. I'm not trying to be pushy. I'm just scared that I won't know how to think about some of the things I might see.

Alice: Point taken, Gurpreet. Last Thursday was a regular Armageddon.

Gurpreet: I don't really know how you made those decisions; I was so busy putting pressure on a wound with Horst barking orders and everything going crazy all around us.

Alice: Well, you kind of go on instinct when it's that bad, or it's like you're just doing what you know from experience. I sort of feel like I'm programmed by my earlier imaginings about what I would do if I was in that kind of a fix.

Gurpreet: Is it too soon to talk about it, Al?

Alice: No, Gurpreet, I've got some distance now. But it's still fresh in my mind. Maybe now is the right time even if there is no good time to talk about it.

Gurpreet: It must be so hard, when you know everybody in town, to make choices like that. I was talking to the mayor yesterday. He said it all started when Terence walked right out on the highway without even looking. He was really very inebriated, the mayor said.

Alice: Terence always was drunk.

Gurpreet: The van full of people heading for the conference swerved to avoid Terence, but hit him and then lost control. They hit Harvey's truck head-on.

Alice: Yeah, that about fits with what I heard. Les saw most of it happen and told me.

Gurpreet: Where was Dr. Anderson?

Alice: Dr. Anderson was already at the Northern Health Conference in Mayville. By the time she got back here, it was all over but the crying.

Gurpreet: By the time they called me in to Emerg it was already chaotic.

Alice: It didn't take long to get that way. They brought Terence in first. He was unconscious with a serious head wound. Right behind him was Aunt Lena. You could have knocked me over with a feather. She was in awful shape. They were both level 1.

Gurpreet: You're really close to Lena, aren't you?

Alice: God, yes. I was emulating Lena when I got into nursing in the first place. She's been my hero.

Gurpreet: Well, she's been a hero to this whole town from what I gather.

Alice: Yes, there's not much good work here that she hasn't had a hand in. Anyway, I saw Lena and did not even think. I took her straight in to see Dr. Horst. Lena told me to let her wait and take care of Terence. I didn't listen. Dr. Horst was sewing up this carpenter who had mangled his hand. He just handed off the carpenter to Jesse to keep the bleeding under control and started right to work on Lena.

Gurpreet: What happened to Terence?

Alice: We had him in the next room, and told Dr. Horst about him. Dr. Horst just said okay and worked furiously on Lena while I went back to call everybody in and tell a level 3 in the waiting room that it was going to be a long time. I could hardly talk.

Gurpreet: Is Lena going to make it?

Alice: Maybe. She's got a lot of internal injuries. Harvey was sitting right beside her in the truck, and he died on impact, they think. She's so tough. God, I hope she'll make it.

Gurpreet: I guess you didn't even have a chance to catch your breath before the others came in.

Alice: You got that right. Those people from the van were not hurt as bad, but we all had somebody to work on. That's when you came in and I put you to work on that young guy who looked like he might bleed out. It was him or that really old man who was unconscious, so I chose the young guy. The old fellow had probably already had a good shot at life at his age. They both pulled through in the end.

Gurpreet: Was Terence still alive then?

Alice: I'm not sure. Jesse was with him. She just said by the time Dr. Horst had Lena stabilized, it was too late for poor old Terence, and I didn't have the heart to ask any more about it.

Gurpreet: Are you okay, Alice?

Alice: Yeah, I feel bad about it, but I think I did the right thing.

Gurpreet: Nobody could have done better, Alice.

DEBATE

Clarifying the Case and Identifying Relevant Facts

Patrick: Well, I think it's pretty clear what happened in this case.

Doran: Yes, but it's a little hard to remember who is who. Aside from the nurses Gurpreet and Alice, there are a great many patients and health care workers to keep track of.

Warren: Maybe a quick review would help. The action takes place in a rural setting where one often finds a scarcity of resources that one would not find in a larger centre. There's Bains, a wealthy dentist and a patient in Emerg. He gets in ahead of other patients because chest pain makes him a level 1. Ashley, a patient in the emergency department with type 2 diabetes, was used as an example by Gurpreet to try to contrast with Bains.

Patrick: Oh yes, that's not something that actually happens in the case. Rather, Gurpreet is just juxtaposing two patients in her imagination. She wanted to consider two level 1 patients competing for resources.

Warren: That's right. Dr. Angela Anderson, an emergency physician, was away during the big accident, leaving all the cases to Dr. Hans Horst, the other emergency physician in this small town. Then there is Terence, a chronic alcoholic, who caused the terrible traffic accident that made him a patient in the emergency department. He gets treated after Alice's Aunt Lena, and he ends up dying. Remember that Alice put Aunt Lena, a pillar of the community, ahead of Terence.

Doran: There was another important decision Alice made, too, but the patients did not have names.

Warren: Yes, a young patient is treated ahead of an elderly man. In addition, there are sundry other characters who do not figure prominently in the story: Harvey, one of the drivers, who died on impact in the accident; Jesse, an emergency department nurse; the carpenter whose wound treatment is put on hold while more urgent patients are treated; and the mayor and Les, who witnessed the accident. Some of the unnamed patients were in the van that swerved to avoid Terence and hit Harvey's truck head-on.

MORAL ISSUES RAISED BY THE CASE

BACKGROUND

"The Canadian Triage and Acuity Scale (CTAS) was introduced during the late 1990s....
The CTAS is now being implemented as a national triage standard for Canada's emergency health care system. Prior to its formulation, hundreds of rural and urban Canadian
emergency departments (EDs) had developed home-grown triage systems to sort patients by urgency. There was, and still is, huge variation in rural ED triage across the
country." The CTAS guidelines were drawn up as a consensus document by the CTAS
National Working Group of nurse and physician specialists in emergency department
triage and have been validated by a number of publications. The CTAS directs triage
nurses and doctors to place patients in emergency departments on a five-point scale,
where patients at level 1 require immediate treatment, patients at level 2 are slightly
less urgent, etc.

CTAS

Acuity	Triage level	Physician assessment	Nurse assessment
Critical	1	Stat	Stat
Emergent	2	<15 min	<15 min
Urgent	3	<30 min	<30 min
Semi-urgent	4	<1 h	<1 h
Non-urgent	5	<2 h	<2 h

Note: Stat is the abbreviation of the Latin statim, "immediately."

The CTAS has been criticized for requiring unrealistic response times, especially for
emergency departments in rural communities, where hospital resources (including per-
sonnel) are in short supply.

Source: Quotation and other information taken/adapted from James M. Thompson and Graham
Dodd, "Ruralizing the Canadian Triage and Acuity Scale," Canadian Journal of Emergency
Medicine 2, no. 4 (2000): 267.[4]

Patrick: The essential problem concerns the treatment of patients in emergency situations, and who should be given priority. The guidelines nurses have just tell them
to take patients in order of medical urgency, but in cases like this one, where the
hospital's emergency department is overwhelmed, questions about these guidelines are bound to arise.

Doran: Sure, we want to know whether other factors besides urgency are morally relevant. We need to know how to make decisions when cases are equally urgent, and yet the patients cannot all be cared for at once. This is the general issue we should investigate.

Patrick: Yes. The specific question we could debate is *whether Alice acted permissibly in our drama.* For example, Alice took other considerations, like age and merit, into account, when deciding on who should be treated ahead of whom. In answering this question, we will no doubt consider the more general issue: *What rules ought to be followed when deciding on the order of care in emergency situations where needed resources are scarce?* But let's begin with Alice. Were her decisions justified?

Stating Our Positions

Warren: I believe we will be able to justify Alice's decisions by appeal to principles people would accept in the original position.

Doran: Although I feel great sympathy for Alice, I believe she made decisions that were not hers to make as a triage nurse. For instance, I am quite uneasy about her decision to take Lena ahead of Terence. Triage nurses should base their treatment decisions impartially on *clinical* factors, and not on personal affection, judgments of guilt or innocence, and so forth.

DEFINITION AND BACKGROUND

Clinical factors are considerations that may affect the proper order of care, arising from an assessment of the medical needs of the particular patients; **non-clinical factors** are those that do not arise from an assessment of the medical needs of the particular patients. An example of a non-clinical factor might be the guilt or innocence of the patients waiting for treatment. Nurses, at least, are sometimes suspicious of rules that allow the use of such non-clinical factors.

Patrick: I'm also a little uncomfortable with Alice's decision to put Lena ahead of Terence. But given her special relationship with Lena, I don't think we can morally blame her for doing this. Indeed, I think that from my virtue ethics perspective, her actions can be shown to be morally permissible. More generally, I believe that acting virtuously requires that we allow *non-clinical* considerations to play a role in prioritizing patients.

MICROALLOCATION RULES: CLINICAL CONSIDERATIONS

Warren's Argument for Fair Microallocation Rules: Worst First, First Come, and Hopeless Second

---

BACKGROUND

"While macroallocation of resources concerns public health policies, microallocation is concerned with selecting which individuals are to receive scarce or insufficient health care resources" (266).

Some use the term *mesoallocation* to refer to allocation at the level of institutions, and *macroallocation* to refer to allocation at the level of governments deciding among health care and other areas needing support. We are looking at the issue of microallocation under conditions of scarcity. The principles we consider and defend in this chapter are not necessarily appropriate to mesoallocation or macroallocation.

Source: Quotation taken from P. A. C. Fortes and E. L. C. P. Zoboli, "A Study on the Ethics of Microallocation of Scarce Resources in Health Care," *Journal of Medical Ethics* 28 (2002): 266–69.

Warren: I think that if we consider what we would accept in the original position we can generate a set of high-level rules governing microallocation.

Before I get to specific rules governing microallocation, though, it seems to me that a reasonable general rule to choose in our own interest as seen from the original position is the rule of **impartiality**: health care professionals should usually be impartial in helping patients.

I say "usually" because the rules chosen in the original position must be consistent with human sympathy. For this reason, we would also accept a rule about making rules I call **sympathy**, the **metarule** that the rules be chosen and interpreted so they can be followed by people with ordinary human sympathies. That is why our first rule, impartiality, must be limited. Indeed, the sympathy metarule imposes a limit on all of our rules.

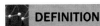

DEFINITION

Impartiality is used here in the ordinary sense, meaning "freedom from bias, favouritism or prejudice."

DEFINITION

A **metarule** is a rule that governs the production, use, and interpretation of other, lower-level rules. Warren explains the sympathy metarule in chapter 3.

Doran: So, you suggest that the justified rules for deciding how to distribute scarce health care resources must be rules that are generally applied impartially, yet consistent with human sympathies. I already have some questions about these claims, but before they are asked, why don't you explain what specific microallocation rules you think would be chosen in the original position?

Warren: We all have a strong interest in reasonable access to care, so we wouldn't want to be bumped by less needy people who have help from insiders. Of course, some of us will need care more urgently than others. That is why we would accept the rule **worst first**: treat the worst cases in the emergency department first.

Patrick: That sounds right, but it may depend on what you mean by "worst." Do you mean, for instance, those who will die without immediate treatment, those who are suffering the most, those with the most to lose if they die, or something else?

Warren: By "worst" I mean those who are most urgently in need of treatment in the medical judgment of the triage nurse. In Canada our CTAS guidelines define five levels of urgency. Within different levels of triage, the worst first rule would still require the triage nurse to make distinctions. For example, at level 1 a patient who is liable to die if not seen immediately would be placed ahead of a patient at level 2, who could wait for more than 15 minutes. At level 3 where both patients could wait for 30 minutes, the one who was likely to be in more pain than the other might be admitted first. Medical judgment will be influenced by both pain and loss of function that the patients may suffer. Permanent loss of function is more serious, of course, than temporary loss.

> **BACKGROUND**
>
> As noted, the CTAS guidelines are a set of rules about how to make medical judgments following, in effect, the worst first rule. The guidelines do not deal with ties, exceptions, and some other things that occupy us in this debate. We want to understand the more general picture, including the exceptions to worst first in a fair system.

Patrick: Okay, that somewhat helps to clarify the worst first rule. What other rules ought to be adopted?

Warren: Once we have taken the worst first, we might think that it would be fair to apply the **first come** rule within a given triage level: first come, first served.

Doran: That idea seems reasonable to me. Respect for persons requires that we take patients who are equally badly off on a first come, first served basis. On its face, at least, there'd be something disrespectful in passing me over and taking you, if I have been waiting longer and we are in equal need of care.

> **THEORY**
>
> The Kantian takes respect for persons as the very foundation of ethics, not something to be justified by appeal to the rules chosen in the original position.

However, a possible exception to the worst first and first come rules might be a case where the patient who arrived first can only survive for a very short period of time, while those behind that person are in urgent need of medical care from which they could substantially benefit.

Warren: Yes, respect for persons would be in all our interests, as seen from the original position. As to the patient who cannot be saved for long, consider, in support, the following claim: If two patients arrive in a terribly overcrowded emergency department, patient A first and patient B second, and both are level 1, the triage nurse should turn aside A, whom the nurse judges to be hopeless in the long term, in favour of B, who might have a chance for a long life if treated.

BACKGROUND

Traditional triage practices on the battlefield and in other emergencies in the field sort patients into a number of categories, depending on considerations of urgency. They also sort patients into the categories of those that can be saved and those that cannot be saved. Those that cannot be saved may be given comfort measures, but priority in terms of life-prolonging measures is given to those that can be saved.

Now we see we should add the first of perhaps many exceptions to worst first and first come—**hopeless second**: do not treat hopeless cases ahead of those where there is hope.

Patrick: By "hopeless in the long term," do you mean something along the lines that the patient won't survive even with treatment?

UP FOR DISCUSSION

Should first come play a role in treatment decisions? Why should those who were lucky enough to get to the hospital first be treated ahead of those who are equally badly off but who took longer to get to the hospital?

Warren: Well, at least the patient won't survive for a significant period of time. We are talking about hours, not days. Someone who can be kept alive with heroic medical efforts for only a few hours is clearly in this category with respect to another patient who can have some months of good-quality life if treated immediately. Hopeless patients are patients for whom comforts only are medically indicated.

Doran: I am not sure if hopeless cases should be defined so narrowly. But we can explore this issue with greater precision later.

Patrick: Right. Are there any more rules that you think we would choose from the original position, Warren?

Warren: Maybe, but let's see what we've got so far: consistent with human sympathy, health care workers should impartially follow the rules of (1) worst first, plus (2) first come. This is the basic set of rules; however, there are exceptions. The first exception is what I've called (3) hopeless second: do not treat hopeless cases ahead of those where there is hope.

Patrick: This looks like a good start. Before we start discussing further exceptions to the basic principles, why don't we see whether there's agreement on the sympathy metarule, which is supposed to govern the interpretation and application of the principles. Doran, do you have any objections to the sympathy metarule?

Doran's Objection to the Sympathy Metarule

Doran: I think I agree with the general microallocation principles, but I'm not sure about the sympathy meta-rule. Isn't it a bit odd for a contrac-tarian like you, Warren, who makes fairness central to morality, to want to restrict impartiality?

> **THEORY**
>
> Impartiality is often thought to be basic to fairness. Think of what we require, for instance, from a judge in the court system. Fairness is the fundamental moral idea in John Rawls's contractar-ian theory.

Warren: Actually, as seen from the original position, it is in our interest to have public servants generally operate impartially. It is, however, also strongly in our interest to promote human sympathy and the bonds of family and friendship. These bonds would be destroyed if we tried to be utterly impartial.

Patrick: I agree that we can't ignore such bonds, given the importance of such virtues as love, friendship, loyalty, and so on.

Doran: Can you give me some examples of when sympathy might play a prop-er role in triage decisions?

> **TECHNIQUE**
>
> Demanding an illustration of a prin-ciple is a technique designed to elicit the strengths and weaknesses of that principle.

Warren: To give you an accurate picture, I will have to give you four kinds of cases. The sympathy metarule might allow for a **mitigation**, an **excuse**, a **justification**, or none of the above. The first three come in increasing order of rarity, with justified actions contrary to normal triage being very rare indeed.

> **DEFINITION**
>
> A **mitigation** shows that a wrong action is not as blameworthy as usual. An **ex-cuse** shows that the person who did the wrong action should not be blamed at all. A **justification** shows that the action was not wrong after all.

Patrick: Let's start with mitigation. When is sympathy acceptable as a mitigating factor?

Warren: If a nurse or a physician gets a close friend somewhat faster treatment in the emergency department than would otherwise be given, then we might well have a case of a wrong action that would be less blameworthy because of the strong bonds of sympathy that motivate it. In the original position, we would recognize the powerful pull of sympathy and not want to rake the nurse or physician over the coals for this. The action would be impermissible, but not the darker sort of offence that, say, quicker service in exchange for a monetary reward would be. Even if a very serious punishment is contemplated in some cases of favouritism, the mitigating factor of strong bonds of sympathy may lessen the punishment in this case.

Patrick: I think I agree with you so far, Warren. The virtuous person would of course be loyal and have a special kind of concern for close friends. This makes it difficult to place much blame on the nurse or physician in the situation you describe. But virtue also requires fairness, so as you say, Warren, her action may still be wrong, since it was unfair to others.

Doran: I'm not so sure I like the direction you guys are going, but carry on. I'd like to see what counts as an excuse.

Warren: Excuses are much rarer since they require that the pull of sympathy be overwhelming. Consider a case in which a triage nurse is very sympathetic to the poor and the downtrodden. A homeless person who evokes great pathos in the emergency department is given a place in the queue that should, by triage rules, have gone to a wealthy businessman who is also waiting and slightly more urgent. In this case, the nurse did the wrong thing, but her action is morally excusable because she was temporarily overwhelmed by sympathy and incapable of exercising normal judgment.

Patrick: That would be a very rare case indeed. But I'm not entirely sure why you see this as a case in which sympathy excuses, rather than merely mitigates. Does it have to do with the fact that the nurse was so *overwhelmed* by sympathy that it impaired her reasoning capacities?

Warren: Yes, the triage nurse would find it emotionally impossible to be impartial in this circumstance. One would not expect this from professionals generally. Most cases that appear to be like this could be subsumed under cases of mere mitigation, because the pity for the homeless patient would not be strong enough to be overwhelming. Nonetheless, if it overwhelmed the nurse's reasoning capacities, it would be excusing.

Doran: Perhaps some people are too kind-hearted to be triage nurses. What I don't expect to see, however, is a genuine case of justification.

Warren: The kind of cases I have in mind rely on the people in the original position recognizing that there are some bonds so strong that it would be foolish to make rules that ignore them. That would result in the rules being ignored. Suppose a triage nurse sees her own small child brought in from a serious incident at the daycare nearby. Several other children are brought in at the same time with similar injuries and urgency. The nurse would be duty bound to let someone else take over. Suppose that can't be done in this circumstance. If the nurse got prompt treatment for her own child simply because it was her own, rather than taking the children at random as she would otherwise have done, could that nurse be said to have done something morally wrong? I think in the original position we would recognize the futility of asking for superhuman impartiality. The nurse's action would be justified.

Patrick: I'm inclined to agree with you, Warren. The virtuous nurse would of course strive to be fair and impartial, but not to the point that she would treat her seriously injured child as just one among many children in need. Since it is *her* child in need, it seems that a special sort of concern and treatment is warranted.

Still, I am trying to get clearer about the limits of the sympathy metarule in your view. Maybe it would help to see a case in which there is no mitigation, excuse, or justification, but sympathy is still present.

Warren: Well, suppose a nurse has strong sympathies for people of his own race and favours them in ways that bend the triage admissions policies. That would be wrong. Sympathies for one's race are sympathies one can and ought to limit severely, unlike the parent's sympathy for the child. In the original position, we would want to avoid the evils we might suffer from racism and would require that the effective sympathies be those that are, like the mother's for the child, part of being human and strongly in our interest. In the original position, we would know we are likely to benefit from strong family bonds, while strong racial affiliations lead to strife that is not in our interest.

Patrick: Right, but we need to tread carefully here. **Nepotism** as well as racism can undermine our interests.

Warren: Yes, to prevent nepotism, those in the original position would insist on rules that require public servants to **recuse** themselves when in a conflict of interest. In some cases, however, that can't be done. Rules that require parents to ignore the ties that bind them to their children would be honoured more in the breach than the observance. It is in our interest to preserve respect for the rules by not making them inhumanly strict.

The sympathy metarule moderates the rules so that where strict adherence is not in our interest as seen from the original position, there is a mitigation, excuse, or justification available depending on the degree and kind of sympathy. Where it is greatly in our interest to promote a particular kind of sympathy, like the bond between parent and child, we must allow exceptions in rare cases where no alternative is available. Too many exceptions would undermine the rules, as would no exceptions. It is a delicate balance.

> **THEORY**
>
> Warren tries to avoid ethical relativism by appealing to human sympathies that are independent of culture, like the bond between parent and child. It is, however, an empirical question what human sympathies exist and what their relative strengths might be. Often, we are forced to make reasonable guesses about empirical matters while we wait for social science to enlighten us about the facts.

Patrick: That's for sure!

Doran: Warren, you described one case where the sympathy metarule allows for partiality—the case where one takes one's own child first, instead of taking equally badly off patients in random order. This is a vanishingly rare case. Are there other circumstances, perhaps slightly less rare, where sympathy would justify partiality? For instance, what if you had two patients, equally in need of urgent care, where the patient second in line was the triage nurse's parent, or sibling, or best friend? Would the triage nurse be justified in acting on her sympathies?

Warren: I think the cases you are imagining may be as rare as my original case of justified partiality. Having said that, I would think that a triage nurse, if and only if he is unable to step aside and delegate responsibilities to others, may permissibly put his mother or sibling ahead of someone else, provided that they were both equally in need of immediate care. In the original position, it will be recognized that people with ordinary human sympathies may not be able to overcome the bonds of immediate family; however, with respect to friends, I think such a decision would be viewed as unjustified, though there are mitigating factors.

Doran: And so sympathy alone would not have justified Alice in putting her mentor Lena ahead of Terence? Sympathy, in her case, would only work to mitigate or excuse the wrong?

Warren: Yes. Sympathy will mitigate or excuse, not justify, Alice's actions.

Patrick: But you don't think Alice acted wrongly, do you? Don't you think it was morally permissible for Alice to put Lena ahead of Terence?

Warren: Yes. I will argue later that other considerations, in addition to sympathy, will render her decision permissible.

Patrick: I see. I think we're in agreement about this case thus far.

Doran: I understand your reasons, and accept overwhelming sympathy as a mitigating factor, but I would not say that a triage nurse acts permissibly if she puts her own child at the head of the queue. Such an act, while highly understandable, is also unprofessional. Just as a judge or a professor ought not to play favourites when evaluating a family member's case or work, and just as an attorney ought to try as hard as she can for her client even if she is repulsed by him, I don't think health care workers should allow their medical decisions to be influenced by family ties.

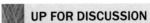

> **UP FOR DISCUSSION**
>
> Do you think a triage nurse could ever be justified in putting their own child ahead of other similarly urgent cases?

Warren: Strict impartiality is, nonetheless, not a reasonable choice from the original position. Humanized impartiality is. We must make exceptions to rules that allow for human sympathies; otherwise we will have rules that will not be followed. This does not mean that we simply follow our sympathies in ordering patients for care. It does, however, allow for these rare exceptions to straightforward application of the CTAS guidelines. Remember that justified exceptions to the guidelines will be very rare indeed.

> **TECHNIQUE**
>
> Warren is "biting the bullet" here. The initially counterintuitive idea that someone concerned about fairness would abandon strict impartiality is accepted but explained.

Patrick's Objection to the Sympathy Metarule

Patrick: I share your concern about allowing sympathy to influence the decisions of medical (and other) professionals, Doran. And I certainly wouldn't accept a general rule that says it's always okay to give one's family and friends special consideration. But, as Warren has been arguing, we cannot ignore the various worthwhile bonds we form with family, friends, and others. In some very special cases, partiality is called for. Nevertheless, although I've expressed general agreement with the role you accord to sympathy, Warren, I also want to raise a question or two about the sympathy metarule and examples of its application.

Warren: Go ahead.

Patrick: What motivates the sympathy metarule is that you want to choose rules in the original position that are consistent with human sympathy. But if that's so, you not only need rules that are consistent with the sympathy of those distributing medical resources, but you also need rules that those of us in the queue for medical services could follow. Do you think that people in general would agree to triage nurses sometimes bumping family members ahead of them?

Warren: As Alice notes in our drama concerning the CTAS guidelines, people may be upset at the application of fair rules. That does not make the rules unfair. The impartiality rule requires that the triage nurse should be as impartial as is humanly possible. That, I think, is a rule we could accept in the original position. It gives us the best we can get within human limits. I am assuming that those in the queue, with occasional exceptions among the ones being bypassed, would generally feel much the same sympathy as the triage nurse in these extraordinary cases. There is a difference of degree that you overlook. From the original position, we would not accept a system in which only insiders and those they favour would be adequately treated. Impartiality has to be strong, just not absolute.

> **BACKGROUND**
>
> There are a variety of practice standards beyond the CTAS guidelines that affect health care providers. For example, each province in Canada has its own practice standards for nurses, and the Canadian Nurses Association publishes a nationally accepted Code of Ethics for nurses.

Patrick: Okay. From my virtue ethics perspective, I would agree that sympathy ought to play a role in allocation decisions. But there's a role for other virtues, too—for example, compassion, benevolence, charity, empathy, loyalty, and so on. So I would like to know why you single out sympathy as a relevant consideration. Or perhaps you construe sympathy more broadly than I do?

Warren: Yes, I seem to be construing sympathy much more widely than you are. Other positive emotions contribute to it. The key idea is that people in the original position are going to see it as in their interest to have rules applied impartially; however, they will also realize that people have various deep personal attachments that cannot always be set aside in the name of impartiality. They will thus agree to rare exceptions to the impartial application of rules—otherwise, the moral rules would be overly demanding and unlikely to be followed.

Patrick: I see. There's one last point of clarification before we move on. You are not merely claiming that we shouldn't require impartiality because people are incapable of it, are you? You are saying that in some special and rare cases, impartiality would be morally inappropriate—that is, partiality is morally called for in those situations. Is that right?

Warren: Right.

Doran: The basic set of rules you have defended so far, Warren, is still not adequate for handling the full range of cases health care workers are confronted with. So why don't we consider some other cases and see whether the rules proposed are able to handle them?

> **THEORY**
>
> A widely accepted dictum in philosophy is that ought implies can. That is, it is absurd to say that something ought to be done when it cannot be done. Warren's claim is not that people cannot be impartial in these triage cases involving close family members; rather, it is that, under special conditions, they need not be impartial, even if they could be.

Objection to the Sufficiency of Hopeless Second

Doran: Earlier you proposed the rule we've called hopeless second: do not treat hopeless cases ahead of those where there is hope. This seems a little too simple.

Patrick: Yes, Warren, what would you say about this case? Suppose we have a not-quite-hopeless patient who arrives at the emergency department in need of immediate medical attention. If this patient receives treatment, he will survive a few months, or perhaps a year or so at best, so he does not qualify as a hopeless case. A few minutes later, another patient arrives who also needs immediate care. Let's suppose that if

> **TECHNIQUE**
>
> Here a hypothetical case is used to suggest the need for either an additional microallocation principle or a modification of the hopeless second principle.

treated, this patient can be expected to live another 50-plus years. Now suppose the emergency department does not have enough resources to treat both of them. It seems to me that, in this case, the patient who will live longer should get priority. But the basic set of rules does not seem to permit this.

Minimize YPLL (Minimize Years of Potential Life Lost)

Warren: I agree that the patient who arrives second should be given priority, so we need to move beyond hopeless second. Let's have a look at a rule explicitly in use in health care. Some physicians would appeal to **minimize YPLL**, the rule that we should bias decisions in favour of minimizing years of potential life lost. It would be in our self-interest in the original position to accept a rule like this. It is a rule that lets us suffer small losses but avoid large ones.

Patrick: I am not at all sure that minimize YPLL would allow us to avoid only small losses. For instance, suppose a 55-year-old is admitted to the emergency department with heart trouble. A few minutes later, a 45-year-old comes into emergency complaining of the same thing. Minimize YPLL seems to imply that we should bump the 45-year-old ahead of the 55-year-old, if the physicians can treat only one of them. The 55-year-old may well have lots to lose in this case. So it seems that bumping the 45-year-old ahead of the 55-year-old would be wrong.

> **BACKGROUND**
>
> **Minimize YPLL** is primarily not a micro-allocation principle as we use it here. Usually it is a principle adopted in epidemiology and the insurance industry. It is used as a way of measuring the impact of a disease or other negative health determinant. As such it operates at the **mesoallocation** (institutional) or **macroallocation** (governmental) level.
>
> As a microallocation principle (operating at the level of individuals), minimize YPLL is somewhat like hopeless second, which tries to minimize potential life lost by passing over patients with little to gain from treatment; however, minimize YPLL goes further than hopeless second in what it would permit.

> **TECHNIQUE**
>
> Notice, again, a counterexample is used to demonstrate that a particular principle is false.

Warren: I agree; that would be wrong.

Doran: Yes. I agree with your intuitions, Patrick, that we should treat the person who is expected to live another 50 years ahead of the person who is expected to live only another 6 to 12 months, especially if the one person has already led a long life while the other has not. The minimize YPLL principle is able to accommodate this intuition; however, it turns out that this principle is too simple, for it implies something that is surely false—that, in cases where only one patient can be treated, we should bump the 45-year-old ahead of the 55-year-old. Given that minimize YPLL is vulnerable to counterexamples, it is clear that we need a different principle to deal with these cases and others like them.

THEORY AND DISCUSSION

One might wonder why we should trust our intuitions about what is right or wrong in these sorts of cases. The answer, in part, is that we are seeking **reflective equilibrium**; that is, we are seeking moral principles that cohere with the moral judgments about cases that we are most confident about. We therefore need to test our proposed moral principles against various cases. See chapter 1 for a discussion of reflective equilibrium.

Substantial Benefit

Doran: Perhaps the principle we are looking for is something like the following: If a patient stands to benefit substantially from being treated first, while the patient ahead of him in the queue will not benefit substantially from being treated, then the patient who will benefit substantially should be treated first. Let's call this principle **substantial benefit**. Notice that this principle would support our judgments that it would be permissible to treat someone who is expected to gain 50 years of good life ahead of someone who is expected to gain only 6 to 12 months of good life. And notice that this principle would support our judgment that it would not be permissible to bump the 45-year-old ahead of the 55-year-old, since the 55-year-old would certainly gain a substantial benefit from treatment.

Warren: That sounds better than minimize YPLL, for it applies only when there is a large difference between patients. From behind a veil of ignorance, we would accept the substantial benefit principle since it would be more likely to serve our interests whatever triage category we might fall into. Where it serves our interests, our interests are strong. Where it neglects them, our interests are slight. Where the gap in interests is not great, we would have to appeal to other rules. Of course, what is a large difference will be context-relative and depend on difficult judgment calls.

Patrick: Substantial benefit looks like a move in the right direction. In order to test this principle, though, we need to spell out the notion of a substantial benefit.

Doran: This is a difficult task. Perhaps substantial benefit should be looked at as a matter of quantity and quality. A year of high quality could be a substantial benefit, but a year or more of poor quality would not be a substantial benefit.

Patrick: What would this principle imply about a case like this? Suppose a person who can walk has a higher quality of life than someone in a wheelchair. If that's true (and I'm not saying it is), is it permissible to bump that person ahead of the one in the wheelchair? Surely that would be wrong.

Doran: Of course that would be wrong. On the one hand, I want to say the benefit has to be health related. But, on the other hand, we need to prevent the able-bodied being put ahead of those who are wheelchair bound. The best way to do that is to just deny that those in wheelchairs have lower-quality lives. Certainly, the wheelchair bound can substantially benefit from life-prolonging measures!

Warren: From the perspective of the original position we don't want to say that someone who is permanently wheelchair bound would automatically be bumped. There's bound to be some vagueness about substantial benefit, but it helps to look at some cases using such a principle.

Patrick: Good. So it seems that substantial benefit is an improvement over minimize YPLL. It allows us to explain why it would be permissible to give priority to the patient who will live 50 years over the not-quite-hopeless patient who will live one year of poor quality. We can also explain why it would *not* be permissible to give priority to the 45-year-old over the 55-year-old. Both would receive a substantial benefit from treatment. But other difficulties remain.

Fair Turn

Warren: I agree. Suppose we have a 77-year-old man admitted to the emergency department with a critical heart condition, and shortly after he arrives, a 5-year-old child comes in with a similar problem. In the original position we would accept a rule that says that if the emergency physicians can treat only one of the patients, then the child should be bumped ahead of the elder. The child would suffer a large loss if left to die. The elder would suffer a relatively small one in terms of years of potential life left to live. These last years of the elder would, nonetheless, be a substantial benefit to him.

Patrick: That's exactly the kind of case I had in mind! It reminds me that Alice put a young man in treatment before a much older man because the elder one had already had "a good shot at life." Both could get a substantial benefit from treatment, so we need another principle to justify putting the younger patient first.

Warren: From the original position, I think we would accept a rule that favours those who haven't had a fair turn at life over those who have. So what I'm proposing is the **fair turn** rule: Patient B can go ahead of patient A (who arrived first) if A has had a fair turn at life and B has not. This rule explains why it is permissible to bump the 5-year-old ahead of the 77-year-old, even when the 77-year-old, if treated, will have a life worth living.

> **BACKGROUND**
>
> Some philosophers call this the "fair innings argument." See, for example, Michael M. Rivlin, "Why the Fair Innings Argument Is Not Persuasive," *BMC Medical Ethics* 1, no. 1 (2000), http://www.biomedcentral.com/1472-6939/1/1.

Doran: The principle is too loose, I think, as it would allow a 1-year-old to bump a 40-year-old. I don't think that would be right, however. The 40-year-old may be in the midst of her life projects—family, career, and so on—and she may have small children dependent on her for care, and so forth. Her "turn at life" is not done, so she should not be passed in the queue by someone else who is no worse off than she is. Likewise, I suppose, if a small child was ahead of the 40-year-old, the small child should not be passed over in the queue either.

Warren: The fair turn rule would allow the 1-year-old to bump the 40-year-old only if we agree that 40 years is a fair turn. But if we think of fair turn as *average life expectancy*, then the principle can avoid your counterexample.

> **TECHNIQUE**
>
> Notice how Warren avoids a counterexample by clarifying how the principle is to be understood.

Patrick: The fair turn principle will still meet with difficulties, even if we base the idea of fair turn on average life expectancy. The average life expectancy of a male in Canada is about 79, while the life expectancy of a female is about 83.[5] Now, suppose patient A is an 80-year-old male, and patient B is a 75-year-old male. Fair turn, if understood in terms of life expectancy, seems to imply that B should be given priority over A. But that doesn't seem right, does it?

Doran: Good point. This is tricky stuff! But perhaps it is not unreasonable to maintain that, other things being equal, the 75-year-old should be able to bump the 80-year-old, since the younger man has not had the benefit of an average life expectancy, whereas the older man has. That's not unreasonable, is it?

Patrick: I'm not sure what to say about this case. The age difference between A and B is pretty small, and B is just two years shy of having had a fair turn. So I'm not sure we'd be justified bumping B ahead of A on the grounds that B has not yet had a fair turn at life. I think we'd have to appeal to other considerations to justify doing this.

Warren: Right. When lifespans are close, the triage nurse could ignore differences or look at other factors like the general health of the candidates. There are many other influences on fairness that the nurse would not

> **BACKGROUND**
>
> In 1961, a committee at the University of Washington, which came to be known in the press as the "God Committee," was formed to determine who would get access to a new life-saving treatment, dialysis. The committee used social circumstances of candidates rather than clinical assessment of need or potential medical benefit. This caused a storm of controversy and helped to give rise to the field of health care ethics.
>
> *Source:* Gregory E. Pence, *Classic Cases in Medical Ethics*, 2nd ed. (New York: McGraw-Hill, 1995), 297–313.

know about, of course. What if the 75-year-old had many unfair social advantages over the 80-year-old? Exceptions to fair turn should be based on purely medical evidence. Health status determines who gets resources. Normally, triage nurses cannot be expected to take account of social advantages one patient may have had over another because they do not know about them.

Patrick: But even then we are met with hard cases. Here's another one. Suppose patient A is 73 and has enjoyed 13 years of retired life. Patient B is 60, and is now looking forward to his retirement. They both stand to benefit substantially from treatment, and neither has had a fair turn at life, if life expectancy is 77 years. Yet I'm inclined to say that it would be okay to bump B ahead of A, because A is much closer to having had a fair turn at life than B. What do you guys think?

 UP FOR DISCUSSION

Do you think it would be permissible to bump a 60-year-old ahead of a 73-year-old in the case Patrick raises?

Doran: We could say that where B has not come close to having had a fair turn, and A has obviously had nearly a fair turn, then B goes ahead of A. Or we could bite the bullet and say that B should not go ahead of A, since neither has had a fair share of life, and since A has been waiting for treatment longer than B. Neither position strikes me as irrational.

Warren: There is going to be some arbitrariness here. Patient A may have been virtuous and B vicious, for instance. There are all sorts of unknowns. The quality of life measure is, for practical purposes, very difficult to make precise. And it may be the case that rules that are general enough to be of use to triage nurses will also be rules that contain some vagueness or arbitrariness. The problem with shrugging this off here is that the decisions of triage nurses may be a matter of life and death.

Patrick: Right. When patients are close in their needs, I think the nurse will perhaps have to consider various *non-clinical factors*—factors like whether the patient has dependents, whether the patient is responsible for their condition, the patient's contribution to society, and so on.

Warren: These justifications of exceptions could go either way. We might admit one patient because of the patient's large family or, instead, admit the other because he is orphaned and has suffered enough from loss of family to merit special treatment.

Doran: I don't think that non-clinical considerations, like those just mentioned, ought to play a role in a triage nurse's decisions about whom to treat.

Patrick: I'm inclined to think they should play a role, at least sometimes. But I'm not entirely comfortable with this position. So why don't we explore the question of whether we should adopt principles that would give a role to these other kinds of factors?

MICROALLOCATION RULES: NON-CLINICAL CONSIDERATIONS

Moral Responsibility

Doran: Okay. Let's first consider this: Should moral responsibility play a role in prioritizing health care? Consider this case. Suppose that Alice knew that Terence caused the accident. He was brought in before Lena, one of the victims of the accident. Both are level 1 and are in serious need of immediate medical care, but only one patient can be treated, while the other must wait. What do you guys think—would it be permissible to give priority to Lena because she is an innocent victim and put Terence second because he caused the accident?

Warren: Normally, the nurse would not know who was who among the accident victims, and the police and ambulance attendants would not say anything. There might, however, be a rare case where the nurse knows or is told. Alice is in that situation because she knows many people in her small town, including some of the incoming patients. Such cases put our principles to the test. Generally, we would expect non-judgmental, impartial triage according to the impartiality rule: health care professionals should usually be impartial when helping patients. That's natural in the original position. We don't want nurses acting as judges and juries. We don't want them distracted by judgments of guilt or innocence or value of persons. It would not be in our interest in the original position to allow access to care to be so clouded with nurses' individual judgments about things outside their training, if such judgments could be avoided, for this could leave any of us out in the cold.

Doran: So you think the patients' moral guilt or innocence should be completely left out of the triage nurse's decision?

Warren: No, triage nurses are human, not superhumanly capable of staying within their area of expertise. Suppose Alice knows Terence is responsible.

UP FOR DISCUSSION

There are, of course, other cases of moral (and non-moral) responsibility that can give rise to questions of proper allocation of health care. For instance, should a person's culpable failure to take adequate care of himself be a consideration when deciding priority of care?

UP FOR DISCUSSION

If two people well known to the triage nurse come into an emergency room, one after the other, suffering from chest pain, and the first patient is someone who has led a life of doughnut-eating sloth, and the second is someone who has taken excellent care of himself, would it be wrong, other things being equal, to treat the second patient ahead of the first?

In such a case, Alice might find it nearly impossible to treat Terence and let his victim die. In some extreme cases, then, we might make exceptions to worst first and first come on the basis of known guilt plus sympathy. Normally, however, we would expect triage nurses to use only clinical factors to make a decision.

Patrick: It's not just that it's nearly impossible to treat Terence ahead of his victims, Warren. It's that it would be *morally wrong* to do this, in the kind of case described. I believe Terence's victims warrant greater compassion and sympathy, and so they ought to be given preferential treatment.

Warren: In rare cases where it is nearly impossible to ignore our sympathies, the rules would be undermined if we required strict impartiality. That is why, in the original position, exceptions to impartiality would be required. Consequently, it is morally wrong to treat the guilty first in some rare cases where there is no doubt who is the perpetrator and who is the victim.

Doran: I have a different take on this. In general, I accept the moral principle that if one of two people should have to suffer more, it should be the person who is at fault for the injury, and not the innocent victim. So, I think it is only fair that Lena be placed ahead of Terence if they both cannot be treated immediately; however, we are talking about the factors a triage nurse should be considering. And I guess I lean toward the view that we want our health care professionals making treatment decisions based on health care considerations, period. As a triage nurse, then, I think Alice ought not to ask herself who was at fault for the accident, but should instead follow the rule that a patient is a patient. Again, the best support I have for this may be an analogy with other professions. Attorneys charged with defending someone they know is guilty would not be justified in failing to vigorously defend their clients, but should follow the standards of their profession. I think the same is true of triage nurses—they ought to stick to clinical considerations.

 UP FOR DISCUSSION

When, if ever, would a triage nurse be justified in putting one patient ahead of another, on the grounds that one of the patients was at moral fault for an accident?

Innocents First

Warren: It seems that Patrick and I accept a principle that we can call **innocents first**: Patient A, who is innocent and who cannot wait for care, ought to be given priority over patient B, who is known to be at fault for the injury and who also cannot wait, other things being equal. The rule of innocents first is one reason I think Alice was justified in treating Lena ahead of Terence in the revised case in which Alice knows for sure that Terence is at fault.

Patrick: Well, I accept it in the same spirit that I accept any principle. That is, it may hold as a general rule of thumb, but like all principles, there are bound to be exceptions.

Doran: What about this sort of case? Suppose a prison vehicle was crushed in an avalanche, and both the driver and a convicted felon, about whose moral fault we have ample evidence, were seriously injured and in need of emergency medical care. Unlike the case of Terence and Lena, neither person did anything to bring about the injury. I don't think considerations of a person's guilt or innocence, virtue or vice, should affect triage decisions. Do you?

Warren: I am not so sure I agree with you, Doran. Suppose, for example, that in the case you imagined, the prisoner that is injured is an infamous child molester and murderer, while the other person who is injured is the police officer assigned to guard him. If both were level 1, would the nurse be required to ignore her abhorrence for the molester and take him first because he came in just ahead of the police officer with whom she strongly sympathizes? I think that's asking too much.

Patrick: I agree. As we've noted, medical professionals will often lack the information needed to make accurate judgments about patients and their guilt or innocence, virtue and vice, and so on. But where they do have this information, I think preferential treatment based on these and other non-clinical factors is sometimes morally justified.

Doran: I don't know. I understand the nurse's temptation to treat the police officer ahead of the criminal, but I am not sure that it is justified. As I said before, we should be reluctant to give nurses the authority to queue people up for care according to their perceived moral worth.

Warren: In reality, the practice is "don't ask, don't tell." Ambulance drivers would not tell nurses about a patient's guilt, innocence, or any other non-medical characteristics. Nurses would not ask. In a case like that of the molester, though, the sympathy metarule allows the nurse to attend to the police officer first. These are extreme cases that rarely come up but which demonstrate the limits on our principles.

> **UP FOR DISCUSSION**
>
> Should the moral responsibility of patients for their own or others' suffering ever influence a triage nurse's decision about whom to treat first when two patients are at the same level of medical urgency? Does your answer change if the patient is not morally responsible for his own or others' injuries but is a felon who was convicted of a crime?

> **UP FOR DISCUSSION**
>
> Worst first clearly takes priority over first come. What about the principles like fair turn or innocents first? Should innocents first come into play before fair turn, for example?

Third-Party Interests

Patrick: Thus far we have been focusing on exceptions to worst first and first come that concern harms and benefits to particular patients. But there seems to be another category of exceptions to these and perhaps other rules that involve harms and benefits to **third parties**.

Warren: Yes, I was thinking the same thing. Indeed, there seems to be an incredibly complex range of cases that may provide exceptions to the combination of the worst first and first come rules as well as to other principles we have begun to contemplate. To see what I have in mind, consider the following three cases:

1. *Childless person versus parent of young child:* Patient A, a childless person, arrives in the emergency department with chest pain. Patient B, a single parent of a young child, arrives in emergency shortly thereafter with chest pain, too. Both are level 1 and are in serious need of immediate medical care, but only one patient can be treated while the other must wait. (We will call this the dependents case.)

2. *Drunk versus doctor:* Patient A, the town drunk, arrives in the emergency department with chest pain. Patient B, the neighbouring town's only doctor, arrives in emergency shortly thereafter, also with chest pain. Both are level 1 and are in serious need of immediate medical care, but only one patient can be treated while the other must wait. (We will call this the public good case.) (Note: This case puts more emphasis on the public good than the case of Lena and Terence, which is focused on gratitude and perhaps the moral fault of Terence for Lena's injuries.)

3. *Person with highly infectious disease versus person without infectious disease:* Patient A arrives in the emergency department with symptoms of a highly infectious disease and needs immediate care. Treatment of this person will put health care workers at significant risk of contracting the disease. Patient B arrives in emergency shortly thereafter with chest pain. Both are level 1 and are in serious need of immediate medical care, but only one patient can be treated while the other must wait. Should A be treated first, or should A be quarantined while B is treated? (We will call this the innocent threat case.)

In each of these cases, the principles of worst first and first come support treatment of patient A, but

 UP FOR DISCUSSION

Some might say that it would be *unfair* to Lena to ignore her exemplary life and let her die to save a wastrel like Terence. Others might say it is unfair to Terence to pass over him to treat Lena, given that he was at the hospital first and equally in need of care. Which view do you agree with more, and why?

common sense suggests that in at least some of these cases it would be permissible to treat patient B first because of the rights or interests of third parties. If this is correct, then we would need to identify some principled reason that explains and organizes our judgments in these third-party cases.

Patrick: These are interesting and tricky cases, Warren. The challenge, of course, is to explain which third-party interests matter and *why.*

Public Interest

Warren: I would say that we can account for some of these cases by appealing to a rule we could call **public interest**: *Where the public interest is great enough, a patient may be given priority over those who came earlier.* This rule leaves open the possibility that not just prevention of great harm but promotion of enormous public benefit might also motivate us to treat a patient ahead of others. What counts as a sufficient public interest depends on balancing the needs of the patient who is passed over against extreme benefits or harms to the community.

Patrick: Aren't you flirting dangerously with utilitarianism?

Warren: Not necessarily; the position seems to be more like **extremitarianism.**

We are not saying that the greatest good needs to be promoted—rather, just that when much greater harm to others will result if B is not treated ahead of A or much greater benefit to others will result, then B may be bumped ahead of A.

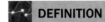

> **DEFINITION**
>
> There is no recognized ethical term **extremitarianism**. This is a word Warren made up playing on **utilitarianism**. For the extremitarian, the harms or benefits have to be extreme before they can justify exceptions to worst first and first come.

Patrick: Okay, but what about the dependents case, then? I'm torn here. I want to say that the virtues suggest we should bump B ahead of A and, in general, give priority to patients with young children. But I'm worried about unfairly discriminating against patients who can't have children or simply choose to remain childless.

Doran: I am inclined to say that B should *not* be put ahead of A in the dependents case, because it would not respect A as a person, and because no general public good will be served by doing so. I worry that allowing the patient with young children to go ahead of those without children would unfairly discriminate against the childless.

Patrick: Right. There's a tricky balance here. The virtuous person would seek to balance fairness against compassion for the parent and child. I think we'd need to know more details to say what considerations are most salient in these cases. There are lots of difficult issues to sort out here. For instance: How much greater benefit is enough to count as sufficient to override the principles of worst first and first come? And does it really make a moral difference that, in the public good and innocent threat cases, the interests being protected are those of individuals in society at large, whereas in the dependents case, the interests being protected are primarily those of the patient's immediate family?

UP FOR DISCUSSION

Should considerations of public interest, or the fact that one patient has dependents and the other hasn't, ever affect triage decisions?

Warren: At least one factor in answering these questions is the application of the public interest rule. Is the public interest in protecting the community's children great enough to justify a preference for patients with dependents?

Patrick: It seems a bit odd to make protection of children subject to public interest. Surely there is more to favouring the interests of kids than just the wisdom of public policies. I would think that if a preference for patients with dependents is justified, it is justified out of direct concern for the patient and their dependents.

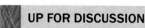

UP FOR DISCUSSION

Consider this rule: *Give special protection to the vulnerable.* Would such a rule help justify putting parents ahead of the childless to help protect children? What theoretical considerations would have us adopt such a rule? Consider objections and replies.

Warren: I agree. Public interest is only one factor in the decision to bump the parent ahead. The other rules we are discussing may also come into play, as well as rules we have not put out for consideration here.

It is worth reiterating, though, that whether we are speaking of the public good or just the interest of an individual third party, only in rare, extreme cases should triage nurses take the public interest into account. Patient B should be bumped ahead of patient A when there is an extreme and obvious difference in guilt and innocence or when, to take another instance, it is obvious that treating B over A would serve a great public good or prevent a great public harm. Extremitarianism rides again.

Medical Interests

Doran: I am going to part company with you again. In the dependents case, I doubt that common sense would suggest that it is okay to bump the childless person in favour of the parent of a young child. It seems to me that triage nurses should not consider things like whether or not a patient has dependents when deciding whom to treat first. The nurse should focus on who needs care most, who was waiting for care longest, whether the patient would substantially benefit from care, and so on. But non-medical considerations, such as whether one person is a parent, or an only child, should not figure into treatment decisions. In part, this is because nurses are almost never going to be in a position to know who has dependents and who hasn't. But it goes deeper than this, for I just don't think that such factors should be relevant to treatment decisions. Parents and non-parents are equally deserving of care. To pass over a person with no kids to save a parent seems to discriminate against those who are childless.

Warren: Yes, it is only in rare cases that nurses are in a position to know about the dependents, but in those rare cases that knowledge could be morally relevant because of the way the sympathy metarule restricts impartiality and because of other rules that may come into play. To say it is never relevant is to make too strong a claim.

Doran: My views on the cases of public good and innocent threat are similar to yours. I agree that the only doctor in town may be treated ahead of the layperson, and the person without the highly infectious disease may be treated ahead of the one whose infectious condition makes him a great threat to the medical staff. But my reasons are different from yours. It is not quite public benefit that justifies this exception to ordinary triage considerations, rather it is something like **medical benefit** that justifies these decisions. This principle can be stated as *Where the medical interest is great enough, a patient may be given priority over those who came earlier.* For it seems what links public good and innocent threat is that if the person second in line is not treated, a great *medical* harm will happen. For instance, a great medical harm will befall the community if the doctor dies, or if the medical staff is incapacitated by some new plague. Triage nurses, as medical professionals, have a legitimate interest in promoting medical well-being, and so in these highly unusual cases they may treat second first so as to prevent medical disaster.

 UP FOR DISCUSSION

Can you think of an example of the public interest requiring that patient B go ahead of patient A while medical interest does not require bumping A?

Patrick: Well, I'm not sure that we can justify the preferential treatment in these cases just by appeal to either the public interest or the medical benefit principle. Each principle seems to capture *part* of what justifies special consideration, but each leaves something out as well. The public interest and the medical benefit justify putting the doctor ahead of the drunk, for instance, but I believe it's also supported by considerations about what kinds of life each is living. The doctor is apparently leading an admirable and worthwhile life, while the same can't be said for the drunk. I know this is a potentially dangerous path to head down, but in the extreme cases we're considering, I think these sorts of considerations are unavoidable.

Doran: As you know, I disagree that nurses should take into consideration the virtue of their patients when making triage decisions.

Warren: In most cases I think that is right, but there are the extreme cases where I would want to reserve room for exceptions. I also think that the attempt to narrow consideration to medical interests, while a good idea generally, will not work in all cases.

UP FOR DISCUSSION

Although Warren and Patrick argue that triage nurses can be justified in allocating resources in ways that are not impartial in some exceptional cases, the issues of what triage rules nurses should be taught, or what rules should be codified as part of official triage guidelines, are separate matters. They are not examined here but rather left for readers to consider.

COLLECTING OUR THOUGHTS

Patrick: There is so much more to be said on this and the other complex issues surrounding third parties. We have hardly broached the subtle distinctions between the problems presented by different third-party interests. I think that a complete account is beyond what we can accomplish now, so let's stop and collect our thoughts.

Doran: Yes, let's stop here. Although there are disagreements, there is a fair amount of consensus among us, despite our coming from different planets with respect to theory.

UP FOR DISCUSSION

Do we need principles to guide triage nurses in cases where the public interest requires treating B ahead of A, but the fair turn principle requires treating A ahead of B? Think of a hypothetical case where these principles could conflict. How would a utilitarian versus a care ethicist prioritize these principles? What about a Kantian, and a social contractarian? How would you decide which principle ought to take priority in this case?

Patrick: I suppose that indicates that we are probably onto something useful with Warren's set of principles. Not surprisingly, we are rather tentative about some of our conclusions, and there is some disagreement over the extent to which non-clinical factors should play a role in prioritizing patients.

Warren: True, we are far from confident in the really hard cases, and some disagreements persist. I am encouraged, however, that our rules manage to address these difficult issues with any success at all. Perhaps we have here the beginnings of a position on matters that seemed barely accessible to reason.

Doran: At the very least, we have raised some challenging issues for others to think through and debate.

UP FOR DISCUSSION

Apply the principles defended by Warren, Doran, and Patrick to Alice's decision to treat Lena ahead of Terence. Given these principles, did Alice act permissibly?

SUMMARY

Here is a summary of the main questions, concepts, and arguments covered in this chapter:

- This chapter focuses on questions of microallocation of scarce health care resources, that is, selecting which individuals are to receive scarce health care resources.
- The main questions explored are the following: Who should be given priority in the treatment of patients in emergency situations when CTAS (Canadian Triage and Acuity Scale) guidelines do not settle the issue? Are other factors besides clinical urgency morally relevant? How are we to make decisions when cases are equally urgent yet patients cannot all be cared for at once? In particular, was it right for Alice to treat Lena ahead of Terence in our drama?
- The rules we arrive at should generally be applied impartially, although we need to recognize that health care workers are only human. Warren employs the sympathy metarule: that normal sympathies need to be taken into account when choosing rules in the original position.
- According to Warren, whether sympathies justify, excuse, or merely mitigate blame will depend on the kind of case. Doran thinks sympathies may mitigate blame, but that the sympathy metarule won't justify violating the impartial application of fair rules.
- Patrick, Doran, and Warren agree on the rule that the worst-off patient should be treated first. In cases where several people are similarly badly off, patients should normally be treated on a first come, first served basis. (These are the worst first and first come rules.) However, there are some exceptions to these rules.
- The hopeless second rule was intended to provide one of these exceptions. It was replaced by a more inclusive rule, substantial benefit: if two patients both need immediate care but the second patient (B) to arrive in the emergency department can benefit substantially from care while the first patient (A) cannot benefit substantially, then B may be treated first.
- Articulating the idea of substantial benefit is very complicated. It involves considerations such as whether A stands to gain only a little in quality of life from the treatment whereas B stands to gain much more; exceptions will depend on whether A has had a fair turn at life but B has not. Quality of life and

fair turn are key notions, although they are difficult to specify in the abstract. Sometimes it may be permissible to take a person who has not had a fair turn at life over someone who has led a full life; the difference in the expected quality of life of the two patients must be large, however. Further, these judgments may be very hard to apply in concrete cases, and so the discretion of health care workers must be relied upon.

- Lastly, we discussed a category of exception to the worst first and first come principles that is based on non-clinical matters. Here Warren and Patrick accepted two rules, innocents first and public interest. These rules state that worst first and first come may be overridden in cases of extreme and obvious moral responsibility for an injury (like Terence's case), or extreme moral vice (like the child molester case), or in cases of great public interest like the public good case (about the town's only doctor).

- Doran, on the other hand, argued for fewer exceptions to the rules of worst first, first come, and substantial benefit. He argued that these principles should not be overridden in cases of moral fault, vice, or public good, or where one patient had young children but the other did not; however, he accepted that triage nurses would be justified in violating these rules in rare cases, where doing so was necessary to promote great medical interests.

REVIEW QUESTIONS

1. What are the impartiality, worst first, first come, and hopeless second rules?
2. State an objection to each rule. Can the rule be revised to meet the objection?
3. What is the sympathy metarule?
4. Distinguish justifications from excuses and mitigations. How are these distinctions significant in the application of the sympathy metarule, according to Warren?
5. What are the minimize YPLL, substantial benefits, and fair turn rules?
6. Why do Doran, Patrick, and Warren reject minimize YPLL in favour of substantial benefit? What problems do they see with the substantial benefit rule?
7. What is the innocents first rule? Why do Warren and Patrick accept this rule, and why does Doran reject it?
8. What is the public interest rule? With what would Doran replace it and why?
9. Why does support of the public interest not require utilitarian moral theory (accepting happiness maximization as what is morally required)?
10. Explain the disagreement that remains among Patrick, Doran, and Warren at the end of the debate.

NOTES

1. In April 2018, a bus carrying 29 people, including the Humboldt Broncos junior hockey team, was struck by a tractor-trailer outside of a small Saskatchewan town. Sixteen people on the bus were killed, including 10 hockey players. Many others on the bus were badly injured. This driver of the tractor-trailer was charged with dangerous driving causing death. First responders were overwhelmed. This tragic incident reminds us, sadly, of the importance of sound triage principles.

2. See, for instance, National Advisory Committee on SARS and Public Health, *Learning from SARS: Renewal of Public Health in Canada* (Ottawa: Health Canada, 2003), http://www.phac-aspc.gc.ca/publicat/sars-sras/naylor/. See also Canadian Institutes of Health Research, *Report on the Pandemic Preparedness Research Initiative: Report on Activities & Outcomes* (June 2006–June 2008), http://www.cihr-irsc.gc.ca/e/32573.html.

3. See, for instance, "Senior's Death Triggers Calls for ER Changes," *CBC News*, April 26, 2006, http://www.cbc.ca/bc/story/bc_er-nanaimo20060426.html. See also Thomas A. Mappes and Jane S. Zembaty, *Biomedical Ethics*, 6th ed. (New York: McGraw-Hill, 2005), ch. 9, "Social Justice and Health-Care Policy."

4. Additional information about CTAS can be found at https://caep.ca/resources/ctas/implementation-guidelines/.

5. Statistics Canada, "Life Expectancy," https://www150.statcan.gc.ca/n1/pub/89-645-x/2010001/life-expectancy-esperance-vie-eng.htm.

10

ALTERNATIVE MEDICATIONS AND PROFESSIONAL RELATIONSHIPS

INTRODUCTION

In recent years, increasing numbers of Canadians have been turning to **complementary** and **alternative medicine** to treat everything from the common cold to cancer. By *complementary and alternative medicine*, we mean the kinds of drugs, therapies, practices, and so on, that are not used in conventional Western medicine. Examples include acupuncture, homeopathy, naturopathy, and herbal therapy. When these drugs and therapies are used together with conventional treatments, they are commonly referred to as complementary or integrative medicine. When used in place of conventional drugs and practices, they are called alternative medicine.[1]

Our drama begins with Mr. Nolle learning that he has a cancerous tumour. Although there is no cure, the standard treatment, which involves chemotherapy and radiation, is expected to prolong his life. Mr. Nolle, however, adamantly refuses the standard treatment. As he is leaving the hospital, his nurse mentions to him the existence of an alternative herbal treatment that appears to have worked for the nurse's friend. Mr. Nolle is excited about the prospects of this herbal treatment, and he finds a physician, Dr. Anderweg, who is willing to administer the herbal injections to him. Dr. Anderweg does not agree that Mr. Nolle's choice is the best for this kind of tumour; however, she respects his decision.

Although this drama raises many interesting ethical issues, our focus is on whether Dr. Anderweg behaves permissibly in administering the herbal injections to Mr. Nolle. The more general question that we explore is whether physicians, in general, are morally permitted to administer scientifically unproven alternative or complementary treatments at their patients' request. At first glance, there may seem to be nothing morally wrong with this, since competent patients have a right to request whatever course of treatment they think is best. But the issue is complicated by the fact that many alternative therapies are scientifically untested and therefore potentially harmful. Moreover, patients who opt for alternative medicine may be forgoing conventional forms of therapy that have been proven to be life-saving or at least life-extending. These considerations (and others) make the provision of alternative medicine by physicians a morally complicated matter. Warren uses social contract theory to argue that Dr. Anderweg acts permissibly in Mr. Nolle's case, and that physicians, in general, should be given ample discretion to administer alternative therapies to their patients. Doran and Patrick take issue with many of Warren's claims.

BACKGROUND

Scientific varies its meaning considerably from one context to another. Here we are concerned to use it in a sense that allows us to distinguish science from mere guesses or speculation or even pseudo-science (fake science). Science makes use of rigorous methods of observation, testing, and logic.

It may be counterintuitive that pseudo-scientists try to prove themselves right while scientists try to prove themselves wrong. Scientists test precise ideas by experiments that will show up any fault in those ideas. That is rigorous testing. Pseudo-scientists may hide flaws in their ideas by using vague language.

For example, suppose a doctor experiments with an herbal remedy *H* on 10 people with cancer, all of whom go into **remission**. For pseudo-science, this study might be considered a proof positive of the vague idea that *H cures cancer.* For a real scientist this rough guess needs to be made into a more precise idea, like this: *H inhibits the growth of cancerous tumours fitting the description serous papillary carcinoma of the endometrium, stage 3.* Now we have an idea that can be shown wrong by experiments designed to test it. If this more precise idea is not shown wrong, then science keeps it as *possibly* true. If an idea fails a good test, science discards it. Only pseudo-scientists claim nothing could disprove their ideas.

For more on the scientific method, see Hanne Andersen and Brian Hepburn, "Scientific Method," *Stanford Encyclopedia of Philosophy* (Summer 2016 Edition), ed. Edward N. Zalta, https://plato.stanford.edu/archives/sum2016/entries/scientific-method/.

In addition to exploring an important ethical issue, one of the primary purposes of this debate is to illustrate how a philosophical position can evolve and improve by responding to criticism. While reading this chapter, you should therefore pay particular attention to Warren's *ample discretion principle*, which specifies what Warren regards as acceptable limits on the kinds of treatments physicians can provide to their patients. You should also note Patrick's and Doran's use of counterexamples in an effort to reveal flaws in Warren's principle. These examples force Warren to revise the ample discretion principle several times over the course of the debate. In the end, Warren arrives at a principle that he thinks is justified and that demonstrates that Dr. Anderweg acts permissibly in Mr. Nolle's case. Doran accepts the final statement of the principle but doubts that it applies to Mr. Nolle's case. Patrick goes further and argues that Warren's principle, even when fully revised, is false.

LEARNING OBJECTIVES

After completing this chapter, you should be able to:

- Explain Warren's, Doran's, and Patrick's views on whether it was permissible for Dr. Anderweg to administer the herbal remedy H to Mr. Nolle, and whether it is permissible, in general, for physicians to administer alternative treatments to their patients who request them
- Define Warren's best interest principle
- Describe Warren's final statement of the ample discretion principle
- Understand why Warren thinks the ample discretion principle would be chosen in the original position
- Distinguish the various versions of the ample discretion principle, and explain how it evolves under pressure from the frog toxin, psychic surgery, and prayer counterexamples
- Describe Doran's view on why it was not permissible for Dr. Anderweg to administer H to Mr. Nolle
- Explain Patrick's reasons for thinking that it was not permissible for Dr. Anderweg to administer H to Mr. Nolle, and why he thinks, in general, that it is not permissible for physicians to administer alternative treatments to their patients

---

DRAMA

Please note: This case is based on various true stories, although names, places, and some uncontroversial elements of the case have been changed to preserve anonymity and confidentiality. Discussions of this and similar cases with health care professionals have also informed this fictional case. Mr. Nolle is presented as a rough-spoken person. This is deliberate: we want to emphasize the distinction between being competent and being educated or cultured. Patients should not be thought to be incompetent merely because of the way they present themselves. The drama merely raises issues. The philosophical arguments are to be found in the debate following the drama.

CHARACTERS

Mr. Nolle: a patient with a cancerous tumour, serous papillary carcinoma of the endometrium, stage 3

Dr. Trad: Mr. Nolle's attending physician

Nurse Einverstand: a nurse caring for Mr. Nolle

Dr. Anderweg: a physician who treats Mr. Nolle at home

Mr. Swan: a quality control administrator at the hospital where Dr. Trad and Dr. Anderweg see patients

---

Scene 1

The scene is a hospital ward. Dr. Trad briskly approaches the bed where Mr. Nolle is recovering from having a tumour removed.

Nolle: You look like grim death, Doctor. What's the bad news?

Trad: (*Taken aback*) Well, in fact, the news is not all that good. I'm afraid you have a serous papillary carcinoma of the endometrium, stage 3, which is…

Nolle: (*Interrupting*) Tell me what I've got—in words I'll understand.

Trad: (*Continuing coolly*) …which is a rather rare cancerous tumour. (*Trad softens his voice*) The prognosis, that is, your outlook is for up to 24 months of life if you accept **chemotherapy** and **radiotherapy** but only about 6 months if you don't take treatment. (*Nolle holds up his hand*) Let me explain these treatments.

Nolle: Nope. Those are two treatments I know all too well. Heather had that stuff done to her before she died. I swore to God they'd never do that to me.

Trad: I am familiar with your wife's case. Yours is different, believe me. If I were in your shoes, knowing what I know, there is no question in my mind that I would take these treatments. Nothing else works.

Nolle: You're not saying it'll cure me.

Trad: No, no, but it will give you some relatively healthy time. Every bit of time is precious.

Nolle: You've got that right. That's why I sure won't spend the last of my time like Heather did. If you haven't got a cure for me, I'm just not interested.

Trad: Don't be hasty. This is an enormously important decision.

Nolle: And I'm the one making it. There's no way I'm getting **chemo**, not over my dead body. (*Laughing heartily at Trad's uncomfortable expression*) I know you don't think I'm taking death serious, but laughter is still the best medicine.

Trad: You don't have to decide right this minute. Please think carefully about this. I'd like you to talk to…

Nolle: Getting resigned to dying would kill me. Ha! You should have seen your face when I said that, Doc.

Trad: Very well. We'll talk again when you're more accustomed to your diagnosis.

Nolle: When hell freezes we will. Look, if you got no cure, forget it. I've made my own decisions all my life. I know enough to know chemo is no good for me. I'm not about to give up and just try to die slowly. Don't waste your time.

Scene 2

In the same ward, Nurse Einverstand is helping Mr. Nolle get ready to leave the hospital after Mr. Nolle's refusal of radiotherapy and chemotherapy for his tumour.

Nolle: Thank you. I don't have much stuff to take home, 'cause I never did intend to stay here long.

Einverstand: Well, I'm so glad you're well enough to go home.

Nolle: Hell, I'm not well at all. Not one bit. I'm just not going to sit around here getting chemo and radio till I drop. There's other stuff to try. I don't know where to find it, but I'll sure as hell look. I'm going to find a cure or die trying. (*Laughs heartily*)

Einverstand: Oh yeah, there are alternative therapies. My friend used one and is doing great two years beyond her expected time.

Nolle: No kidding! What's she taking?

Einverstand: Oh, it's this new herbal thing that she gets injected. I don't know much about it except that it's not a medically accepted treatment.

Nolle: I knew it. Natural cures, that's the stuff.

Einverstand: Oh—well, I shouldn't get your hopes up…

Nolle: Why the hell not? Hope is all I've got. Now you tell me where I can find out about getting some of this herbal stuff.

Einverstand: I'll call my friend and call you with the information.

Nolle: Cross your heart and swear to God?

Einverstand: (*Laughing*) Yes, of course.

Scene 3

Six months have passed. Nurse Einverstand waits in a meeting room. Dr. Anderweg enters. Dr. Anderweg has been administering injections of an herbal remedy to Mr. Nolle at home. His condition has worsened, there has been much growth in the tumour, and he has been readmitted to hospital. He wishes to continue the herbal treatment in the hospital.

Einverstand: Dr. Anderweg?

Anderweg: Call me Kendra. Nice to meet you.

Einverstand: He's such a neat old man. What a shame it didn't work for him.

Anderweg: Well, there was only a snowball's chance.

Einverstand: What? You've been giving Mr. Nolle the injections. Don't you believe in this therapy?

Anderweg: I believe a patient has a right to choose, but I told him that if I had a **radiosensitive tumour**, I would not be trying something untested on it instead of radiotherapy. But you know Mr. Nolle. It was alternative therapy or nothing.

Einverstand: It seemed to work on Marjorie.

Anderweg: "Seemed" is the operative word here. Maybe your friend just got lucky and had a remission. Maybe the herb only works for certain cancers. It was worth a try. When medicine has no cure, I don't mind patients trying anything if they've got little or nothing to lose. Mr. Nolle joked with me that his cure might not be 100 percent effective, but resignation is 100 percent fatal.

Einverstand: Actually, the treatment gave him something and still does. He told me when he came in that he probably would have died months ago without your treatment. He wants you to keep injecting him. He says it's his only hope.

Anderweg: Hope is a gift. He got six good months at home, too. He might have done no better with chemo and radiotherapy.

Trad: (*Entering the room, grim-faced*) He might have had that with nothing. He might have had two years with proper treatment. I'm surprised you aren't dancing around his bed with a rattle and feathers.

Einverstand: Dr. Trad!

Trad: (*Turning to Einverstand*) Nurse, if you ever again persuade one of my patients to give up medically approved treatment for…

Einverstand: (*Interrupting*) Don't take that tone with me. I didn't persuade Mr. Nolle of anything. I doubt anyone ever has. He is very strong willed. He asked me for information and I gave it to him.

Trad: Sure. *Information!*

Anderweg: This won't get us anywhere. Don't you believe in honouring patient autonomy and a patient's right to choose his own therapy, when we have no cure?

Trad: Therapy! Since when have double-blind controlled studies been done on this stuff?

Einverstand: The patient thinks it's working and he wants to continue treatment.

Trad: If you two get up to your quackery in here, I'll have you up before the appropriate disciplinary bodies so fast your heads will spin. (*Trad storms out*)

Scene 4

In an administrator's office. Einverstand and Anderweg sit across from Mr. Swan, a hospital administrator dealing with quality control.

Swan: I have taken your request and the patient's request to our legal counsellors and I have spoken with Dr. Trad.

Anderweg: Did you get the recommendation of the Ethics Committee?

Swan: Oh yes, and I have given it careful consideration, as have our legal counsellors, but we cannot agree with it.

Einverstand: So it's a no?

Swan: To allow this treatment would make the hospital particularly vulnerable. Dr. Trad has warned us that the injections could perhaps worsen the patient's condition by spreading the cancer.

Anderweg: Given that he will never take chemo or radiotherapy, he has nothing to lose with this alternative.

Swan: I'll let you and Dr. Trad argue the merits of that, but I can tell you that this hospital has a great deal to lose.

Einverstand: Surely you are being overcautious. If all we can give him is **palliation**...
(*The phone rings*)

Swan: (*Picking up the phone*) Excuse me. Hello. I can't talk now ... ah. I see. (*Putting down the phone with exaggerated care*) Mr. Nolle is dead.

Einverstand: Oh, that's awful news. It's too bad the herbal therapy didn't work for him... Well, we did try to respect his wishes.

Swan: This hospital takes patient autonomy seriously. Still, I will be guided by legal advice.

Anderweg: Tell me, what is the Ethics Committee for?

Swan: Now, Dr. Anderweg, you know as well as I do that it is a subcommittee of the Quality Committee, which is a subcommittee of the Board and, as such, has a purely advisory function. We accept most of the advice of the Ethics Committee, but in this case it took patient autonomy a little too far.

Einverstand: You'll be hearing from my association. We nurses have a very different view of the matter.

Anderweg: So, I hope, does the College of Physicians and Surgeons. We'll do what we can to bring this institution into this century.

DEBATE

Clarifying the Case and Identifying Relevant Facts

Patrick: Let's begin by making sure that we're clear on the relevant facts of the case. Many are spelled out, but key pieces of information are missing.

Warren: Well, just to summarize, Mr. Nolle was a strong-willed elderly man whose wife had died an unpleasant and lingering death while getting the standard treatment. He refused to even consider that treatment for his cancerous tumour. Nurse Einverstand mentioned to him an alternative therapy, H—herbal injections that a friend of Einverstand had used with apparent success. Nolle chose H over standard therapy, even though he was told that his case was different from his wife's. Mr. Nolle wanted to try treatments that were intended to be cures, not merely ways of delaying death. Dr. Anderweg agreed to give him these injections, although she said that she herself would have taken the standard treatment. Mr. Nolle died after six months of treatment.

Doran: Dr. Trad mentioned that there was a risk that the injections of H could cause the cancer to spread. Did Dr. Anderweg advise Mr. Nolle of this risk, and any others?

Warren: There was a small chance that injections could dislodge cells from the tumour that would spread the cancer to other sites. Since Mr. Nolle's chances were slim in any case, this was not a significant risk, in Dr. Anderweg's opinion. There was also a danger of bleeding or infection from the injections. These were more serious risks, but Dr. Anderweg was confident that she could control them or deal with them if they arose. She did not discuss these risks with Mr. Nolle.

Doran: So Dr. Anderweg didn't discuss these risks with Mr. Nolle. Hmmm.

Patrick: Warren, I was wondering about the following. Given Dr. Anderweg's skepticism about H, why didn't she just refer Mr. Nolle to a **naturopath**— someone who specialized in the sort of medicine Mr. Nolle requested?

Warren: Even if Dr. Anderweg could have found a naturopath, I suspect that she was worried about having someone without her training giving the injections because of the chance of bleeding and infection. Still, there might well be some very skilled

> **TECHNIQUE**
>
> It is always important to try to establish the relevant facts before beginning the debate. Factors such as whether Mr. Nolle was informed; whether the alternative medication, H, had been scientifically tested; the likely effects of conventional treatments; and others, all make a difference to the moral evaluation of Dr. Anderweg's, and others', behaviour.

> **BACKGROUND**
>
> "Practitioners other than physicians and dentists who may enroll and provide benefits under MSP [Medical Services Plan] include midwives, nurse practitioners, optometrists and other supplementary benefit practitioners. The Supplementary Benefits Program assists premium assistance beneficiaries ... and others, to access the following services: acupuncture, massage therapy, physiotherapy, chiropractic, naturopathy, and podiatry (non-surgical services). The program contributes $23.00 towards the cost of each patient visit to a maximum of ten visits per patient per annum summed across the six types of providers."
>
> *Source:* Health Canada, *Canada Health Act Annual Report 2016–2017* (Ottawa: Health Canada, 2018), https://www.canada.ca/en/health-canada/services/publications/health-system-services/canada-health-act-annual-report-2016-2017.html.

naturopaths in the area. Dr. Anderweg was also concerned about the cost to Mr. Nolle, thousands of dollars, if a naturopath took the case. The province would cover the treatment if Dr. Anderweg gave it, but would at best cover a small fraction of the costs if given by a naturopath.

Doran: Was Mr. Nolle offered any counselling to help him think through his decisions about treatment? It seems that this would have been a good idea.

Warren: I don't think anyone considered counselling. The tumour was progressing rapidly. Mr. Nolle was anxious to get started. Also, he was the type to dismiss counselling. He wasn't likely to listen to anybody's advice but his own.

Doran: What was Dr. Anderweg's opinion about the likely effect of traditional therapy if Mr. Nolle received it?

Warren: Dr. Anderweg thought Mr. Nolle had no chance in any case, and the standard treatment could only delay death. She knew she could not guarantee Mr. Nolle that he would not have nasty side effects from standard treatment. She thought H would be innocuous as far as side effects were concerned.

Doran: Thanks for providing these details, Warren. I think have a better handle now on the relevant background facts. Patrick, do you have any other questions for Warren?

Patrick: Yes. I was wondering whether there is any research at all on H that suggests that it could actually help Mr. Nolle's physical condition, aside from a possible **placebo effect**. Was H undergoing clinical testing?

UP FOR DISCUSSION

Should our public health insurance cover unconventional and alternative health care services?

THEORY

Kantian respect for persons is typically taken to require informed consent in order to treat a person always as an **end**, and never merely as a **means**.

Defenders of an **ethic of care** would also encourage extensive counselling and open discussion by the entire medical team with a patient, so as to reach the solution that best responds to the patient's needs.

BACKGROUND

"The prevalence of complementary and alternative medicine (CAM) use has been estimated to be as high as 65% in some populations. However, there has been little objective research into the possible risks or benefits of unmanaged CAM therapies."

Source: Tyler C. Smith, Besa Smith, and Margaret A. K. Ryan, "Prospective Investigation of Complementary and Alternative Medicine Use and Subsequent Hospitalizations," *BMC Complementary and Alternative Medicine* 8, no. 19 (2008), http://www.biomedcentral.com/1472-6882/8/19.

Warren: There was some **anecdotal** evidence suggesting that H may be effective in treating cancer, but H had not been scientifically tested.

Patrick: Okay. If there are no more questions for now, I think we can move on.

MORAL ISSUES RAISED BY THE CASE

Patrick: One interesting question raised by the drama is whether competent patients have a right to choose their course of treatment. I suppose most of us would agree that they do. A related and more difficult question is what it takes for a patient to qualify as competent. But this is a question we explore in chapter 4, so we can set it aside here.

Doran: We have an MD, in this case, giving unproven herbal medicine, and we have a nurse recommending an alternative treatment that he knows little about to a patient that he scarcely knows. There is a gigantic range of alternative medicine being marketed. Some of it may have merit; much of it is pure charlatanism. Given this, we could consider debating whether it was reckless for Nurse Einverstand to suggest H to Mr. Nolle and unprofessional for Dr. Anderweg to administer it. This raises important moral questions about the professional responsibilities of health care workers.

Warren: The case also raises the more general question of whether it is morally permissible for doctors in general to administer unproven alternative therapies.

Patrick: Yes, that seems to be the main general question raised by the case. And given the increasing demand for alternative medicine, discussing that issue would be very timely.

Doran: Right. But let's begin with the more specific question of *whether it was morally permissible for Dr. Anderweg to administer H, given that Mr. Nolle requested it.*

> ### UP FOR DISCUSSION
>
> The Canadian Nurses Association Code of Ethics (2017) contains the following rule: "Nurses provide education to support the informed decision-making of capable persons. They respect the decisions a person makes, including choice of lifestyles or treatment that are not conducive to good health, and continue to provide care in a non-judgmental manner."
>
> Does this rule determine whether Nurse Einverstand should inform Mr. Nolle about alternative medications? Do you think Einverstand acted inappropriately when he mentioned unproven therapies to Mr. Nolle? What role should nurses play in recommending therapies?
>
> *Source:* Canadian Nurses Association, *Code of Ethics for Registered Nurses* (Ottawa: CNA, 2017), https://www.cna-aiic.ca/~/media/cna/page-content/pdf-en/code-of-ethics-2017-edition-secure-interactive.

Patrick: Sure. We can use this as a spring-board to the more general question Warren noted: *Is it morally permissible for doctors, in general, to administer scientifically unproven alternative therapies if their patients request them?*

Warren: Sounds good to me. Let's get going.

Stating Our Positions

Warren: I believe that it was permissible for Dr. Anderweg to administer H. It was in Mr. Nolle's best interest.

Doran: I would say Dr. Anderweg's actions were probably not morally permissible. Mr. Nolle needed to receive more information about his treatment options, and he needed to receive counselling to ensure that he was making the best choice for him. I also think that it may have been better for Dr. Anderweg to refer Mr. Nolle to a competent naturopath if one was available.

Patrick: As an MD, Dr. Anderweg should, in general, stick to treating patients with drugs that have undergone, or are currently undergoing, rigorous clinical testing, or at least have been proven effective over the course of time and have been generally accepted by medical professionals. Because H does not fall into these categories, I believe it was irresponsible and reckless of Dr. Anderweg, as an MD, to give it to Mr. Nolle. If Mr. Nolle really wanted H, Dr. Anderweg should have referred him to a naturopath or some other specialist in alternative medicine.

Doran: So it looks as if Patrick and I are inclined to think that Dr. Anderweg should not have given Mr. Nolle the alternative treatment, whereas you see nothing wrong with her doing this, Warren.

Warren: That's right. I think Dr. Anderweg could've administered almost any therapy that Mr. Nolle chose.

Patrick: Really? That seems like an excessively permissive position. But I suppose much depends on what you mean by "almost," so perhaps you could clarify. Is there *any* therapy it would be wrong for Dr. Anderweg to administer to Mr. Nolle, assuming that he requested it? What if he was ill informed and chose badly?

THE BEST INTEREST PRINCIPLE

Warren: Of course, few of us are as well informed as the experts in health care we consult, so bad choices might happen on a regular basis. Let me propose the following principle: *If a treatment is in a patient's best interest, and the patient requests it, then that treatment is permissible.* This principle is too simple, but let's use it as our starting point and refine it as problems emerge.

TECHNIQUE

Warren is starting with an idea with which he is not completely satisfied, but by inviting questions and objections he will be able to test it until he can reject or strengthen the idea. We can often clarify our ideas by putting them under stress in this way.

Patrick: Warren, the notion of a patient's best interest is central to your principle. Are you thinking of *best interest* just in terms of a patient's physical condition, or do you have something more general in mind, something like the patient's overall condition, where this includes mental well-being?

Warren: I mean to take *best interest* very generally so as to include the use of medically useless treatments that have a useful placebo effect on the patient; so the patient's psychological, physical, and any other kind of well-being can be promoted. The idea is that a treatment is in a patient's best interest if the net benefit to the patient, judged in terms of their overall well-being, is higher than with any other treatment.

Doran: So, since you think it was permissible for Dr. Anderweg to administer H to Mr. Nolle, I assume that you think H was in Mr. Nolle's best interest, even though the standard therapy could offer him up to 24 months of life instead of just 6?

Warren: Yes, he seems to have had 6 months of good life in lieu of 24 months of misery.

Doran: Why do you assume Mr. Nolle would have had 24 months of misery if he received the standard care?

Warren: My assumption is based on what he and others said in the case.

Doran: Dr. Trad says that the prognosis is for up to 24 months of life, if Mr. Nolle accepts the chemotherapy and radiation. Also, he says that Mr. Nolle's case is different from his wife's case. So I don't think you can assume that he would have experienced 24 months of misery if he went with the standard treatment.

Warren: Mr. Nolle would probably have been miserable with a treatment that he viewed as horrifying, even if his course was different from his wife's. It is not the physical effects of chemo and radiotherapy that would necessarily have undermined his well-being, but his resignation and hopelessness. He clearly preferred a life, even a short one, with hope, over the longer, less appealing life offered by Dr. Trad. As Dr. Anderweg said, hope is a gift. She also said that for Mr. Nolle it was alternative therapy or nothing. So the standard therapy was not a live option for him.

Doran: Well, I can agree with you, Warren, that *if* Mr. Nolle had six quality months on the alternative therapy, this could be better than a longer life of poor quality. What I question, however, is your claim that he would have been miserable if he had taken the standard treatment. We just don't know that. Perhaps if Mr. Nolle received counselling and support, he would have had a longer, better life with the standard care. We just don't know. So I have doubts about your claim that the alternative therapy was in his best interest.

Warren: Doran, you are right to raise doubts. It is possible that, over time, he might have been better off with the standard therapy because he had come to accept it as his best option, but from what I know about the case that was very unlikely. The evidence suggests that the alternative treatment alone gave him hope during six months of life and that was better than resignation, which he said was "100 percent fatal."

Patrick: But what were the various alternatives? We seem to be assuming that Mr. Nolle had just three options: the standard treatment consisting of chemotherapy and radiotherapy, the herbal treatment, or nothing. But perhaps there were experimental cancer treatments that would offer him more hope, and more months of life, than H. Warren, do you know whether Dr. Anderweg looked for any experimental cancer drugs or treatments that she could have offered to Mr. Nolle?

 UP FOR DISCUSSION

Do you think that H was in Mr. Nolle's best interest? Suppose you do not. If Mr. Nolle would not take the conventional therapies, and given that there were no experimental treatments, was H in his best interest then?

Warren: She looked for other treatments, but for that particular kind of cancer there were no experimental drugs that she thought would help.

Patrick: Okay. I acknowledge Mr. Nolle's right to choose the course of treatment he thinks is best. So, although I think he acted foolishly, I recognize his right to refuse the standard course of treatment and seek an alternative therapy. What troubles me about this case is that a *medical doctor* provided an untested and unproven alternative therapy. Even if we grant your claim that H was in Mr. Nolle's best interest, I'm not at all convinced that it was permissible for Dr. Anderweg to give it to Mr. Nolle.

Warren: Why?

Patrick: You based your position on the best interest principle: *If a treatment is in a patient's best interest, and the patient requests it, then that treatment is permissible.* But I believe this principle is false, and I have a **counterexample** that I believe proves this.

Doran: What's the counterexample, Patrick?

TECHNIQUE

Recall that a **counterexample** is an example that purports to counter a general claim, principle, analysis, argument, and so on. Patrick's aim is to show that Warren's best interest principle is false. His counterexample is intended to show that some treatments might be impermissible even when patients request them and they are in those patients' best interest.

Patrick's Frog Toxin Counterexample to the Best Interest Principle

Patrick: Suppose that Mr. Nolle had been raised among a group of religious extremists who believed in the miraculous healing power of minute doses of the toxin secreted by a particularly rare species of frog. Now, suppose that instead of H, Mr. Nolle asked Dr. Anderweg to give him injections of the toxin. I'm assuming that the injections of the toxin would be small enough that they would pose no greater risk of harm than H. I'm also assuming that the injections of the toxin would give him hope, just as I I did. So, I'm imagining a case that mirrors the actual case in all relevant respects, except that it involves an unproven toxin therapy instead of herbal therapy. My intuitions are that it would be morally wrong for Dr. Anderweg to comply with Mr. Nolle's request for the frog toxin. If I'm right, then your principle is mistaken, Warren. Can you provide us with a strong argument in support of your view—one that would show that my intuitions about the frog toxin case are incorrect?

> **BACKGROUND**
>
> Many animal toxins appear to have clinically proven medical applications. See, for example, Chan and colleagues' "Snake Venom Toxins: Toxicity and Medicinal Applications," *Applied Microbiology and Biotechnology* 100, no. 14 (2016), https://www.ncbi.nlm. nih.gov/pubmed/27245678. Patrick is here imagining a toxin that has no clinically proven medical benefits.

Doran: I think this is a convincing counterexample, Patrick. I share your intuition that it would be wrong for Dr. Anderweg to comply with such a request.

Warren: Interesting example, Patrick; however, I am willing to bite the bullet on this one. I maintain that Dr. Anderweg's treatment of Mr. Nolle with herbal injections, or with any other treatment that is in his best interest and that he requests (possibly even frog toxin), is morally permissible. I'll argue for this by way of what I will call the **ample discretion principle**—a rule that would be chosen in the original position.

> **TECHNIQUE**
>
> When confronted with a counterexample, one can attempt to show that the example does not in fact counter the claim, principle, etc., in question. That is what Warren tries to do. Warren will accept the strange view that even frog toxin injections, under extremely restricted circumstances, could be permissible. He will then try to convince Doran and Patrick that it is strange but true.

THE AMPLE DISCRETION PRINCIPLE

Warren: It would be in the interest of the rule choosers in the original position to accept the ample discretion principle: *Physicians may exercise ample discretion to decide whether or not to use any treatment that the patient chooses, provided that it is in the patient's best interest.* Like computer graphics, medicine is an art based on sciences. To limit physicians to scientifically proven treatments would be to rule out possible help from physicians that might be critically important to the choosers of rules once they are patients in the real world. If you don't know what shape you might be in, you need the right to **autonomy** to protect your interest if you get into a tough situation, for example, a situation where normal medicine cannot help you.

> **THEORY**
>
> Here is an example of Warren's use of his **social contract** ethical theory. To understand this, you need to remember what the original position is and how it is used in contractarian ethics. You can see this at length in the statement of Warren's theory in chapter 3.

> **DEFINITION**
>
> Warren's argument for the ample discretion principle employs the concept of autonomy. **Autonomy** is often understood as self-determination, making one's own uncoerced choices.

Autonomy in the medical context, however, is a poor thing if some of the very people who are best equipped to help you exercise autonomy, namely physicians, are prevented from helping. I think it is clear that, in the original position, we would reject any rule that forces us and forces our doctors in the real world to stick to what is scientifically confirmed.

Limiting discretion would, moreover, limit medical research and discovery. That is clearly contrary to the interests of patients who reject or have run out of standard options. In the original position we would protect our interest by providing for the ample discretion of physicians. It's hard to say exactly how much is *ample*, but Dr. Anderweg was within reasonable limits.

Doran: So, in short, your argument is that whatever rules parties choose in the original position are justified, and that they would choose a rule that gave physicians ample discretion in hopeless cases, provided that the therapy is in the best interest of the patient. Is that right? Mr. Nolle's case was hopeless anyway, so anything goes when Dr. Anderweg prescribes.

Warren: That's not exactly it. You are right that I treat rules as justified if they would be accepted in the original position. As to the second point, however, we come to ample discretion through autonomy. First, we need to establish that a strong right to autonomy would be chosen in the original position. Ample discretion is then needed to allow people to exercise autonomy. The case, moreover, does not have to be hopeless, although that is the clearest kind of case. The choice of the rule or principle of ample discretion is dependent on the patient's strong interest in autonomy when the patient is choosing a treatment. It is Mr. Nolle's strong right to choose that would wither if willing physicians like Dr. Anderweg were prevented from honouring his choice.

> **UP FOR DISCUSSION**
>
> What do you think are the appropriate limits on patient autonomy? Do you think that people in Mr. Nolle's dire straits should have the option of requesting and receiving from physicians any treatment, however unconventional, that is in their best interest?

Patrick: I agree, Warren, that physicians ought to have the liberty to try out new drugs and therapies. But this should be done in the right sort of setting. This is what clinical trials are for. If H were part of a clinical trial, and the risks were clearly laid out for Mr. Nolle, then I would have no objection to Dr. Anderweg complying with his request for H. But that is not the case in this situation. Your ample discretion principle gives physicians too much liberty. For that reason, I think the principle would not be chosen in the original position.

Doran's Indeterminacy Objection to Warren's Principle

Doran: I agree. It's not clear to me why people in the original position would choose the ample discretion principle rather than some other competing principle. Perhaps people in the original position will choose a rule that instructs physicians to do what is in their best interest and protects patients from taking reckless decisions, or perhaps they will choose a rule that instructs physicians to do whatever the patient chooses, or a rule that instructs physicians to do whatever the patient chooses provided it is not too harmful. Your contract argument does not conclusively prove that a principle of ample discretion is justified.

Warren: Actually, I think that "conclusively prove" is too strong a phrase. One can be persuasive short of a conclusive proof. In fact, I don't think that any ethical theory is capable of providing us with moral certainties or absolutes that would come from a conclusive proof. It is enough if we can give good reasons for why people in the original position would choose more or less discretion for physicians, without knowing for sure what they would choose.

> **THEORY**
>
> Although Warren's views have some distant Kantian heritage, notice how different they are with respect to conclusive proof. If Kant thought that a principle expressed a **categorical imperative**, he would believe that it tells us our duty with absolute certainty.

Doran: Fair enough, but my problem remains. I just do not see what reasons people in the original position would have for selecting your preferred rule, ample discretion, over some other seemingly plausible rule—for example, *Do what is in the patients' best interests, while protecting patients from their ill-informed choices.* So I am not convinced that your way of thinking about the case gives us a strong reason to accept the ample discretion principle and to say that Dr. Anderweg did what was permissible.

Patrick: I'm with Doran on this one, Warren. Can you say more about why you believe the ample discretion principle would be chosen over competing principles?

Warren: Okay, let's see how ample discretion can be defended against competing principles. You suggested an alternative principle a moment ago, Doran, namely, *Do what is in the patients' best interests, while protecting patients from their ill-informed choices.* This is a highly paternalistic principle, one that gives too much power to the physician, so I do not think it could be considered in their interest by the choosers of rules. That principle would let Dr. Trad tell Mr. Nolle what to do. The other principles you suggest are just not sufficiently restricted to protect patients' interests. Protection of our interests is what we consider in the original position.

Doran: But using your contract argument, wouldn't patients want to protect themselves from their poor choices? I might request some inefficacious therapy over a proven treatment because I am desperate for a miracle cure, or because I am simply afraid of some aspect of the standard treatment. Surely, doctors should not be given the discretion to act on these choices. In Mr. Nolle's case, the concern is that he is motivated by misunderstanding and desperation.

> **DEFINITION**
>
> **Paternalism** is the interference with a person's liberty for that person's own good. For an excellent introduction to the concept of paternalism, see the *Stanford Encyclopedia of Philosophy's* entry at http://plato.stanford.edu/entries/paternalism/.
>
> Utilitarians have no objection to paternalism when it maximizes happiness. In contrast, Kantians would generally reject paternalism for rational adults, since it violates their autonomy. Warren seems to be siding with Kantians on this point.

> **TECHNIQUE**
>
> Doran and Patrick are chipping away at the plausibility of the ample discretion principle to undercut one of the premises of Warren's argument that Dr. Anderweg acts permissibly. If one of Warren's premises is not true, his argument is unsound. His conclusion about Dr. Anderweg might follow logically from the ample discretion principle (and so the argument would be logically valid), but following from a falsehood is no recommendation for his conclusion about Dr. Anderweg's action.

Patrick: Right. And parties in the original position may want to protect themselves from not just their own bad judgment, but also from the poor choices of their doctors.

Warren: I take your points. I agree that parties in the original position will want to make sure that physicians are not given the discretion to act on their own or their ill-informed patients' whims.

Doran: But what if the patient is incapable of making rational choices, for instance? Can the doctor just go ahead and do whatever he thinks is in the patient's best interest even if it is a very weird treatment? Suppose Dr. Anderweg thinks Mr. Nolle is **incompetent** to choose?

 UP FOR DISCUSSION

Do you think that people in the original position would accept the principle of ample discretion, or would they choose a more paternalistic principle—say, one that ensured that doctors gave only the medically recommended treatments?

Warren: There is an important difference between the rules that would be chosen affecting **competent** and incompetent patients. Incompetent patients require protection that is much more paternalistic, and the discretion of the physician would be much less. Since incompetent patients cannot protect themselves or decide to take big risks that might help them achieve their goals, very conservative care is warranted.

BACKGROUND

Competence comes in degrees. Someone could be more or less competent to perform some task. Beyond that, we may be more willing to deem someone competent as the risks one runs by exercising autonomy become smaller.

Rules set in the original position would honour only adventurous choices made with the **valid consent** of competent persons.[2] Dr. Anderweg would, of course, still be required to pursue the best interest of an incompetent Mr. Nolle, but within stricter limits. She could not do anything experimental or too strange at her own discretion, like using H. If Mr. Nolle is deemed incompetent, then Dr. Anderweg should just play it safe. If we are going to support autonomy with ample discretion, then it must be for competent patients or their surrogate decision-makers to validly consent to treatment.

THE AMPLE DISCRETION PRINCIPLE REVISED: VALID CONSENT OF COMPETENT PATIENTS ONLY

Doran: Okay, Warren, so it seems you would like to replace the initial statement of the ample discretion rule with the following: *Physicians may exercise ample discretion to decide whether or not to use any treatment to which a competent patient gives* *valid consent, provided that it is in the patient's best interest.*

Warren: Yes, that's right.

Patrick: Warren, I have a couple of questions about the revised principle. First, what exactly do you mean by *competent?*

My second question is this: Now that you have restricted the application of the ample discretion rule to competent patients, I'm not sure why you need the further clause that the chosen treatment is in the patient's best interest. Why not just say this: *Physicians may exercise ample discretion to decide whether or not to use any treatment to which a competent patient gives valid consent.* This principle would seem to be more consistent with the goal of protecting autonomy.

 UP FOR DISCUSSION

Do you think physicians should be free to give *competent* patients unconventional and scientifically unproven treatments if they are in the patients' best interests and the patients validly consent to them?

Ample Discretion, Patient Competence, and Valid Consent

Warren: Let me answer your first question. Patient competence is an exceedingly complicated issue that we cannot fully address here.[3] But perhaps we can agree on the following: competence involves a capacity to make choices based on comprehension of relevant information and the consequences of one's choices. A person can be competent in one area, but not other areas. For instance, a person can be competent to make health care decisions, but not competent to make important decisions about financial matters because of a phobia about money. To be competent to make health care choices, it seems one must be capable of understanding one's condition, treatment options, the probable consequences of each treatment, and their respective risks and benefits. One must then be able to make a decision based on this information. When I speak of patients being competent or incompetent, I am speaking of their having or lacking this ability.[4] Before she agrees to Mr. Nolle's request for H, then, Dr. Anderweg must ensure that Mr. Nolle is competent in this sense.

Patrick: I agree with most of your remarks about competence. But how do we tell whether Mr. Nolle is competent?

Warren: In legal and medical contexts, persons are generally assumed to be competent unless there is good reason for doubting this. So the question is whether we have a good reason for doubting Mr. Nolle's competence. He is requesting a non-standard course of treatment over a more conventional treatment that has been clinically tested. But that, by itself, does not show that he's incompetent.

Patrick: I agree that the mere fact that he requests an unconventional treatment is not sufficient to show that he's incompetent. But we have good reason to question Mr. Nolle's competence, given his complete refusal to seriously consider the course of treatment that

> ## BACKGROUND
>
> "Legal standards for decision-making capacity for consent to treatment vary somewhat across jurisdictions, but generally they embody the abilities to communicate a choice, to understand the relevant information, to appreciate the medical consequences of the situation, and to reason about treatment choices."
>
> *Source:* Paul S. Appelbaum, "Assessment of Patients' Competence to Consent to Treatment," *New England Journal of Medicine* 357 (2007): 1834–40, doi:10.1056/NEJMcp074045.

the medical community in general thinks is best. His experience with his wife, who did not do well with the standard course of treatment, prevented him from being able to think rationally about his own situation. He wouldn't even allow Dr. Trad to explain the relevant differences between his own condition and his wife's. This leads me to question whether he is competent to make decisions about his course of treatment.

Doran: I am not sure that the problem is that Mr. Nolle is incompetent. I don't think he lacks the capacity to make his health care decisions; my concern is that he does not give valid consent.[5] In this case, in order to give valid consent, Mr. Nolle needs a better understanding of his treatment options and the likely effects of his choices. He then needs to deliberate about them in a way that is consistent with both his goals and the facts at hand. My concern is that because Mr. Nolle will not even consider all of his treatment options, he does not really understand the likely effects of the conventional therapies and alternative therapies as they relate to his circumstances. Because he lacks the relevant information, his consent to H is not valid.

> ### TECHNIQUE
>
> Here, Patrick and Doran are not disagreeing with the revised ample discretion principle; instead, they are questioning whether this principle applies to Mr. Nolle's situation.

Warren: He knows enough about the risks to know how to pursue his goal of living in hope of a cure. Mr. Nolle prefers a short life of hope to a longer life of resignation. He knowingly chooses to take a chance on non-standard treatment that gives him hope instead of resignation. So his consent to be treated with H is valid. He is not ignoring evidence relevant to his goal of maximizing hope. He is ignoring evidence relevant to the medical view about his chances, but he does not want the evidence for the medical view in case it undermines hope. "Where ignorance is bliss, 'tis folly to be wise." It would be different if Dr. Trad had offered him a cure or a means that supported hope. Since hope makes his life worthwhile to him, Mr. Nolle would be a fool to abandon hope and accept resignation by becoming informed about the improbability of his long-term survival.

Doran: It is not that I necessarily disagree with his final decision, Warren, but he should have seriously considered his options. Dr. Anderweg should have made sure he was properly informed. Perhaps with more discussion with Dr. Anderweg, and perhaps even with Dr. Trad, Mr. Nolle could have come to see that there were advantages offered by the standard therapy, or perhaps they could have found a way to encourage Mr. Nolle to choose *both* the standard therapy and H.

Patrick: I wonder whether it is responsible for a physician to encourage hope in competent patients when the situation is known to be hopeless (or nearly hopeless). If Mr. Nolle truly was competent, Dr. Anderweg should have been honest with him; she should have made it clear to Mr. Nolle, while being as sympathetic as possible, of course, that the odds of survival were heavily stacked against him, and that taking H would likely do nothing to change that.

In any case, as Doran notes, if Mr. Nolle had seriously considered his options, he would have seen that it didn't have to be a choice between H and the standard therapy, between hope and resignation.

Warren: Mr. Nolle did consider his options seriously and with sufficient information. His options were to live in resignation or to live in hope. Nothing Dr. Anderweg could have told him could have made any difference to his goal of living in hope unless it was to make it more difficult to achieve that goal. For him, accepting standard treatment would be an admission of defeat, engaging death with delaying tactics. One cannot give up and maintain hope at the same time, and the standard treatment, with its likely unpleasant side effects, was, for him, giving up. That is why Dr. Anderweg withheld the details concerning standard treatment and arguments for standard treatment that Mr. Nolle did not want or need to hear. She respected his choice of hope. Physicians often leave out the gory details that we do not need to hear when knowing them cannot help us.

Ample Discretion and Patient Autonomy

Patrick: What do you have to say in response to my second question, Warren? Now that you have limited the application of the ample discretion principle to the valid consent of competent patients, why do you need the best interest clause? Why not just say this: *Physicians may exercise ample discretion to decide whether or not to use any treatment to which a competent patient gives valid consent.*

Doran: Right. Warren, you argued that parties in the original position would choose the ample discretion principle in order to protect their autonomy. But wouldn't the version of the principle Patrick just suggested give patients greater autonomy than your principle when it comes to health care decisions?

Warren: In the original position we would want to have autonomy with safety precautions built in. Unlimited autonomy is not in our interest, although a very strong right to autonomy is. Finding the balance is difficult, but we would accept certain limits on our autonomy, like being required to wear seat belts, for example, that would prevent us from sacrificing our lives or well-being because of a moment of temporary carelessness or because we had insufficiently understood the information about the possible outcomes. Similarly, we want autonomy with some safety precautions in our medical decision-making. We need physicians to be good advisers and guides to our medical decisions.

The restriction on physicians is a safety precaution to prevent a competent patient from being granted a request that could be harmful because, for instance, that patient does not fully understand a complicated set of medical facts the doctor has explained. It allows the patient much choice and the physician a great deal of latitude in fulfilling patient choices. It would allow all sorts of alternative medications to be used by physicians. Patients, however, sometimes need physicians to talk them out of bad decisions, not just accept them because they are the patients' choice. When the patient has very little to lose by treatment, the treatments may be quite strange, but the physician is still restricted to pursuing the best interest of the patient.

Patrick: Okay, but now I don't see autonomy as having any real significance, in your view. The ample discretion principle says that doctors can provide any treatment a competent patient validly consents to, provided that the treatment is in the patient's best interest. But how is this any different from just saying that MDs can administer any treatment provided that it is in the patient's best interest? Adding the bit about what a competent patient requests doesn't seem to add anything of significance to the principle. Ultimately, it is the physician, not the patient, who determines the course of treatment.

Warren: The piece about the valid consent of competent patients does add much. Patients can request and get many things that physicians would not think to provide if physicians were guided only by their own knowledge and their patients' best interest. A physician might, for example, realize that a traditional cure that a patient requests, previously unknown to the physician, would be a powerful placebo for that particular patient. An innumerable variety of treatments is added.

Patrick: I'm not sure, Warren. To illustrate my point, consider the following example. Suppose that patient A is ill and requests treatment *x*. Suppose also that A's doctor thinks that *x* would help A, but, all things considered, treatment *y* is in A's best interest. So A wants *x*, and *x* is beneficial, but A's doctor is not permitted to administer *x*, according to your principle, because another treatment, *y*, is in A's best interest. It seems, then, that your principle does not give patient autonomy much teeth, since it doesn't allow competent patients to determine their course of treatment, unless what they want is also what their doctor thinks is in their best interest.

Warren: Treatments are rarely so well evidenced that all physicians agree on what is best. The patient can get a second opinion. The patient can, furthermore, refuse treatment. The physician may, in such a situation, offer a second-best treatment that has now become the one in the patient's best interest because the patient adamantly refuses what would have been best. In that way, the patient may get *x* rather than *y*.

I say *may*, rather than *will*. The physician may refuse to offer certain treatments if they pose enough risk of harm or the physician thinks the patient does not really understand the choice, for instance. There may be allocation issues as well. Suppose an 80-year-old demands a triple bypass which would be indicated if the patient were younger. The physician may think it is too likely to kill the 80-year-old and should be given instead to a 40-year-old. Autonomy gives us the right to refuse, and the right to choose, some treatments without the interference of narrow ideas about physicians' roles. It does not let us have anything on the shelf to which we take a fancy.[6]

Patrick: Okay, I think I now have a better handle on your principle and how it preserves patient autonomy. Patient A can in fact get *x*, which is the treatment she wants, by refusing to take *y*, which is the treatment her doctor thinks is genuinely best. But then I don't see how the best interest clause helps to protect patients from their bad choices. When a patient refuses to take the three best treatments, for instance, the fourth then becomes the treatment that is in the patient's best interest. That is a very unusual way of thinking about which therapy is in a patient's best interest.

Warren: It is not unusual in practice. In a rare case in which a patient will accept only a really poor treatment, the physician should refuse to give it; patients will usually come to a reasonable decision with education. In some cases, like Mr. Nolle's, the treatment serves other interests of the patient than medical ones, and the physician should be allowed to help the patient to pursue such powerful interests as hope. But let's move on—I can see that Doran is eager to ask a question.

THE AMPLE DISCRETION PRINCIPLE REVISED (AGAIN): HARM AVOIDANCE

Doran: Let's return to the proposed principle: *Physicians may exercise ample discretion to decide whether or not to use any treatment to which a competent patient gives valid consent, provided that it is in the patient's best interest.* We disagree about whether Mr. Nolle was sufficiently informed to give valid consent, and so we disagree about whether this principle would justify Dr. Anderweg's behaviour. But beyond this disagreement, I think the principle itself is flawed. Even if a competent patient validly consents to a certain treatment that is in their best interest, it may be wrong for the doctor to administer the therapy. One reason it might be wrong is that the chosen treatment would harm **third parties**. For instance, the principle, as it now stands, seems to allow patients to receive, and MDs to provide, unfair distributions of medical resources.

Warren: If you call Mr. Nolle's consent invalid, you will have few valid consents. I have more sympathy with your second point about third parties, though. Can you give an example to illustrate your point, Doran?

Doran: Sure. If I need a kidney, it might be rational for me to request that my doctor provide me with the next matching kidney that becomes available. But there might be someone else who is entitled to the kidney, perhaps because he has been waiting longer, and his condition is worse. I don't see anything in your principle that would prohibit my doctor from allowing me to receive the kidney. To avoid such counter-examples, we can revise the principle as follows: *Physicians may exercise ample discretion to decide whether or not to use any treatment to which a competent patient validly consents, provided that it is in the patient's best interest, and that it is consistent with the equal opportunity of all who are seeking medical resources.*

Warren: I was assuming physicians would not exercise discretion in ways that would harm people other than the patient, but you are right that we need to make some explicit condition in the ample discretion principle.

Patrick: That principle may not go far enough, since we want to ensure against other harms besides violations of equal opportunity. We want to guard against certain harms to third parties in general. Part of my concern about Dr. Anderweg administering H to Mr. Nolle is that this could harm the reputation of doctors in general, and undermine public confidence in the medical profession, if it became public knowledge. That may also be part of Dr. Trad's worry about Dr. Anderweg prescribing H.

Warren: Yes, but the danger of damage to the reputation of the profession in Mr. Nolle's case would come mainly through public misunderstanding of the discretion that must be allowed physicians in such cases. Dr. Anderweg took a calculated risk, exercised discretion, and did what turned out to be best for Mr. Nolle. It was not publicized. It was not harmful.

Doran: When these remarks are applied to the specific case of Patrick's frog toxin example, Warren, your view implies that it is permissible for doctors to administer the toxin only if they could keep this course of treatment secret, or take other steps that would prevent harm to the medical profession and to third parties more generally. Is that right?

Warren: Yes, that's my view. Dr. Anderweg might say that she gave the injection of H because it served Mr. Nolle's goal of hope and because hope might have a strong placebo effect. It would be much harder to justify frog toxin, however. Frog toxin may be a reasonable choice in some extreme circumstances, but it may only be administered when, on balance, no harm to others results. In any case, we need to take into account, as your examples show, more harms than just the harm of unfair access to resources.

Here, then, is my revised rule: *Physicians may exercise ample discretion to decide whether or not to use any treatment to which a competent patient gives valid consent, provided that it is in the patient's best interest and harmless to others on balance.* This broader restriction against harm works against unfair practices like lack of equal opportunity and disrepute, as well as other harms. Yet these restrictions still allow the principle to protect our interests. The principle prevents excessive conservatism in medicine, thereby allowing progress to be made.

TECHNIQUE

It is typical for principles to become more complex as qualifications are added to reply to objections. If too many qualifications are added, philosophers start to speak of death by a thousand qualifications.

 UP FOR DISCUSSION

What kinds of harms are serious enough to serve as harms that we must avoid when applying the ample discretion principle?

Patrick: There are many perfectly acceptable treatments that harm others, in some sense, that this principle would seem to rule out. For instance, if there's one kidney available, and two people need it, then there's a clear sense in which the person who doesn't get it is harmed by the first person's getting the kidney. But this kind of harm is allowed, because it's not unfair. So, I think you need to add something to the effect that the harms to others that your principle doesn't allow are *unfair* harms.

Warren: I intended to capture that by "harmless to others on balance," which would rule out a patient's being given a treatment in a way that denied equal opportunity to other patients. There may be a sense in which another patient who is second in line for it is harmed, if someone gets the only kidney, but this is not unwarranted harm or unfair harm of the sort the principle is intended to oppose.

Patrick: Well, I have another concern. You speak of excess conservatism in medicine that this principle will avoid. Yet a medical establishment that is conservative with regard to the adoption of strange and unproven treatments can still make significant progress. What medical advances are promoted by ample discretion?

Warren: What if H had cured Mr. Nolle? Physicians need some leeway to practice experimental medicine, like the neurosurgeon who recently went against most of his colleagues to induce **hypothermia** in a comatose patient, for example. The neurosurgeon saved a life and revealed a hypothesis worth researching by using a totally non-standard treatment. The treatment was untested, but the patient had nothing left to lose. Cutting-edge medicine is, necessarily, not yet accepted by most physicians nor scientifically confirmed.[7]

Patrick: I don't know, Warren. As I mentioned earlier, I'm not at all against the use of unproven experimental drugs when they are part of legitimate trials and tests, and when the patient has been fully informed of the risks. But this case is different. H is not part of any clinical studies, and Mr. Nolle was not informed of the risks involved in taking it. So it seems it was irresponsible for Dr. Anderweg, as an MD, to administer H, even if it would not harm Mr. Nolle or anyone else.

Doran: I might be persuaded to agree with you, Patrick, if there was a medically acceptable treatment that could offer meaningful benefit. This may have been the case for Mr. Nolle, given what Dr. Trad says. But in cases where patients have no good options, and where the unconventional therapy is in the patients' best interest and harmless on balance to others, I think there may be nothing wrong with physicians honouring their patients' mental well-being—provided, of course, that patients are informed and counselled about their options.

UP FOR DISCUSSION

If patients who have nothing left to lose are willing to try a new potential cure, what are the limits on administering experimental medications? Would you say that Mr. Nolle's situation was one where he had nothing left to lose?

AGAINST THE REVISED AMPLE DISCRETION PRINCIPLE: THE DIVISION OF LABOUR OBJECTION

Patrick: Well, I suppose that at least part of what's bothering me about H, frog toxin, and other untested and unconventional therapies is the following. There seems to be a kind of division of labour in the health services industry. The boundaries aren't sharp, but we have different kinds of health care professionals responsible for different kinds of services.

Medical doctors in our part of the world are trained in conventional Western medicine. The relevant governing bodies, such as the various provinces' Colleges of Physicians and Surgeons, require the practice of medicine to be informed by scientific evidence.[8] Thus, when I go to see a medical doctor, I expect to be treated with medicine that has undergone clinical testing, or is currently in an experimental phase (as is the case with many of the drugs used to treat HIV/AIDS, for example), or is in some other way supported by scientifically valid testing and evidence.

BACKGROUND

The Canadian Medical Association's (CMA) policy statement on the use of complementary and alternative medicine notes that "the CMA's position is based on the fundamental premise that decisions about health care interventions used in Canada should be based on sound scientific evidence as to their safety, efficacy and effectiveness—the same standard by which physicians and all other elements of the health care system should be assessed."

Source: Canadian Medical Association, *CMA Policy: Complementary and Alternative Medicine* (Ottawa: CMA, 2015), http://policybase.cma.ca/dbtw-wpd/Policypdf/PD15-09.pdf.

Other health professionals are trained in other, less conventional, forms of health care where the standards of practice are not so strictly based on scientific evidence. Consider, for instance, homeopaths and naturopaths. Many of the treatments that homeopaths and naturopaths administer have undergone little, if any, formal clinical testing. When we go to see health care professionals in these fields, the expectation is that we will be treated with non-conventional medicine that may not be scientifically proven.

Given these considerations, I think it is generally morally irresponsible and reckless, and therefore wrong, for medical doctors to administer untested and scientifically unproven alternative therapies such as H or frog toxin, even if a competent patient requests this.

In saying this, I'm not, of course, claiming that it would be wrong for *all* health care professionals to administer strange and unusual therapies. I might not have any objection, for instance, if a shaman administers frog toxin therapies. That's the kind of therapy I would expect a practitioner of that sort to administer. Even some naturopaths might do that. So, if Mr. Nolle wanted H, Dr. Anderweg probably should have referred him to a naturopath or someone who practiced alternative medicine.

Doran: Warren, do you think the fact that the Canadian Medical Association and the College of Physicians and Surgeons forbid doctors from using scientifically untested treatments is enough to conclude that Dr. Anderweg acted unethically in giving H to Mr. Nolle?

Warren: No. We cannot determine ethical permissibility merely by consulting current professional guidelines. For these guidelines are themselves fallible. In the past, doctors have been forbidden by their profession's ethical codes from performing abortions and euthanasia, and they were instructed to do whatever they thought was in the best interest of their patients even if this involved breaches of confidentiality and lying to their patients about their health status. So, we cannot determine right and wrong just by looking at what a professional code permits or forbids.

UP FOR DISCUSSION

Do you accept the view that there should be a division of labour among health care professionals? If so, under what conditions are there allowable exceptions?

Patrick: I agree with you about that, Warren, but in this case, I do think the guideline that doctors stick to tested treatments is ethically correct.

Doran: I also agree with you, Warren, that a profession's code of conduct is not morally decisive. I believe it gives a practitioner a *prima facie* moral obligation to follow it, but that, like other moral obligations, it can be overridden by other moral considerations. I share your thoughts about the division of labour, Patrick. And you might be right that the best thing to do is for Dr. Anderweg to refer Mr. Nolle to a naturopath, if one is available. But let's suppose one is not available, or the one who is available is likely to botch the job, or that access to naturopaths is prohibitively expensive for the patient. Then, all things considered, it may not have been wrong for Dr. Anderweg to administer the alternative therapy if Mr. Nolle was competent and informed of his options.

I think physicians have a variety of *prima facie* obligations—obligations that both of you have already touched on. They include duties to promote their patients' health and well-being (physical and psychological), to respect their patients' autonomy, to promote the health of other patients, to safeguard the reputation of their profession, and so forth. In a case such as Mr. Nolle's, I'd judge that the duties to promote his autonomy and his physical and psychological well-being would win out *if* he was competent and informed. In other cases, though, the circumstances may be different, and my judgment may be different.

> **BACKGROUND**
>
> Here Doran is following a Rossian approach to Mr. Nolle's case. This is similar to the approach known as principlism that was popularized by Beauchamp and Childress. The principles include beneficence, non-maleficence, autonomy, and justice. See chapter 2 for a brief discussion of *principlism*.

Warren: Well, at least on those conditions we would come up with the same verdict in Mr. Nolle's case, but I think Patrick has some further arrows in his quiver for my principle and our conclusion. Before we go on, however, I should say that the division of labour is, in my view, merely an artifact of the ample discretion principle, since it is usually in the best interest of patients if practitioners stay within the scope of their practice. Division need not be morally required, however, when it is in the patient's interest that different kinds of practitioners share the labour.

The Psychic Surgery Counterexample

Patrick: Yes, even if there were no naturopaths available, then it would probably still be wrong for a doctor to administer the frog toxin therapy. You must admit that the toxin example gives you pause. Let me try another even more extreme example. Suppose that Mr. Nolle was raised in a cult that believed in psychic therapies and psychic phenomena in general. And suppose that Mr. Nolle was convinced that his only hope of beating cancer, or at least getting the most out of his remaining time, was to have someone perform **psychic surgery** on him.

Now suppose also that there was no one available to perform this kind of "surgery" except Dr. Anderweg. As an MD, Dr. Anderweg has a dim view

> 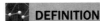 **DEFINITION**
>
> **Psychic surgery** is a magician's trick, although some patients have faith in it and see the magician or trickster who performs it as a saviour. The trickster appears to pull something out of a person's abdomen (often a chicken liver that has been palmed). Then the trickster announces that the tumor has been removed.

of this sort of thing, of course, but she sees that it would give Mr. Nolle hope, just like H, and would not harm him. Finally, suppose that Dr. Anderweg could "perform" psychic surgery without any harm to the medical profession. Warren's view seems to imply that it is permissible for Dr. Anderweg to perform psychic surgery in this situation. I think it would be irresponsible and dishonest, among other things, and therefore wrong ... very wrong! Physicians have a responsibility, I believe, to uphold certain standards concerning the treatments they provide to their patients.

Warren: I think the doctor would have to look at all who are affected by this person's treatment, not just the patient. What if other members of the cult who did have better options than the patient might be influenced to try psychic surgery rather than a curative treatment? If, in a vanishingly rare circumstance, only the doctor and the patient would ever learn of it, and it was in the patient's best interest, then the doctor would be morally permitted to perform psychic surgery. As long as only the patient's interests are affected, then the doctor should still have ample discretion to choose treatments that include weird treatments, if those serve the patient's best interest as placebos, for example. We would be bound to choose that if we were in the original position. How else could we protect our interests in the real world? Division of labour for its own sake does not protect them. Those in the original position would look at their chances in the real world and say, "If it can do some good and won't do harm, then go for it." The cases where such tricks as psychic surgery do no harm are, however, so few as to be negligible. Patients are bound to talk about their treatment and physicians know this. Confidentiality is often breached and physicians know this. The division of labour will not be total but will remain largely in place for that reason alone.

Doran: I do admit that the frog toxin example gives me pause. And I agree with Patrick that it would be wrong for Dr. Anderweg to perform psychic surgery. I suspect that is because a patient could not be competent and fully informed and still give valid consent to psychic surgery (or frog toxin, for that matter). I also think that physicians have a *prima facie* duty to uphold the standards of their profession whether or not anyone finds out about it. Taken together, these constitute powerful conditional reasons against a doctor giving a patient psychic therapy. But the actual case of Mr. Nolle is a bit different, given that reasonable people believe in herbal therapies, and given that some herbal therapies almost certainly work.

THEORY

A Kantian who thought that a physician was bound by their oath to uphold certain standards of practice would think that this perfect duty must be done no matter who knew or what were the consequences of doing that duty. In contrast, a utilitarian would permit a physician to use any therapy provided that it had the best consequences, all things considered, for everyone concerned.

Warren: I'll take Doran's help here and say that my view does not license psychic surgery *if* a competent person could not validly consent to psychic surgery.

Patrick: Given what was argued earlier regarding Mr. Nolle's request for H, I'm not sure we need to regard the patient who requests psychic surgery as incompetent or inadequately informed. If, for example, the person was raised in a culture that practiced this sort of thing, and was suspicious of Western medicine, and if she believed that psychic surgery was her best and only hope, then I'm not sure we could regard the patient's request for psychic surgery as invalid. If I'm right, then Warren's principle implies something that seems clearly to be false: that it is permissible for a medical doctor to perform psychic surgery in certain cases.

 UP FOR DISCUSSION

Do you agree with Doran that there is only a *prima facie* obligation for doctors to give treatments that are medically approved or undergoing clinical trials? Or, do you agree with Patrick that there should be a more absolute division of labour between physicians and other medical professionals? Is there a third option that you would endorse?

Warren: Don't forget that the cases in which such things are allowed are vanishingly rare because of third-party harms. When can a physician be sure that the patient will keep such a wild secret as having had psychic surgery?

More Counterexamples to the Ample Discretion Principle: Prayer and Other Unconventional Treatments

Doran: Here's a different example that may present a problem for your view, Warren. Unlike the psychic surgery case, this example does not raise the question of whether the person gives valid consent, nor is the kind of case I have in mind vanishingly rare. Suppose Mr. Nolle refuses treatment but just asks Dr. Anderweg to pray with him once a week. Is that permissible, or should the doctor refer him to a minister? My initial reaction is that the doctor ought to refer, although I am not sure about this. But what would the ample discretion principle say?

Warren: Well, I'm an atheist. Still, I have to say that if all the conditions were met, the principle would license the prayer treatment. If there really were no harm to MDs or others, nothing better the physician could do, and it really gave the patient hope, as in Mr. Nolle's case, then it would be okay, but only then. Prayer would not be a rational choice for me, but it would for many.

BACKGROUND

A 2018 poll found that 48 percent of patients wanted their physicians to pray with them.

Source: Dana E. King and Bruce Bushwick, "Beliefs and Attitudes of Hospital Inpatients about Faith Healing and Prayer," *Journal of Family Practice* 39, no. 4 (1994): 349–52.

Patrick: Good example, Doran. As you two might have guessed, I don't think physicians ought to administer a "prayer treatment." But just to clarify, I'm not claiming that it is always wrong for a doctor to pray with a patient. For instance, suppose a patient has become good friends with his doctor over the years, and the patient and doctor belong to the same church. Then I do not see anything wrong with the doctor praying with his patient. But this must be done as his friend, not as his doctor. Since prayer is not a recognized course of treatment, medical doctors should not be in the business of offering prayer *as a course of treatment*, even if competent patients request it.[9] If a competent patient wants a course of treatment that involves prayer or psychic surgery, her doctor should refer her to a minister or psychic surgeon. Warren, your principle seems much too liberal to me. It would allow doctors to treat people using all kinds of crazy things!

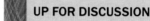

UP FOR DISCUSSION

Is it morally permissible for physicians to pray with their patients if their patients request it? Does it matter if the patient thinks prayer will help cure them, but the physician thinks that prayer has no medical benefit? Does your view change if what the patient wants is not prayer, but psychic surgery?

Warren: Doctors do in fact prescribe *comforts* to patients in palliative care. These comforts may, in rare cases, include some strange and unusual things. These are ways of showing compassion to patients, and they are very much in the interest of those who choose the rules in the original position. The frog toxin case is much more troubling, however, because it is harder to reply to the charge that people other than the patient will be harmed. But that is why we had to explicitly bring out the restriction on harming others in the ample discretion principle. Together with the valid consent restriction, these limit the permissible range of weird treatments.

UP FOR DISCUSSION

Do you think that it is permissible for physicians to engage in non-standard treatments that have no therapeutic value but only symbolic value to patients, or do you think that a physician's role should be limited to more traditional therapies?

FINAL THOUGHTS

Patrick: Well, there's a lot more to discuss. Unfortunately, however, we're out of time, so why don't we wrap up our debate with some last words for now on the subject?

Doran: Doctors need to make sure that they are respecting the informed choices of their patients. They do not want to be acting on patient requests when the patients do not adequately understand their predicament or their options. Dr. Anderweg, therefore, had a duty to make sure Mr. Nolle was relevantly counselled about his illness and options before acting on his request for alternative therapy. I think I agree with the final statement of the ample discretion principle, but I do not think it supports Dr. Anderweg's behaviour, given my understanding of the facts about the case. We want health care workers to respond with care and concern for their patients, to look out for their best interests, and to respect their informed choices, while not treating others unfairly and without damaging the medical profession. This is a difficult balancing act. The first steps were to talk with Mr. Nolle and to help him see that his situation was different from his wife's, and to explain to him compassionately and patiently why the standard therapies were likely to promise better outcomes in his case than the alternative therapies. If he still insisted on the alternative therapy, then he should have been referred to a competent naturopath. If a competent naturopath was not available, then perhaps Dr. Anderweg would have been justified in administering H.

Patrick: Competent patients have a right to choose whatever course of treatment they would like. And physicians ought, in general, to respect the health care choices of their competent patients. It does not follow from this, however, that medical doctors are always morally permitted to comply with their competent patients' requests, even when those requests are in the patients' best interest and do not unfairly harm others. There are recognized limits to the kinds of tools medical doctors can and should use to treat their patients, and physicians should generally stick within those limits. There are likely exceptions to this, but I don't think Mr. Nolle's case is one of those exceptions. Certain herbal therapies may be, or may soon be, within those limits. But frog toxin, psychic surgery, prayer, and so on, are currently not within those limits, and likely never will be. If Warren's ample discretion permits doctors to administer such things, then I believe that his principle is false.

I am certainly not against progress in medicine. Nor do I oppose physicians' use of new and unconventional drugs and therapies—provided that the drugs and therapies are part of legitimate tests and trials. Mr. Nolle, however, asked his physician to inject him with an untested and unproven herbal therapy. I do not think this choice was informed. But even if it was an informed choice, it was reckless and irresponsible, and therefore it was wrong for Dr. Anderweg, as an MD, to comply with Mr. Nolle's request.

Warren: The principle does not justify harmful or irrational choices, so it is hard to come up with real cases of things like psychic surgery that this principle would, in fact, justify. In general, we should not unnecessarily tie doctors' hands because of intuitions about division of labour or weirdness of treatments. In reality, division of labour is also often preserved by the conditions on the principle. In extraordinary circumstances, that division may be crossed or weirdness allowed, but only very rarely would frog toxin or psychic surgery plausibly be a treatment to which there is valid consent, and which is in the patient's best interest and not harmful, on balance, to others. Dr. Anderweg did no harm and did some good with H, which was a reasonable choice for someone with Mr. Nolle's goal of living in hope.

Think like those in the original position. We are all behind a veil of ignorance with respect to the circumstances of our future medical care. If some day you are in a situation where you have only a snowball's chance, wouldn't you want a physician you know and trust to be the one to help you with a long-shot cure? And what about experimental medicine? Many currently accepted treatments were once weird alternatives. Consider the maverick neurosurgeon's successful induced hypothermia cure. We must allow discretionary weirdness as a part of accountable medical practice. That does not mean that anything goes. We must allow ample discretion but not unlimited discretion.

As to informed consent and counselling, Dr. Anderweg respected Mr. Nolle's adequately informed choice of hope by keeping information from Mr. Nolle that would have been worse than useless to him. She knew that Nolle understood that the information he was refusing was only good for the choice of resignation. Dr. Anderweg's treatment of Mr. Nolle was therefore morally permissible.

 UP FOR DISCUSSION

After consideration of the arguments advanced in the debate, do you believe it was permissible for Dr. Anderweg to administer H to Mr. Nolle? Why or why not?

SUMMARY

Here is a summary of the main questions, concepts, and arguments covered in this chapter:

- The main questions explored are whether it was morally permissible for Dr. Anderweg to give an alternative therapy, H, to her patient, Mr. Nolle, and whether it is morally permissible, in general, for physicians to administer alternative therapies to their patients who request them.
- Warren argues that it was morally permissible for Dr. Anderweg to give H to Mr. Nolle, and he believes that it is morally acceptable for physicians, in general, to administer alternative therapies to their patients, provided certain conditions are met.
- Specifically, Warren defends the ample discretion principle: *Physicians may exercise ample discretion to decide whether or not to use any treatment to which a competent patient gives valid consent, provided that it is in the patient's best interest and harmless to others on balance.* Warren thinks this principle is justified because it would be chosen by people in the original position.

- Doran agrees with the ample discretion principle; however, he does not think that Dr. Anderweg acted permissibly in Mr. Nolle's case. This is because, unlike Warren, Doran does not think that enough was done to ensure that Mr. Nolle understood his treatment alternatives so that he could give valid consent.
- Patrick agrees with Doran that Dr. Anderweg acted impermissibly in Mr. Nolle's case. But Patrick goes further and argues that the ample discretion principle is false because it is vulnerable to counterexamples. Instead, Patrick defends the existence of a division of labour, where physicians administer treatments that are scientifically tested, or are undergoing scientific trials, or are part of accepted medical practice, while practitioners of alternative medicine treat patients who choose alternative therapies.

REVIEW QUESTIONS

1. Why does Warren believe it is permissible for Dr. Anderweg to administer H to Mr. Nolle?
2. What is the best interest principle? What is the response to Patrick's question about the nature of best interest?
3. Explain Patrick's frog toxin counterexample and what it purports to show. What is Warren's reply?
4. What is the ample discretion principle? What is Warren's argument for this principle?
5. Briefly explain Doran's initial objection to the ample discretion principle and the reply to this objection.
6. Explain Patrick's concern about whether the ample discretion principle protects patient autonomy. Why does Warren think that autonomy is, nonetheless, preserved?
7. What considerations motivate the first revision of the ample discretion principle?
8. What considerations motivate the second revision of the ample discretion principle?
9. Briefly explain Patrick's division of labour objection. How does Doran respond to this objection?
10. Briefly explain Patrick's psychic surgery counterexample and Doran's reply.
11. Describe Doran's prayer counterexample and what it purports to show. How is this example different from the psychic surgery example? Is the reply different as well?

NOTES

1. See the National Center for Complementary and Integrative Health, "Complementary, Alternative, or Integrative Health: What's in a Name?" https://nccih.nih.gov/health/integrative-health.
2. To say that a patient consents is just to say that *the patient willingly accepts the treatment.* Since Mr. Nolle demands H, *a fortiori*, he willingly accepts H. But, of course, to say that a person consents to treatment does not guarantee that this consent is valid.

3. We focus more explicitly on the issue of competence in chapter 4.

4. An excellent discussion of competence and of informed consent can be found in chapter 3 of Tom L. Beauchamp and James F. Childress, *Principles of Biomedical Ethics*, 5th ed. (New York: Oxford University Press, 2001), 57–112.

5. We focus more explicitly on the issue of valid consent in chapter 4.

6. Warren's example of the 80-year-old who demands a triple bypass raises questions of fair allocation of scarce medical resources in emergency situations, an issue we discuss at length in chapter 9.

7. According to a CBC television news report in December 2006, Dr. Joseph Varon at St. Luke's Hospital in Houston saved Dan O'Reilly from almost certain death after O'Reilly was knocked out by a wave in Ixtapa, Mexico. O'Reilly, who went 45 minutes without oxygen, spent 72 hours in induced hypothermia following coma—a treatment the physician had never tried before. O'Reilly continues to surprise his physiotherapist ("Frozen Man," *The National,* CBC TV, December 6, 2006).

8. See, for example, the College of Physicians and Surgeons of British Columbia practice standard regarding the use of complementary and alternative medicine: https://www.cpsbc.ca/files/pdf/PSG-Complementary-and-Alternative-Therapies.pdf.

9. A large study on the effectiveness of prayer revealed no clinical benefits. See "Prayers Don't Help Heart Surgery Patients; Some Fare Worse When Prayed For," *Science Daily,* April 3, 2006, https://www.sciencedaily.com/releases/2006/04/060403133554.htm.

GLOSSARY

abortion: The intentional termination of a pregnancy with the intent and result of killing the prenatal organism.

absolute moral truth: A moral truth that applies to all persons, at all times, in all situations.

act utilitarianism: The ethical theory that says the right action in a situation is the one that maximizes happiness and minimizes unhappiness, where everyone's happiness and unhappiness is given equal consideration.

active euthanasia: Directly causing an individual's death—for instance, by administering a lethal injection—for that individual's own health-related good.

ad hominem: A Latin expression meaning "against the man," a **fallacy** in which one tries to refute an **argument** by attacking the one who offered the argument, rather than the argument itself.

advance directive: A document in which one states one's wishes in the event one is no longer able to make health care decisions. It comes into effect when one is no longer **competent**. There are two types: *Instructional directives* (living wills) may give specific instructions or set out general principles to follow. *Proxy directives* (durable powers of attorney for health care) specify who is to make health care decisions for a person who is no longer able to make them. (Adapted from the End of Life Law and Policy in Canada, Health Law Institute, Dalhousie University, http://eol.law.dal.ca/?page_id=221).

all-things-considered duty: The duty that is most pressing after all *prima facie* duties are weighed in a situation, according to W. D. Ross's **pluralistic deontology**.

alternative medicine: The kinds of drugs, therapies, practices, and so on, that are not a part of conventional Western medicine. Examples include acupuncture, homeopathy, naturopathy, and herbal therapy.

AMA: Stands for "against medical advice." Patients who leave hospital when their doctors tell them to stay are asked to sign a form certifying that they know their physician wants them to stay. It gives legal certitude that the patient was warned against leaving.

amnesiac: Afflicted by amnesia, the loss of memory of past experiences.

amnestic anesthetic: A drug that causes temporary amnesia but is designed to temporarily take away sensations.

amniocentesis: A procedure in which the uterus (the womb) is perforated to obtain amniotic fluid—fluid from the membranes enveloping the **fetus**. The fluid contains skin cells from the fetus, which are analyzed to detect abnormality in fetal development.

ample discretion principle: Warren's view that physicians may exercise ample discretion to decide whether or not to use any treatment that a competent patient chooses, provided that it is in the patient's best interest and harmless to others on balance.

anecdotal: Said of evidence that is not the result of research but of stories or anecdotes about the efficacy of certain treatments.

appeal to emotion: The **fallacy** of using emotionally charged, biased language in order to persuade someone to accept a **conclusion** without having to think carefully about the issues involved.

applied ethics *or* **practical ethics:** A part of **normative ethics** concerned with specific moral issues; for example, Is it ever permissible for a woman to have an **abortion**? Is it always wrong for medical professionals to lie to their patients?

argument: A set of at least two claims, one of which is the **conclusion**. Any other claims in the set are **premises**. The conclusion is the claim that one is trying to establish, and the premises are the reasons offered in support of the conclusion.

asphyxia: A deadly condition caused by oxygen deprivation.

autonomous: Having **autonomy**, self-determining.

autonomy: Self-determination.

begging the question (circular argument): A **fallacy** in which the truth of the **conclusion** is presupposed by one or more **premises**. (All valid **arguments** do this, but circularity is a problem when the conclusion you are arguing for occurs as one of your premises, or is offered as a reason for accepting one of your premises, and you intend to convince someone of the conclusion.)

blended private/public care: Health care that includes both publicly funded care and care for which people pay privately.

breech presentation: *Breech* means "buttocks," and breech presentation is the presentation of the buttocks or feet in labour.

Caesarean section *or* **C-section:** The delivery of a **fetus** by surgical incision through the abdominal wall and uterus.

categorical imperative: A command that states what one ought to do regardless of one's desires or goals. For Kant, these imperatives are the rules of morality. Kant has, however, a particular principle called *the* **categorical imperative.** It comes in several forms, including the **universal law version** and the **humanity version.**

chemotherapy (short form, **chemo**)**:** A cancer treatment using chemical means.

circular argument: See **begging the question.**

classical act utilitarianism: See **utilitarianism.**

clinical factors: Considerations that may affect the proper order of care, arising from an assessment of the medical needs of the particular patients.

codifiable: Expressible as a set of rules with priorities for their application.

cognitivism: In **metaethics,** the view that our moral claims are descriptions of the moral features of actions, persons, and so on. As such, moral claims are the kind of thing that are true or false, and that we believe, know, assert, doubt, and deny.

comforts: Whatever is prescribed for a patient that has no medical use but is merely intended to make the patient more at ease. See also **palliation.**

competent: Capable of rational self-determination; in this context, capable of rationally choosing one's own medical treatment. Individuals may be competent relative to some tasks, but not others.

complementary medicine: The use of **alternative medicine** in conjunction with standard Western medicine.

conclusion: The claim one is trying to prove through an **argument.**

conclusion indicator: Verbal clue which signals that a **conclusion** is being offered, for example, *therefore, thus, hence,* and *so.*

consequentialism: The view that the right act is entirely determined by its consequences, which are the promotion of the greatest amount of good or the least amount of bad.

conservatives: In the context of the abortion debate, those who generally oppose abortion—claiming that abortion is wrong in all, or virtually all, cases.

contractarianism: See **social contract theory**.

contradiction in conception: A result pertaining to Kant's **universal law version of the categorical imperative**. It occurs when one is not able to will a **maxim** as a **universal law** because the practice would be self-defeating or self-contradictory if it were practiced by everyone all the time. It signals the violation of a **perfect duty.**

contradiction in will: A result pertaining to Kant's **universal law version of the categorical imperative**. Kant admits that one can conceive of a **maxim** as a **universal law,** but still not be able to will it because a contradiction will arise between the universal law and what a person will (later) want. It signals a violation of an **imperfect duty.**

counterexample: An example that is intended to counter a given claim or **argument.**

CSBC: Caesarean section by choice; Caesarean delivery in the absence of medical indications at the choice of the mother.

CTAS: The Canadian Triage and Acuity Scale, introduced during the late 1990s. The CTAS is now being implemented as a national triage standard for Canada's emergency health care system.

cultural imperialism: A phrase used to object to the imposition of the beliefs of one culture on another.

cultural relativism: The ethical theory that says there are no objective truths in ethics, and the correct moral rules are determined by each culture.

deductive argument: An **argument** intended as one in which it is necessary that if the **premises** are true, so is the **conclusion**.

dementia: A loss of intellectual function.

deontology: A category of ethical theory that sees right action as doing one's duty.

descriptive ethics: A part of ethics that seeks to describe what is the case rather than what ought to be the case; for instance, it seeks to describe what people actually believe about particular moral issues. Descriptive ethics also is concerned with questions of why people believe what they believe about ethics, and how they come to hold their particular moral beliefs and attitudes.

difference principle: John Rawls's view that there should be social and economic equality, unless inequality benefits everyone, especially those in the worst-off group.

dilemma: An argument that shows that one's opponent is faced with only two or more logical alternatives, none of which the opponent would accept.

diminishing marginal utility: Said of money, it expresses roughly the idea that an extra portion of income is unlikely to benefit a person above a certain level of wealth as much as it would benefit someone below that level of wealth. After you get a certain amount, money is worth less to you (diminishes in utility) as you get more of it.

dispositional properties: Roughly, properties that objects, persons, and so on, have in virtue of their being disposed to behave in a certain way under certain conditions.

dispositional view of moral properties: The view that moral properties are **dispositional properties**; for example, an action is morally right in virtue of its tendency to elicit certain responses (e.g., approval).

doctrine of the mean: Aristotle's doctrine that the **virtues** exist as a mean between two extremes—one of excess and the other of deficiency.

double jeopardy: The name of a legal rule that prohibits being tried twice for the same crime on the same set of facts. Warren applies the term to health care, saying that a patient should not be required to prove their competence twice in a short period of time.

Down syndrome *or* **Down's syndrome:** A condition in which an extra chromosome causes birth defects, notably slow, incomplete physical development and mental retardation.

duty, all things considered: See **all-things-considered duty**.

dysphagia: A potentially very dangerous condition causing one to be prone to choke.

egalitarian: A term with multiple meanings, often said of philosophers who emphasize equality above such values as liberty.

embryo: A developing organism prior to birth. In humans this stage runs from conception until about the end of the eighth week.

end *or* **end in itself:** In Kant's usage, a **rational being** deserving of respect.

epistemic problem: A philosophical problem concerning knowledge.

epistemology: The philosophical study of knowledge.

equal consideration: The principle that no one's good is to be counted as more important than anyone else's.

equivocation: The **fallacy** of equivocation occurs when a term slides, without acknowledgement, between two or more different meanings within a single **argument,** so as to make an argument which is not **valid** appear valid.

ethical objectivism: The view that there is **objective truth** in ethics. By saying that a statement is objectively true, we mean (roughly) that the statement is true independently of whether anyone happens to believe that it is true or desires it to be true.

ethical relativism: Also called **moral relativism,** the view that there is no **objective truth** in ethics. Instead, it is suggested that moral truths are simply *relative* to a given individual or group.

ethics of care: The view that rather than using principles to arrive at the solutions to moral problems, one needs to adopt a perspective of caring. Here the focus is on maintaining and improving one's relationships.

eudaimonia: A Greek term roughly translated as "flourishing" or "happiness."

euthanasia: An act or omission, intended by one or more individuals, to bring about the death of another individual for that individual's own (health-related) good.

excusable: Said of wrong acts for which there is an **excuse.**

excuse: A reason for wrong action that removes blame by removing the responsibility of the one who did the action.

extremitarianism: There is no recognized ethical term "extremitarianism." This is a word Warren made up playing on **utilitarianism.** For the extremitarian, the benefits have to be extreme before they can justify exceptions to **worst first** and **first come.**

fair turn rule: (a proposed **triage** rule) Patient B can go ahead of Patient A in the queue for life-saving treatment if A has had a fair turn at life and B has not.

fallacy: A mistake in reasoning.

false dilemma: A **fallacy** in which fewer options are presented than are actually available in a way that is misleading.

feminism: The view that women (and girls) have been, and in various ways continue to be, oppressed; it seeks to understand the nature of the oppression and to determine how best to overcome this oppression.

fetus: A stage of a developing organism; in humans, from about the end of the eighth week until birth.

first come: (a proposed **triage** rule) Those who arrive first get treated first, other things being equal.

genetic code: Information encoded in the DNA of an organism that determines what kind of organism it is. Each species has a unique genetic code that distinguishes it from all other species.

good will: (Kant's conception) If one does an act out of respect for morality—out of respect for a **categorical imperative**—then one is said to have a good will, and so one's act has moral worth.

hard paternalism: The interference with a competent person's liberty for that person's own good.

health care ethics: An area of inquiry within **normative ethics,** or more narrowly, **practical** (or **applied**) **ethics,** which deals with ethical problems that arise in and around the practice of health.

hedonism: The view according to which the sole intrinsic good is pleasure and the sole intrinsic bad is pain.

hopeless second: (a proposed **triage** rule) Do not treat hopeless cases ahead of those where there is hope.

humanity: The term that Kant uses to mean the set of **rational beings**.

humanity version of the categorical imperative test: Kant's principle that one must treat **humanity**, whether in one's own person or that of another, always as an **end** and never merely as a **means.**

human-sympathy metarule: A part of Warren's favoured ethical approach. It is a rule about making rules in the **original position** that requires the choosers of rules to choose rules that can be followed by those with ordinary human sympathy.

hypothermia: A low body temperature usually caused by cold weather but sometimes induced as a way to decrease metabolism and use of oxygen by a patient.

hypothetical imperative: A command that states what one ought to do given the presence of a desire or goal.

hypoxia: A reduction of oxygen to tissue in spite of adequate blood circulation. If it is not remedied immediately, the brain is deprived of oxygen, causing damage.

hysterectomy: An operation in which the uterus (the womb) is removed.

ideal social contract: The ideal set of rules to govern moral relations of people in a community, e.g., rules chosen in the **original position.**

impartiality rule: (a proposed **triage** rule) Health care professionals should usually be *impartial*, i.e., free from bias, favouritism, or prejudice, in helping patients.

imperfect duty: According to Kant, a duty that one must sometimes follow, but which need not be followed all the time (e.g., the duty to be charitable).

incompetent: Not **competent.**

inconsistent: Rationally incompatible. A set of sentences is inconsistent if and only if not all of them can be true at once. We say a set of desires, preferences, or wishes are inconsistent if and only if a person could not satisfy the whole set. See **rationality.**

inductive argument: An **argument** intended as one in which it is probable that if the **premises** are true, so is the **conclusion.**

informed consent: Consent given with a satisfactory understanding of treatment options and the likely effects of treatments if those effects are known.

innocents first rule: (a proposed **triage** rule) Patient A, who is innocent and who cannot wait for care, may be given priority over patient B, who was at fault for the injury and who also cannot wait, other things being equal.

instrumental value: Value as a means to something else.

instrumentally good: Good as a means to something else. See also **instrumental value**.

internalism: The view that reasons or motives are somehow "built into" the fact, or judgment, that an action is morally right (or wrong).

intrinsic value: The worth that something has in itself, and not because of its utility or usefulness.

intrinsically good: Good that is valuable for its own sake. See also **intrinsic value**.

intuitionism *or* **ethical intuitionism:** Within ethics, a term that generally refers to the view that there is a plurality of fundamental moral principles that are known through a special faculty of intuition—i.e., these basic moral principles are self-evident or apprehended directly, rather than through inference or demonstration. In some instances, however, those who accept only one self-evident fundamental principle are called "intuitionists." The term may also be applied to those who think we intuit moral properties.

invalid argument: An **argument** intended to be deductive but with **premises** that fail to guarantee that the **conclusion** is true. In an invalid argument the conclusion could be false even if all the premises are true.

involuntary active euthanasia (IAE): Active euthanasia of a **competent** patient without her consent.

involuntary euthanasia: Euthanasia of a **competent** patient without her consent.

involuntary passive euthanasia (IPE): Passive euthanasia of a competent patient without her consent.

jump the queue *or* **queue jumping:** What people are said to do when they unfairly get ahead of others in line for medical care. Also used for getting ahead unfairly in other contexts.

justice as fairness: The name of John Rawls's **social contract theory** of justice.

justification: A reason for something that shows that it was permissible. Contrast **excuse** and **mitigation**.

Kantianism: The philosophy of Immanuel Kant.

libertarian: Said of philosophers who emphasize liberty above such values as equality and beneficence. In political philosophy it is associated with the view that the state may restrict citizens only to protect them against violence, theft, or fraud.

liberty principle: See **principle of maximal equal basic liberties**.

macroallocation: Large-scale distribution of resources such as those with which public health policies are concerned.

magnetic resonance imaging (MRI): A technique for scanning for muscle and joint injuries. Both the scans and the machines that scan are referred to as MRIs.

MAID: Stands for "medical assistance in dying." It includes **euthanasia** and physician-assisted suicide. MAID is legal, though strictly regulated, in Canada.

maxim: As used by Kant, the principle behind one's action.

maximin: According to Rawls, a strategy that one should adopt in the **original position**, namely choose in such a way so that you will be doing maximally well if you should turn out to be in the minimum (or worst-off) position.

means only: In Kant's usage, a mere **thing**, as opposed to a rational person.

means to an end: A way to achieve a goal. When people are used merely as a means to an end they are treated as tools or **things** rather than as **rational beings** who have their own goals and are able to make their own decisions.

medical benefit: (a proposed **triage** rule) Where the medical interest is great enough, a patient may be given priority over those who came earlier.

medicalize: To turn a natural process into a medical procedure. This is a term of medical jargon not in common use.

mesoallocation: Medium-scale allocation of resources, distribution of resources at the level of institutions.

metaethics: A part of ethics concerning the rational investigation into the nature of morality. Here, the focus is on questions *about* morality, rather than questions *within* morality; for example, "Are moral judgments capable of being true or false?" and "What are the meanings of moral terms?"

metaphysical problem: A philosophical problem concerning reality.

metaphysics: The philosophical study of reality.

metarule: A rule that governs the production, use, and interpretation of other, lower-level rules. It is a rule about making rules rather than a rule about what to do.

MI *or* **myocardial infarction:** A heart attack.

microallocation: Distribution of resources at the level of individuals, selecting which individuals are to receive health care resources.

minimize YPLL: (a proposed **triage** rule) Minimize years of potential life lost.

mitigation: A reason for an action that does not excuse or justify a wrong done but lessens blameworthiness.

moral antirealism: The view that (i) moral claims are *not* descriptive at all, or (ii) that moral claims are (partly) descriptive, but none of these descriptions are true. So moral antirealists deny that there are any moral truths or facts.

moral argument: An **argument** in support of a **substantive moral claim.**

moral pluralist: One who believes there is no single basic moral principle that explains all of our moral obligations, but instead, that there are many general moral principles.

moral realism: The view that (i) moral claims are (at least partly) descriptions or reports of the moral features of actions (persons, etc.), and (ii) that some of these claims are true. The moral realist therefore holds that there are moral facts.

moral relativism: See **ethical relativism.**

morbidity: The lack of health in a population represented as the ratio of diseased or injured persons to healthy persons; hence, maternal morbidity is the rate of ill-health of new mothers. Said of an individual, morbidity means being unhealthy or morbid.

motility: The ability to move spontaneously. If this ability is lost in the parts of the body used to swallow, **dysphagia** results.

multiple sclerosis (MS): Scarring of nervous tissue throughout the body, sometimes including the brain, leading to damage to the covering (myelin sheath) of the nerves. It can lead to weakness, loss of coordination, and visual complaints. It may be mild or severe and is usually prolonged with remissions and relapses over many years. Only in rare cases does it lead to serious loss of intellectual function.

naturopath: A practitioner of health care based on **alternative medicine** that emphasizes natural healing methods, while avoiding surgery and drugs.

negative rights: Rights to non-interference, such as the right not to be physically harmed. Negative rights are contrasted with **positive rights**.

nepotism: Showing favouritism to relatives or close friends when impartial, objective criteria should be used.

non-clinical factors: Those that do not arise from an assessment of the medical needs of the particular patients. An example of a non-clinical factor might be the guilt or innocence of the patients waiting for treatment.

non-consequentialism: The view that the right act is not entirely determined by its consequences.

non-voluntary active euthanasia (NAE): **Active euthanasia** on individuals who lack the competence to make a decision about **euthanasia**.

non-voluntary euthanasia: **Euthanasia** on individuals who lack the competence to make a decision about euthanasia.

non-voluntary passive euthanasia (NPE): **Passive euthanasia** on individuals who lack the competence to make a decision about **euthanasia**.

normative: Normative principles are generally contrasted with descriptive principles.

normative ethics: A part of ethics concerned, in large part, with general theoretical questions such as what makes acts morally right or wrong, which states of affairs are desirable or undesirable, what constitutes a good life for the person who leads it, which character traits are virtuous and which are vicious, and, most generally, how one ought to live.

objective truth: There is no single, universally accepted definition of the concept of *objective truth*. Most would agree, however, that an objective truth is a truth that is independent of whether people happen to think, believe, or feel that it is true. For instance, if it is an objective truth that water is H_2O, then it is true whether or not anyone happens to believe it or desire it to be true. Morality is sometimes said to be objective, meaning that the rightness and wrongness of actions is independent of the thoughts, beliefs, and feelings people happen to have toward those actions. This makes moral claims about right and wrong actions objective truths.

optimific: Maximum good consequences; an optimific act is the one that does the *most net good*, or the *least net bad*.

original position: John Rawls's conception of a hypothetical situation from which people are to choose the principles of justice to regulate the major social institutions. Unlike Rawls, Warren uses the original position to generate all moral rules. In the original position, people are equally powerful, equally intelligent, self-interested, and ignorant of their own advantages and disadvantages in the real world.

palliation: Easing a patient's pain or the severity of a patient's disease without removing the cause. See also **comforts**.

passive euthanasia: Allowing an individual to die—for example, by withholding life-prolonging treatment—for the sake of the individual's (health-related) good.

paternalism: Interference with a person's liberty for that person's own good. See **hard paternalism**, **soft paternalism**, **strong paternalism**, and **weak paternalism**.

perfect duty: According to Kant, a duty that must always be followed.

physician-assisted suicide: Occurs when a physician provides a hopeless, usually terminally ill patient with the means (such as a prescription for a lethal dose of a drug) to commit suicide.

placebo effect: The healing effect of a treatment that works only because the patient believes it will work.

pluralistic deontology: W. D. Ross's view that morality consists in many conditional duties which will sometimes conflict. In cases of conflict, one must study the situation carefully and try to reach a considered judgment about which duties are most pressing in that situation. Whatever the strongest duties recommend in that situation constitutes the right thing to do in that situation.

positive rights: Rights whose satisfaction requires the provision of some action, good, or service. Positive rights are contrasted with **negative rights.**

practical ethics: A part of **normative ethics** concerned with specific moral issues; for example, Is it ever permissible for a woman to have an **abortion**? Is it always wrong for medical professionals to lie to their patients?

premise: Reasons provided in support of a **conclusion.**

premise indicator: Verbal clue which signals that a **premise** is being offered. E.g., *because, since, given that, for.*

prescriptive: Said of language that tells people what they ought to do in contrast to merely describing what people do.

presumptively, morally permissible: Presumed to be not morally wrong.

prima facie **duty:** The usual translation of the Latin phrase *prima facie* is "on the face of it." For W. D. Ross, however, *prima facie* duties should be understood as *conditional* duties. Conditional or *prima facie* duties can then be contrasted with **duties, all things considered**.

primary social goods: As defined by John Rawls, goods, under the control of society, that everyone, or almost everyone, can be presumed to want, regardless of their plans in life. For Rawls, these include rights and liberties, opportunities and powers, income and wealth, and the bases of self-respect.

principle of charity: Principle according to which an author's claims and **arguments** are to be interpreted in the best possible light. The general aim is to arrive at a fair and sympathetic understanding of the author's position in order to evaluate it critically.

principle of fair equality of opportunity: A principle of John Rawls's **social contract theory**. It holds that each person should have a meaningful opportunity to attain employment, education, and positions of power.

principle of maximal equal basic liberties: A principle of John Rawls's **social contract theory**. It holds that each person is to have maximal equal basic liberties such as freedom of expression, thought, assembly, religion, and so on.

principlism: The theory that moral problems (especially in health care) are to be solved by weighing a set of widely agreed upon moral principles, such as respect for autonomy, benevolence, and justice.

prolapse: A falling or sinking down of part of the body. In chapter 7, it refers to a downward displacement of the uterus.

psychic surgery: A magician's trick in which the magician appears to remove tissue from a person's body without surgery. Typically, this is used to dupe the gullible into thinking they have had a growth removed from inside their bodies.

public interest: (a proposed **triage** rule) Where the public interest is great enough, a patient may be given priority over those who came earlier.

quadriplegic: A person who is paralyzed so as to be without the use of all four limbs.

queue: A line of people waiting for service or admission. This is used metaphorically to refer to the fair ordering of patients awaiting medical care in Canada. See **jump the queue**.

radiosensitive tumour: A tumour that will respond to **radiotherapy** (radiation therapy).

radiotherapy: The use of ionizing radiation to treat an illness.

rational being: In Kant's conception, a being that can freely set goals for itself and then determine the various means to accomplish those goals (**hypothetical imperatives**), and can also recognize and choose to follow (or not to follow) moral rules (**categorical imperatives**).

rational intuition: A faculty or sense that enables one to "see" moral truths directly, without the need for inference, **argument**, etc.

rational nature: The ability to freely make one's own decisions and to freely set goals for oneself.

rationality: A perennially contested term referring to the capacity of people to choose actions, beliefs, goals, plans, inferences, and other things on the basis of reasons. It is generally thought to include, but not to be limited to, the capacity to employ rules of reasoning that make up correct logic.

reasonable person test: A test of acceptability. Appeals to what a reasonable person would believe are used by philosophers as a common-sense, intuitive test to clarify concepts, determine right and wrong, and so on.

recuse: Disqualify oneself as a judge; by extension, said of other public officials making decisions where they excuse themselves from decision-making on grounds of a conflict of interest.

redistributive taxation: Taxation that redistributes wealth to modify the ways in which it is distributed in society through the forces of commerce. Usually it is aimed at making citizens' advantages more equal than they would be without the tax.

reflective equilibrium: For many, it is the end point of a process of philosophical deliberation. It involves going back and forth between principles and what they imply about specific cases to attain a state of coherence or consistency among the moral principles we accept and our considered moral beliefs.

remission: A period during (or a stage of) a disease in which the patient does not show any symptoms.

right to self-determination: Right to **autonomy,** right to self-government.

robust advantage principle: A part of Warren's ethical approach. It says that we should bias our decisions about allowing social and economic differences so as to provide a robust advantage to the least advantaged. This should be distinguished from John Rawls's **difference principle,** which is much more **egalitarian.**

rule utilitarianism: The ethical theory that says the right action is the one that is done according to a set of rules that maximizes happiness and minimizes unhappiness if consistently followed.

Sanctity of Life principle: The view that it is wrong to kill human beings because human life is sacred. This principle is subject to various interpretations, for example, it may protect only *innocent* human life or it may prohibit only the intentional killing of (innocent) humans. We also consider a Kantian version: the sanctity of *rational* life.

secondary quality: Roughly, powers of objects to produce certain sensations in us. Colours, tastes, and sounds, e.g., are commonly regarded as secondary qualities. Many philosophers take secondary qualities to be **dispositional properties.**

situational ethic: The view that whether an act is right or wrong will depend on the particular situation.

social contract theory: A type of ethical theory that takes a hypothetical agreement among a group of people under special constraints to be the source of the correct moral rules. Social contractarians differ in the details of their theory, but they share the fundamental belief that justified moral rules are the ones that rational individuals would agree to for their own benefit. See **original position** and **veil of ignorance.**

soft paternalism: The interference with an **incompetent** person's liberty for that person's own good.

sound argument: A valid **argument** where all of the **premises** are true.

standard form: The form of an **argument** presented as a numbered list with the **premises** above a horizontal line and the **conclusion** below the horizontal line.

state of nature: A hypothetical time and place where there is no organized society, no recognized social rules, in which everyone is free to do as they please. This concept is a central part of many **social contract theories.**

straw man: The **fallacy** of misrepresenting one's opponent's **argument** or view so that it is easily shown to be **unsound** or weak.

stress incontinence: The inability of the bladder to retain urine under stress, usually because the bladder neck is weakened.

strong inductive argument: An **inductive argument** where the **premises**, if true, make the **conclusion** probably true. The more support provided by the premises of an inductive argument, the stronger the argument.

strong paternalism: The interference in a competent person's liberty for that person's own good, in order to prevent that person from attempting to realize irrational or mistaken goals.

subjective truth: Truth dependent on whether a person happens to think, believe, or feel it is true. In morality, the view that the rightness or wrongness of actions is dependent on individuals' personal attitudes and feelings toward the actions makes moral truth subjective. This view is given the name *subjectivism*. For example, a speaker's claim that abortion is wrong is true if and only if the speaker sincerely believes that abortion is wrong (or disapproves of abortion).

substantial benefit rule: (a proposed **triage** rule) If a patient stands to benefit substantially from being treated first, while the patient ahead in the queue will not benefit substantially from being treated, then the patient who will benefit substantially should be treated first.

substantive moral claim: A claim made directly about the moral status of acts, policies, persons, and so on. Examples of substantive moral claims include "Jones is a bad person" and "**Involuntary euthanasia** is morally wrong."

surface grammar: Superficial grammatical and idiomatic aspects of language that convey apparent meaning.

sympathy metarule: See **human-sympathy metarule**.

the **categorical imperative:** Kant's test for determining whether a particular action is morally permissible or morally wrong. It comes in several forms, including the **universal law version** and the **humanity version**. See also **categorical imperative**.

thing: in Kant's usage, "not a **rational being**." Things are not capable of following both **hypothetical imperatives** and **categorical imperatives**.

third parties: People other than the two main people in a situation. In this context, people other than the patient or the health care provider.

thought experiment: An example developed to prove or disprove a particular claim or **argument** or to persuade us of the plausibility of a thesis.

thromboembolism: The obstruction of a blood vessel with particles carried by the blood from another site.

triage: Sorting patients by degree of urgency in order to allocate treatment. See **CTAS**.

Trojan Horse: By analogy to the fabled statue of a horse in the siege of Troy, a device used to surreptitiously introduce something.

two-tier health care: A system in which one tier or level is publicly funded and one tier is privately funded.

universal care: Care that is provided to every citizen (and lawful resident) regardless of that individual's financial means.

universal law: A principle that states that everyone follows a particular **maxim** all the time, as if it were a law of nature.

universal law version of the categorical imperative: Kant's principle "Act only on those **maxims** that you can, at the same time, will as a **universal law**."

unsound argument: An **argument** that either contains a false **premise**, or is logically **invalid**, or both.

utilitarianism: An ethical theory that takes many forms, but in its classical formulation, as articulated by Jeremy Bentham and John Stuart Mill, is the view that right actions, laws, or policies promote the greatest net amount of pleasure, or the least net amount of pain, where everyone's pleasures and pains receive equal consideration.

valid argument: An **argument** in which it is impossible for all of the **premises** to be true and the **conclusion** false. In other words, *if* all of the premises are true, the conclusion *must be* true.

valid consent: Acceptable consent. When we speak here of valid consent, it means something different from "valid" as applied to **arguments**. See **valid argument**.

veil of ignorance: A central feature of the **original position**, a barrier that prevents people from knowing any particular facts about themselves. For instance, they do not know their race, gender, class, natural abilities, religious convictions, specific values, goals in life, and so forth.

virtue: A character trait needed for being a good person and living well. These traits include the moral virtues (e.g., courage, honesty, industriousness, trustworthiness, compassion, and loyalty). These are deep and stable character traits that dispose those who possess them to take certain actions and have certain feelings. Honest people, for instance, are disposed to act honestly and to feel disapproval toward persons who are dishonest.

virtue ethics: Roughly, an approach to ethics that focuses on *moral (virtuous) character*, rather than on principles of right action.

voluntary active euthanasia (VAE): Active euthanasia on a **competent** person with that person's consent.

voluntary euthanasia: Euthanasia on a **competent** person with that person's consent.

voluntary passive euthanasia (VPE): Passive euthanasia on a **competent** person with that person's consent.

weak inductive argument: An **inductive argument** where the **premises**, if true, provide little support for the **conclusion**.

weak paternalism: The interference in a person's liberty for that person's own good, in order to prevent that person from behaving in ways that are likely to defeat their own goals.

worst first: (a proposed **triage** rule) Treat the worst cases in the emergency department first.

xenotransplantation: The transplantation of nonhuman organs into humans.

zygote: A single diploid cell that results from the merging of a sperm and ovum through a process of fertilization. The developing organism, from the moment of conception until about the end of the eighth week, is called an **embryo**. From that point until birth it is called a **fetus**.

INDEX

A

abortion
  see also abortion (case); fetus
  bodily integrity, right of, 179
  Canadian law, 161
  debate over, 161–162
  early abortions, 189–190
  genetic vs. moral humanity, 169–172
  legal landscape, 161
  and rape, 182, 197n6
  sex-selective abortion, 179
  as vicious act, 184
abortion (case)
  arguments against morality of abortion, 169–185
  arguments for the morality of abortion, 185–196
  clarification of the case, 165–167
  conservative arguments, against abortion, 162, 169–185
  contraception objection, 174–175
  discrimination against the disabled, 177–180
  equivocation objection, 175–177
  focus of debate, 161–162
  genetic code, 169–172
  identification of relevant facts, 165–167
  life criterion, 186–187
  Marquis's argument against abortion, 173–177
  moral issues raised, 167–169
  more rational vs. less rational individuals, 192–193
  necessity of sentience, for right to life, 191–192
  Noonan's argument against abortion, 169–172
  objections to sentience criterion, 187–196
  opening scenes, 163–165
  original position, 168, 179
  "party hard" lifestyle, 184
  principle of charity, 171
  protection of worthwhile goods, 180–181
  rational non-humans vs. non-rational humans, 194–195
  rational vs. non-rational individuals, 193–194
  rationality, and sentience, 188–190
  rationality criterion for a right to life, 185–186, 192–195
  right to life vs. virtues, 181–185
  sentience criterion, 187–196
  social contract theory, 168, 194

  statement of positions, 168–169
  sufficiency of sentience, for right to life, 190–191
  Thomson's violinist example, 181–185
  virtue-based argument for abortion, 180–181
  virtue ethics, and vegetarianism, 195–196
absolute moral truth, 86–87
abusive relationships, 60
access to medical services. See two-tier MRI (case)
ACOG. See American College of Obstetricians and Gynecologists (ACOG)
act utilitarians, 71, 110
  see also classical act utilitarianism
active euthanasia, 132
  and intention, 138
  non-voluntary active euthanasia (NAE). See non-voluntary active euthanasia (NAE)
  vs. passive euthanasia, 132, 138–139
  voluntary active euthanasia (VAE). See voluntary active euthanasia (VAE)
ad hominem, 14–15
against medical advice (AMA). See AMA ("against medical advice")
agreement, facilitation of, 50
all things considered, duty, 44
allocation of health care. See microallocation of scarce resources (case)
alternative medicine, 304–305
  see also alternative medicine (case); ample discretion principle
alternative medicine (case)
  ample discretion principle, 317, 318–334
  anecdotal evidence, 313
  best interest principle, 314–317
  clarification of the case, 310–313
  competency vs. incompetency, 321
  counterexamples, 305, 316, 331–334
  division of labour objection, 329–334
  final thoughts, 334–336
  frog toxin counterexample, 317
  harm avoidance, 326–329
  identification of relevant facts, 310–313
  indeterminacy objection, 319–321
  moral issues raised, 313–314
  moral permissibility, 304–305
  opening scenes, 306–310
  paternalism, 320

patient autonomy, 318–319, 324–326
placebo effect, 312
prayer, 333–334
psychic surgery counterexample, 331–333
statement of positions, 314
valid consent, 321
valid consent of competent patients only, 321–326
AMA ("against medical advice"), 102, 107
  see also right to refuse treatment (case)
American College of Obstetricians and
  Gynecologists (ACOG), 205, 206, 224
American health care system, 267
amnesiac, 84
amnestic anesthetic, 84
amniocentesis, 161
ample discretion principle, 317, 318–334
  competence, 321
  division of labour objection, 329–334
  harm avoidance, 326–329
  incompetent individual, 321
  indeterminacy objection, 319–321
  paternalism, 320
  patient autonomy, 318–319, 324–326
  prayer, 333–334
  psychic surgery counterexample, 331–333
  valid consent, 321
  valid consent of competent patients only, 321–326
analogy, argument by, 217–219, 254
analyses, 9
anecdotal evidence, 313
animals, non-human. *See* non-human animals
antirealist theory, 75
appeal to emotion, 13–14
arguments, 1–8
  acceptance of premise, for sake of argument, 109,
    213
  analogy, argument by, 217–219, 254
  bad argument, 3–4
  in the broad sense, 170
  circular argument, 11–12, 16n3, 79
  deductive argument, 4–5
  defined, 1
  derivation, 170
  different purposes, 16n1
  dilemma, 151
  evaluation of, 3–8
  inductive argument, 6–7
  intuitive appeal, 246
  invalid argument, 5, 175
  logic, 4–5
  moral argument, 7–8
  in the narrower sense, 170

revised statements, 144
sound argument, 5
standard form, 2, 3
strong argument, 6
underlying rationale, 144
unsound argument, 5
valid argument, 4–5, 175
weak argument, 6–7
Aristotle, 54–55
Aristotle's virtue theory, 54–57
articles of peace, 47–48
artificial blood, 225
asphyxia, 202
assisted suicide. *See* MAID (medical assistance in
  dying) (case)
autonomy, 85
  alternative medicine (case), 318–319, 324–326
  Autonomy and Best Interest argument, 142–145,
    152
  and C-section by choice, 199, 223–224
  defined, 227
  free choice, 120, 123
  limits on, 74, 85, 86, 211
  meaning of, 104, 318
  and medical model of childbirth, 224
  and patient safety, 128–129
  respect for, within medical context, 92
  right to refuse treatment. *See* right to refuse treat-
    ment (case)
  self-determination, 105, 318
  social safety net, 249–250
  and voluntary active euthanasia, 142–145, 152
Autonomy and Best Interest argument, 142–145, 152
average life expectancy, 291–292

B

background assumptions, 16n4
bad argument, 3–4
Bartky, Sandra, 60
BC Civil Liberties Association, 135
Beauchamp, Tom, 46, 331
because (premise indicator), 2
begging the question, 11–12, 176
  see also circular argument
Beloved (Morrison), 136
beneficence, 67n42, 331
Bentham, Jeremy, 24
  see also utilitarianism
Bergeron, Véronique, 224
best interest
  see also ample discretion principle
  alternative medicine (case), 314–317

Autonomy and Best Interest argument, 142–145, 152
  and euthanasia, 136, 142–145, 152
  frog toxin counterexample, 317
  never-best-interest objection to NAE, 157–158
  and non-voluntary active euthanasia, 153–155
  and passive euthanasia, 143
  use of term, 315
  and voluntary active euthanasia, 142–145, 152
"biting the bullet," 286
blended private/public health care system, 232
  see also two-tier MRI (case)
bloodless surgery, 225
bodily integrity, right of, 179
Boonin, David, 182–183
breastfeeding, 219
breech presentation, 222

C
C-section. *See* Caesarean section
Caesarean Delivery on Maternal Request (CDMR), 205, 208
  see also Caesarean section by choice (CSBC) (case)
Caesarean section, 199
  see also Caesarean section by choice (CSBC) (case)
Caesarean section by choice (CSBC) (case)
  argument by analogy, 217–219
  autonomy, 199, 223–224
  clarification of the case, 205–210
  driving to school analogy, 218–219
  economic costs of delivery, 209–210, 225
  fast food analogy, 217–218
  global statistics, 205–206
  good reason requirement, 215–216, 220–221
  harms to the baby, 215–222, 230n19
  harms to the mother, 222–224
  harms to others, 224–226
  home birth example, 219–220
  identification of relevant facts, 205–210
  informed consent, 224
  medicalization of safe, natural process, 214
  moral issues raised, 210–212
  moral permissibility, argument for, 212–214
  National Institute for Health and Care Excellence (NICE) guidelines, 208–209
  opening scenes, 201–205
  original position, 215, 223
  placenta accreta, 207
  potential harms, implications of, 214–226
  safety of modes of delivery, 206–208, 229n9
  statement of positions, 210–212
Canada Health Act, 232

Canada's current public health care system, 264
Canadian Medical Association (CMA), 137, 329
Canadian Nurses Association, 286, 313
Canadian Triage Acuity Scale (CTAS), 277, 280
cancer
  see also alternative medicine (case)
  chemotherapy, 307
  radiotherapy, 307
  remission, 305
categorical imperative, 319
the categorical imperative, 36
categorical imperatives, 34–36
  humanity version, 38–40
  universal law version of the categorical imperative, 36–38
CDMR. *See* Caesarean Delivery on Maternal Request (CDMR)
Chamberlain, Wilt, 244–245
charity, principle of. *See* principle of charity
chemotherapy, 307
childbirth. *See* Caesarean section by choice (CSBC) (case)
childless person, interests of, 296
Childress, James, 46, 331
circular argument, 11–12, 16n3, 79
clarification of concepts, 121
  see also specific cases
classical act utilitarianism, 24–32, 64n11
  see also utilitarianism
clinical factors (microallocation rules), 278, 279–292
  fair turn, 290–292
  fairness of microallocation rules, 279–282
  first come rule, 280–281
  hopeless second rule, 281, 287–288
  minimize YPLL (years of potential life lost) rule, 288–289
  substantial benefit, 289–290
  sympathy metarule, 282–287
  worst first rule, 280
code of ethics, Canadian Nurses Association, 286, 313
codifiability of morality, 80
cognitivism, 76
Colleges of Physicians and Surgeons, 329
comatose individuals, 191–192, 328
comforts, 334
common human sympathy. *See* sympathy metarule
compassion objection, 251–253
compassionate society, 248
competence
  ample discretion principle, 321
  and capacity to choose and understand, 123

hard paternalism, 108
and inability to communicate, 140
meaning of, 111–112
and patient autonomy, 92
presumptively morally permissible decisions, 213
psychiatric evaluation, 116–120
and right to refuse treatment, 111–113
valid consent, 321–326
complementary and alternative medicine (CAM), 312, 329
see also alternative medicine (case)
complementary medicine, 304
see also alternative medicine; alternative medicine (case)
conceptual analysis, 135
conclusion, 1–2, 4, 12, 170
conclusion indicators, 2
conditional contract, 183
consciousness, 167, 187–188
consent
and C-section by choice, 224
consensual private incest, 152
decision-making capacity, and legal standards, 323
informed consent, 39, 92–93, 120, 123, 224
meaning of, 337n2
right to refuse treatment, 92–93, 119–124
tacit consent, and abortion, 182
valid consent, 92–93, 119–120
voluntary euthanasia, 139
consequentialism, 24, 25, 27–28, 31, 56, 65n13
consequently (conclusion indicator), 2
conservative arguments, against abortion, 162, 169–185
contraception, 197n7
contraception objection, 174–175
and early abortions, 190
contractarian theory. *See* social contract theory
contractarianism, 249
contradiction in conception, 36
contradiction in will, 36
contrarian ideas, 82–84
cortex, 188
counterexamples, 9–11, 74, 143, 149, 152, 186, 288, 291, 305, 316, 317
see also specific cases
Cowart, Donald (Dax), 124
Criminal Code, 161
criticism, responding to, 305
CSBC. *See* Caesarean section by choice (CSBC) (case)
CTAS. *See* Canadian Triage Acuity Scale (CTAS)
CTAS National Working Group, 277
cultural imperialism, 87

cultural relativism, 87
culture, and sympathy, 284
cutting-edge medicine, 328–329

D
debate, 212
deductive arguments, 4–5
defining the issue, 205
delay, and doubt, 126–129
deontology, 34
derivation, 170
descriptive ethics, 18
empirical study, 19
vs. normative ethics, 18
descriptive moral claims, 75
difference principle, 50, 52–53, 244
A Different Voice (Gilligan), 58
dilemma, 151
diminishing marginal utility of money, 247
disability, discrimination against, 177–180
disaster scenarios. *See* microallocation of scarce resources (case)
discrimination
against the disabled (abortion case), 177–180
reverse discrimination, 274
unjust discrimination, 177–178
wrongfulness of, 177–178
dispositional view of moral properties, 76, 77, 81
division of labour objection, 329–334
doctrine of the mean, 55, 68n57
"don't ask, don't tell," 295
Doran's pluralistic approach to ethics, 70–75
double jeopardy, 118
doubt, and justification of delay, 126–129
Down's syndrome, 161, 162, 179
see also abortion (case)
drunk persons, 296
duty
all things considered, 44
of beneficence, 67n42
dysphagia, 92

E
early abortion, 189–190
Edwards, Jonathan. *See* right to refuse treatment (case)
egalitarian argument, 248
self-respect argument, 255–257
two-tier MRI (case), 253–257
embryo, 166, 172
emergency departments. *See* microallocation of scarce resources (case)

empirical matters
  and moral reasoning, 207
  reasonable guesses, 284
end, 38, 39
the environment, 62
epidemics, 271–272
epistemic problem, 80
epistemology, 89
equal consideration, 24, 26–27, 29–31
equal treatment, 26–27
equality. *See* egalitarian argument
equivocation, 13, 175–177
ethical inquiry, 18–21
ethical objectivism, 23
ethical relativism, 21–23, 64n8, 284
ethical subjectivism, 64n8
  see also ethical relativism
ethics
  vs. morality, 64n1
  types of ethics. *See* specific types of ethics
ethics of care, 58–62, 73
  caring relationships, 60–61
  difficulties with, 60–61
  health care ethics, application to, 59–60
  moral knowledge, 59
  partiality, implications of, 118, 128
  perspective of caring, 59
  and relationships, 60–61
  and right to refuse treatment, 118, 126
  status-oriented feminist approaches, 61–62
euthanasia, 132
  see also MAID (medical assistance in dying);
    MAID (medical assistance in dying) (case)
  active euthanasia, 132, 138–139
  best interests, 136
  CMA definition, 137
  definition of, 134–137
  etymology of, 134
  involuntary euthanasia, 139–140
  kinds of euthanasia, 137–140
  vs. MAID, 140
  moral permissibility of, 141
  non-human animals, 135, 153–154
  non-voluntary active euthanasia (NAE). *See* non-
    voluntary active euthanasia (NAE)
  non-voluntary euthanasia, 139
  passive euthanasia, 132, 138–139
  use of term, 132
  voluntary active euthanasia (VAE). *See* voluntary
    active euthanasia (VAE)
  voluntary euthanasia, 139
exceptions, 144, 284

excusable behaviour, 268
excuse, 282
experience machine, 29
experimental medicine, 328–329, 338n8
  see also alternative medicine (case)
experts, ignoring, 104–111
  see also right to refuse treatment (case)
exploitative relationships, 60
extremitarianism, 297

F
fair equality of opportunity, principle of, 50
fair innings argument, 290
fair turn, 290–292, 295
fairness
  humanized impartiality, 285–286
  impartiality, 279, 282, 285–286
  justice as fairness, 49–53
  microallocation rules, 279–282
  strict impartiality, abandonment of, 285–286
fallacy
  ad hominem, 14–15
  appeal to emotion, 13–14
  circular argument, 11–12, 79
  common fallacies, 11–15
  defined, 11
  equivocation, 13, 175–177
  false dilemma, 13
  straw man, 14
false dilemma, 13
feminism
  and Caesarean section by choice (CSBC), 211
  defined, 57
  ecofeminists, 62
  and ethics of care, 61–62
  feminist ethics, 57–58
  and justice as fairness, 51
  and power, 57
  status-oriented feminist approaches, 61–62
  and traditional ethical approaches, 58
feminist ethics, 57–58
fetus, 166
  see also abortion; abortion (case)
  and consciousness, 167, 187–188
  cortex, 188
  defined, 166
  development of, 166–167
  future of value, 174
  and genetic code, 169–172
  pain, ability to feel, 167, 188
FIGO. *See* International Federation of Gynecology
    and Obstetrics (FIGO)

first come rule, 280–281
Foot, Philippa, 156–157
for (premise indicator), 2
fraud, 250–251
free choice, 120, 123
frog toxin counterexample, 317
Frye, Marilyn, 62

G

gametes, 192
genetic code, 169–172
genetic humanity, 172
Gilligan, Carol, 58, 211
given that (premise indicator), 2
glossary of terms, 339–358
God arguments
 God's creation argument, 150–151
 sacredness of human life, 145–146
"God Committee," 291
Golden Rule, 67n36, 149
good reason requirement, 215–216, 220–221
good will, 35
governmental-level allocation. *See* macroallocation
The Groundwork of the Metaphysics of Morals (Kant),
 248

H

hard paternalism, 108
Hare, R. M., 148
harm
 harm avoidance, 326–329
 non-human animals, 41–42
 potential harms, and CSBC, 214–226
 serious harms, 328
 and two-tier MRI, 256–258
 unfair harms, 328
harm avoidance, 326–329
health care
 see also two-tier MRI (case)
 allocation of health care. *See* microallocation of
  scarce resources (case)
 blended private/public health care system, 232
 Canada's current public health care system, 264
 investment in, 260
 "jumping the queue," 237
 as positive right, 243
 private health care, 233
 public health care, 233
 in United States, 267
health care ethics, 17, 18
 ethics of care, application of, 59–60
 reasoning, and solutions, 20

hedonism, 24
 and classical utilitarianism, 26
 objections against, 28–29, 30–31
 and well-being, 65n16
hence (conclusion indicator), 2
Hobbes, Thomas, 47–49, 82
home birth, 219–220, 226
hopeless second rule, 281, 287–288
human-sympathy metarule, 83–84
 see also sympathy metarule
humanity, 38, 39
humanity test, 39–43
humanity version of the categorical imperative,
 38–40
humanized impartiality, 285–286
Humboldt Broncos, 303n1
hypothermia, 328
hypothetical cases, 287–288
hypothetical imperatives, 34–35
hysterectomy, 206

I

ideal observer theories, 242
illustration, of principle, 282
impartiality, 279, 282, 285–286
imperatives (commands) of morality, 35
imperfect duty, 36
incest, 152
incompetent individual
 ample discretion principle, 321
 and non-voluntary active euthanasia, 158
 and right to refuse treatment, 114–116
 soft paternalism, 108
inconsistency, 23
indeterminacy objection, 319–321
individual-level allocation. *See* microallocation of
 scarce resources (case)
inductive arguments, 6–7
infectious diseases, 296
informed consent, 39, 92–93, 120, 123, 224
innocents
 counterexamples, 147
 innocents first principle, 294–295
 moral guilt or innocence, 293–294
 rule against killing, 25–26
 Sanctity of Life principle, 145
innocents first principle, 294–295
institutional-level allocation. *See* mesoallocation
instrumentally good, 26
insufficient resources. *See* microallocation of scarce
 resources (case)
internalism, 77

International Federation of Gynecology and
    Obstetrics (FIGO), 206, 208
intrinsically good, 26
intuitionism, 45
    see also pluralistic deontology
intuitive appeal of arguments, 246
invalid argument, 5, 175
involuntary euthanasia, 139
irrational rule worship, 34
IVF (in vitro fertilization), 172

J
Jehovah's Witnesses, 225
"jumping the queue," 237
justice as fairness, 49–53
justice principles, 249
justification, 282

K
Kant, Immanuel, 34, 82, 248
    see also Kant's ethics
Kantians, 71–72
    see also Kant's ethics
Kant's ethics, 34–43
    the categorical imperative, 36
    categorical imperatives, 34–36, 319
    contradiction in conception, 36
    contradiction in will, 36
    end, 38, 39
    humanity, 38, 39
    humanity test, 39–40
    hypothetical imperatives, 34–35
    imperatives (commands) of morality, 35
    imperfect duty, 36
    means, 38, 39, 42, 248–249
    moral worth, 34–35
    objections to, 40–43, 72
    perfect duty, 36
    physician's duty, 332
    rational beings, 38–39, 39
    rational nature, 39
    rationality, and possession of moral rights, 198n17
    sanctity of human life, 146, 147
    things, 39
    universal law test, 37–38, 40–43
    universal law version of the categorical impera-
        tive, 36–38
killing
    rule against killing innocents, 25–26
    Sanctity of Life. See Sanctity of Life principle
King, Martin Luther, Jr., 255
Kohlberg, Lawrence, 58

L
Lamb, Julia, 135
Latimer, Robert, 139
Latimer, Tracey, 139
laws, 141
legal principles, 323
legal rights, 141
Level 1, 273
libertarian argument
    compassion objection, 251–253
    complicity objection, 250–251
    intuitive appeal, 246
    negative rights, 243
    objections raised by, 247
    positive rights, 243
    redistributive taxation, 245–250
    two-tier MRI (case), 242–253
    Wilt Chamberlain example, 244–245
liberty
    individual liberty, 105
    interference with, and autonomy, 106–107
    liberty principle, 106
life criterion, for right to life, 186–187
lifespans, 291–292
Lindemann, Hilde, 57, 58
Locke, John, 82
logic, 4–5, 175–177
lorry driver counterexample, 148–149
Lutherans for Life–Canada, 146

M
macroallocation, 279, 288
magnetic resonance imaging (MRI), 232
    see also two-tier MRI (case)
    costs of, 237–238
    government investment in, 238
    wait times, 233, 238
MAID (medical assistance in dying)
    see also MAID (medical assistance in dying)
        (case); voluntary active euthanasia (VAE)
    defined, 132
    vs. euthanasia, 140
MAID (medical assistance in dying) (case)
    Autonomy and Best Interest argument, 142–145,
        152
    counterexamples, 143–144, 152
    description, 133–140
    different kinds of euthanasia, 137–140
    euthanasia, definition of, 134–137
    God's creation argument, 150–151
    Hare's lorry driver counterexample, 148–149,
        156–158

issues in debate, 141
MAID *vs.* euthanasia, 140
moral reasons against killing, non-application of, 150
morality of NAE, 152–158
morality of VAE, 141–152
original position, 141
Sanctity of Life principle, 145–147
suicide counterexample, 148
Marissa and Don case. *See* abortion (case)
Marquis, Don, 173–177
maternal mortality, 222
maxim, 36
maximal equal basic liberties, principle of, 50
maximin, 50, 68n54
mean, doctrine of the, 55
means, 38, 39, 42, 248–249
medical assistance in dying. *See* MAID (medical assistance in dying)
medical benefit, 299
medical interests, 298–300
Medical Services Plan (MSP), 311
medicalization, 214
Medicare. *See* two-tier MRI (case)
mesoallocation, 279, 288
metaethics, 18, 20, 75, 76–77
metaphysical problem, 80
metaphysics, 89
metarule, 279
  see also sympathy metarule
microallocation of scarce resources (case)
  Canadian Triage Acuity Scale (CTAS), 277, 280
  clarification of the case, 276
  clinical factors, 278, 279–292
  closing (collecting our thoughts), 300–301
  counterexample, 288
  fair turn, 290–292, 295
  fairness of microallocation rules, 279–282
  first come rule, 280–281
  "God Committee," 291
  hopeless second rule, 281, 287–288
  humanized impartiality, 285–286
  hypothetical case, 287–288
  identification of relevant facts, 276
  innocents first, 294–295
  medical interests, 298–300
  minimize YPLL (years of potential life lost) rule, 288–289
  moral issues raised, 277–278
  moral responsibility, 293–294
  nepotism, 284–286

non-clinical factors, 278, 292, 293–300
  opening scenes, 272–276
  original position, 279, 281
  practice standards, 286
  public interest, 297–298
  reflective equilibrium, 289
  statement of positions, 278
  substantial benefit, 289–290
  sympathy metarule, 279–280, 282–287
  third-party interests, 296–297
  traditional triage practices, 281
  use of term, 279
  virtue ethics perspective, 286–287
  worst first rule, 280, 295
midwives, 219–220, 225, 311
Mill, John Stuart, 24, 105, 110
  see also utilitarianism
minimization of overall suffering, 10–11
minimize YPLL (years of potential life lost) rule, 288–289
mitigation, 282
money, diminishing marginal utility of, 247
moral antirealism, 75
moral arguments, 7–8
moral claims, 77
moral coding, 80
moral development, 58–59
moral equivalency, the problem of, 22
moral humanity, 172
moral infallibility, the problem of, 21
moral knowledge, 59
moral loss, 176
moral pluralism, 71, 73–75
  see also pluralistic deontology
moral principles, 8
  evaluation or testing of, 9
  vs. legal rights, 141
  and normative ethics, 19–20
  qualifications, 328
moral realism, 75
moral relativism, 21
  see also ethical relativism
moral worth, 34–35
morality
  codifiability of morality, 80
  vs. ethics, 64n1
  first-order issues, 76
  objective morality, 76–77
  and rationality, 198n17
morbidity, 207
Morrison, Toni, 136

MRI. *See* magnetic resonance imaging (MRI)
multiple sclerosis (MS), 92
  see also right to refuse treatment (case)
myocardial infarction (MI), 273

N
NAE. *See* non-voluntary active euthanasia (NAE)
Nancy B. case, 138
National Institute for Health and Care Excellence (NICE), 208–209
natural advantages, 176
natural birth, 202, 203, 215
  see also Caesarean section by choice (CSBC) (case)
nature, state of, 47–49
naturopath, 311
negative rights, 243
nepotism, 284–286
neutral loss, 176
never-best-interest objection, 157–158
non-clinical factors (microallocation rules), 278, 292, 293–300
  innocents first, 294–295
  medical interests, 298–300
  moral responsibility, 293–294
  public interest, 297–298
  third-party interests, 296–297
non-consequentialism, 34
non-hedonistic utilitarianism, 30–31
non-human animals
  ecofeminism and, 62
  and ethics, 87–89
  euthanasia, 135, 153–154
  harm to, 41–42
  and Hobbes's social contract theory, 48–49
  and humanity test, 41
  Kant's ethics, 41
  moral obligations to, 18
  practical social contract theory, 87–89
  rationality criterion, 186, 192–193
  right to life, 189, 193–195
  social contract theory, 49, 51, 72
  utilitarianism, 65n17
  vegetarianism, 78, 195–196
  virtue ethics, 72–73, 81
  xenotransplantation, 171
non-interference, rights to, 243
non-maleficence, 331
non-moral claims, 77
non-voluntary active euthanasia (NAE), 132
  Foot's objection, 156–157
  and incompetence, 158

morality of, 152–158
never-best-interest objection to NAE, 157–158
slippery-slope objection, 153
non-voluntary euthanasia, 139
Noonan, John T., Jr., 169–172
normative ethical theory, 17, 24, 70–71
normative ethics, 17, 18–21, 64n2, 75, 78–79
  vs. descriptive ethics, 18–19
  evaluation of, 19–20
  first-order issues, 76
  good reasoning, 19
  key concepts, identification of, 19
  vs. metaethics, 20, 75–76
  and moral principles, 19–20
  relevant facts, 19
Nowell-Smith, Patrick, 148–149
Nozick, Robert, 29, 244–245

O
objective intrinsic goods, 30–31
objective moral truths or facts, 75
objective morality, 76–77, 79
objective truth, 21
objectivity, concept, 64n6, 91n
observations, 9
On Liberty (Mill), 105, 110
optimific act, 25, 32
optimific rule, 32
organ transplants, 171
original position, 49–50, 51, 83–86
  see also sympathy metarule
  abortion (case), 168, 179
  Caesarean section by choice (CSBC) (case), 215, 223
  MAID (medical assistance in dying) (case), 141
  microallocation of scarce resources (case), 279, 281
  right to refuse treatment (case), 104, 106
  two-tier MRI (case), 241, 255–256
"ought implies can," 252, 287
ova, 174

P
pain
  ability to feel pain, 167, 188
  and medical judgment, 280
palliative care, 334
parents, interests of, 296
passive euthanasia, 132
  vs. active euthanasia, 132, 138–139
  and best interest, 143

and intention, 138
Nancy B. case, 138
paternalism, 320
hard paternalism, 108
justification of, 108
right to refuse treatment (case), 103, 106–107,
108, 125
soft paternalism, 108
strong paternalism, 125
weak paternalism, 86, 125
patient safety, 128–129
perceptual capacity, 78–79
perfect duty, 36
permanent coma, 192
perspective of caring, 59
philosophical methodology, 9–11
philosophy, *vs.* debate, 212
physician-assisted suicide, 137
see also MAID (medical assistance in dying);
MAID (medical assistance in dying) (case);
voluntary active euthanasia (VAE)
placebo effect, 312
placenta accreta, 207
placenta percreta, 207
plague victims, 146–147
Plato, 82, 89
pluralism, 43
pluralistic deontology, 43–46, 74
duty, all things considered, 44
prima facie duties, 43–44
rational intuition, 44
politicians, and two-tier health MRI, 264–266
positive character traits, 54
positive rights, 243
potential
harms, and CSBC, 214–226
and value, 174
power, 57
practical ethics, 18
practical social contract theory, 82–89
choosing moral rules, 82–84
committee metaphor, 84–86
cultural relativism, 87
ethics regarding non-humans, 87–89
human-sympathy metarule, 83–84
original position, 83, 84–86
veil of ignorance, 83, 84–85
video game metaphor, 86
Warren's use of social contract theory, 86–87
prayer, 115, 333–334, 338n9
preferences, informed, 30

preferential treatment. *See* microallocation of scarce
resources (case)
premise indicators, 2
premises, 1–2
prescriptive ethics, 18
see also normative ethics
prescriptive moral claims, 75
presumptively morally permissible decisions, 213
prima facie duties, 43–44, 332–333
primary social goods, 51–52, 241, 261–263
principle of charity, 66n33, 171
principle of fair equality of opportunity, 50
principle of maximal equal basic liberties, 50
principlism, 46, 331
private, for-profit health care. *See* two-tier MRI (case)
private education, 254–255
private health care, 233
the problem of moral equivalency, 22
the problem of moral infallibility, 21
prolapse, 202
pseudo-science, 305
psychiatric evaluation, as proof of competence,
116–120
psychic surgery, 331–333
public health care, 233
public interest rule, 297–298

Q
quadriplegic, 139
qualifications, to moral principles, 328
queue, 143, 237

R
radiotherapy, 307
rape, and abortion, 182, 197n6
rational beings, 38–39, 188–190, 192–195
rational intuition, 44
rational nature, 39
rationality, 89
less rational individuals, 192–193
and non-human animals, 186, 192–193
non-rational individuals, 193–195
and possession of moral rights, 198n17
rationality criterion, for right to life, 185–186,
188–190, 192–195
rationing health care, 138
Rawls, John, 49–53, 82, 106, 249
realist theory, 75
reasonable person test, 113, 221
recusal, 284
redistributive taxation, 245–250

reflective equilibrium, 10, 90n4, 195, 289

refusal of treatment. *See* right to refuse treatment (case)

Regan, Tim. *See* MAID (medical assistance in dying) (case)

relevant facts, 30

  see also specific cases

religion. *See* God arguments

remission, 305

revised statements, 144

rhythm method, 197n7

right to ignore experts, 104–111

right to life. *See* abortion (case)

right to refuse treatment (case)

  clarification of premises, 105–108

  competence, and psychiatric evaluation, 116–120

  competence of Edwards, 111–113

  doubt, and justification of delay, 126–129

  gangrenous foot example, 113–114

  health care team, error of, 108–111

  identification of relevant facts, 100–102

  incompetence to refuse medical care, 114–116

  informed consent, 92–93, 120, 123

  liberty principle, 106

  moral issues raised by the case, 102–103

  objections to premise, 111–129

  opening scenes, 94–99

  original position, 104, 106

  paternalism, 108, 125, 339

  reasonable person test, 113

  right to ignore experts, argument for, 104–111

  right to self-determination, 104–107

  skepticism without reason, 114–116

  social contract theory, 104

  standard form, 104–105

  statement of positions, 102–103

  valid consent, 92–93, 119–124

  validity of refusal, 119–124

  virtue, *vs.* right to refuse, 124–126

right to self-determination, 104–107

robust advantage principle, 259, 266

Rodriguez, Sue, 137

Ross, W. D., 43–46, 331

Rousseau, Jean-Jacques, 82

rule utilitarianism, 32–34

rules, 33–34, 194, 265

S

sacredness of human life, 145–146

Sanctity of Life principle

  counterexamples, 146–149

  God's creation argument, 150–151

Lutherans for Life-Canada, 146

  and voluntary active euthanasia, 145–147

scarce resources. *See* microallocation of scarce resources (case)

scientific, meaning of, 305

seat belt legislation, 86, 107

secondary quality view, 76

  see also dispositional view of moral properties

self-defence, 146, 151

self-determination. *See* autonomy; right to self-determination

self-interest, 47, 223

self-regarding duties, 223

self-respect argument, 255–257

sentience

  fully sentient, 188

  necessity of, for right to life, 191–192

  objections to sentience criterion, 187–196

  and rationality, 188–190

  sentience criterion, for right to life, 187–188

  sufficiency of, for right to life, 190–191

September 11 terrorist attacks, 148

sex-selective abortion, 179

Shafer-Landau, Russ, 41

Sherwin, Susan, 57, 58, 61, 62

since (premise indicator), 2

situational ethic, 25

skepticism without reason, 114–116

slippery-slope objection, 153

so (conclusion indicator), 2

social contract theory, 46–54, 72

  abortion, 168, 194

  cultural relativism, 87

  difference principle, 50, 52–53

  ethics regarding non-humans, 87–89

  Hobbes's social contract theory, 47–49

  human-sympathy metarule, 83–84

  ideal social contract, 83

  justice as fairness, 49–53

  maximin, 50

  moral obligations, 48–49

  objections to, 48–49, 51–53, 72

  original position, 49–50, 51, 83–86

  practical social contract theory, 82–89

  and rationality, 89

  Rawls's social contract theory, 49–53

  right to refuse treatment (case), 104

  robust advantage principle, 259

  self-interest, 47, 50

  state of nature, 47–49

  sympathy metarule, 194

two-tier MRI, 259–260
veil of ignorance, 50, 83, 84–85
Warren's use of, 86–87
social institutions, 242
social safety net, 249–250, 259–260
Society of Obstetricians and Gynaecologists of
Canada, 208
soft paternalism, 108
sound argument, 5
special relationships, 29–30
speculation, 305
sperm, 174
sports, participation in, 239
standard form, 2, 3, 104–105, 213
Stangl, Fritz, 60
Stangl, Teresa, 60
state of nature, 47–49
status-oriented feminist approaches, 61–62
straw man fallacy, 14, 66n33
stress incontinence, 202
strict impartiality, 285–286
strong argument, 6
strong paternalism, 125
subjective moral truths or facts, 75
substantial benefit, 289–290
substantive moral claim, 7
suicide, 136–137, 148
Supplementary Benefits Program, 311
surface grammar, 76
sympathy metarule, 194, 265, 279–280, 282–287

T
temporary coma, 191–192
theft, 250–251
theological views. *See* God arguments
therefore (conclusion indicator), 2
things, 39
third-party interests, 296–297, 326
Thomson, Judith Jarvis, 181–185
thought experiment, 9–11
thromboembolism, 222
thus (conclusion indicator), 2
tolemin, 68n54
Tong, Rosemarie, 61
treatment, refusal of. *See* right to refuse treatment
(case)
triage, 271
see also microallocation of scarce resources (case)
triage nurses. *See* microallocation of scarce resources
(case)
Trojan Horse, 91n17
Tuskegee syphilis experiments, 22–23

two-tier health care. *See* two-tier MRI (case)
two-tier MRI (case)
see also magnetic resonance imaging (MRI)
argument by analogy, 254
benefits to public health care system, 258
Canada's current public health care system, 264
clarification of the case, 236–240
closing arguments, 266–268
compassion objection, 251–253
complicity objection, 250–251
effect of, 256
egalitarian argument, 248, 253–257
harm to public health care system, 256–258
ideal observer theories, 242
identification of relevant facts, 236–240
individual perspective, 264–266
"jumping the queue," 237
libertarian argument, 242–253
means, treatment of people as, 248–249
moral issues raised, 240–242
moral permissibility of, 233–234
opening scenes, 234–236
original position, 241, 255–256
political perspective, 264–266
primary social goods, 261–263
redistributive taxation, 245–250
robust advantage principle, 259, 266
self-respect argument, 255–257
social contract theory, 259–260
sympathy metarule, 265
two-tier arguments, 257–263
virtue-based view, 260–263
Wilt Chamberlain example, 244–245

U
unconventional health care services. *See* alternative
medicine (case)
unequal access to health care. *See* two-tier MRI
(case)
unfairness, 176
United States, health care in, 267
universal care, 232
see also two-tier MRI (case)
universal law, 36
formulation of the categorical imperative, 36–38
test, 37–38, 40–43
unnecessary medical procedures, 225
unsound argument, 5
US Public Health Service, 22–23
utilitarianism
bad, defined, 27
classical act utilitarianism, 24–32

consequentialism, 24, 25, 27–28
equal consideration, 24, 26–27, 29–31
good, defined, 27
hedonism, 24, 26, 28–29
non-hedonistic utilitarianism, 30–31
objections, 27–30, 71
redistributive taxation, 247
responses to objections, 30–32
rule utilitarianism, 32–34
theory of right action, 64n12

V

VAE. *See* voluntary active euthanasia (VAE)
vaginal delivery, 206–208
    see also Caesarean section by choice (CSBC) (case)
valid argument, 4–5, 175
valid consent, 92–93, 119–120, 321–326
valid refusal, 119–124
vasectomies, 225
vegetarianism, 78, 195–196
veil of ignorance, 50, 83, 84–85
violation of rights, 250–251
violence, 250–251
violinist example, 181–185
virtue, 54
virtue ethics, 54–57
    abortion, 180–181
    Aristotle's virtue theory, 54–57
    compassion objection, 251–253
    and consequentialism, 56
    defended, 79–82
    doctrine of the mean, 55
    Foot's objection to NAE, 156–157
    ideal observer theories, 242
    moral character, 54
    moral claims, 75
    objections, 79–82
    objections to, 55–57, 72–73
    Patrick's approach to ethics, 75–82
    perceptual capacity, 78–79
    right to life *vs.* virtues, 181–185
    right to refuse treatment, 124–126
    rights in, 252
    and social institutions, 242
    sympathy metarule, and microallocation rules, 286–287
    two-tier MRI, 260–263
    vegetarianism, 195–196

virtue theory, 72–73
    virtuous character, 54–55
    virtuous person. *See* virtuous person
virtue theory, 72–73
    see also virtue ethics
virtuous person, 55–56, 58, 72, 76, 81–82, 183
virtuous society, 251–252
Vital Signs/True Sport Foundation study, 239
voluntary active euthanasia (VAE), 132
    see also MAID (medical assistance in dying);
        MAID (medical assistance in dying) (case)
    advance directives, 158
    Autonomy and Best Interest argument, 142–145
    Christian-inspired argument in support of, 149
    God's creation argument, 150–151
    Kantian-inspired argument in support of, 149
    moral permissibility, 141–142
    and moral reasons against killing, 150
    morality of, 132–133, 141–152
    Sanctity of Life principle, 145–147
    slippery-slope objection, 153
voluntary euthanasia, 139–140
vulnerable people, protection of, 215

W

Warren, Mary Anne, 172
weak arguments, 6–7
weak paternalism, 86, 125
Wendy's CSBC case. *See* Caesarean section by
    choice (CSBC) (case)
will, 36
Williams, Nancy, 61
women
    see also abortion (case); Caesarean section by
        choice (CSBC) (case)
    bodily integrity, right of, 179
    breastfeeding, 219
    mother's right to autonomy, 199
    rape, and abortion, 182, 197n6
World Trade Center, 148
worst first rule, 280, 295

X

xenotransplantation, 171

Z

zygote, 166, 174, 192